In Western industrialized societies at least one in 800 of the population is affected by multiple sclerosis (MS). If the disease is recognized early and treated adequately the prospects are now better than ever for improving both the quality and length of life for people with MS.

This concise, abundantly illustrated text provides a complete overview of MS for the internist, general neurologist and therapist. Including recent research findings in genetics, immunology and pathophysiology, the authors provide reliable and up-to-date guidance on the epidemiology, diagnosis, prognosis and treatment of MS.

Of particular interest to neuroscientists and neurologists will be the reviews of experimental models of MS, pathology of the demyelinated plaque, HLA associations and the role of immune mechanisms. Environmental factors in the etiology of MS are examined, including the possible role of infectious agents. The clinical sections of the book include discussion of neurological, sexual, psychological and cognitive disturbances, and rehabilitation measures are given special attention.

Multiple sclerosis

Multiple sclerosis

Edited by

Jürg Kesselring

Head of the Department of Neurorehabilitation
Rehabilitation Center
Valens, Switzerland

Foreword by Professor W. I. McDonald
National Hospital for Neurology and Neurosurgery, London

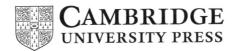

PUBLISHED BY THE PRESS SYNDICATE OF THE UNIVERSITY OF CAMBRIDGE
The Pitt Building, Trumpington Street, Cambridge CB2 1RP, United Kingdom

CAMBRIDGE UNIVERSITY PRESS
The Edinburgh Building, Cambridge CB2 2RU, United Kingdom
40 West 20th Street, New York, NY 10011-4211, USA
10 Stamford Road, Oakleigh, Melbourne 3166, Australia

First published 1997

An updated and adapted translation of the German edition
published by W. Kohlhammer GMBH, D-70549, Stuttgart, Germany,
as *Multiple Sklerose*, second edition, by Jürg Kesselring.

Printed in the United States of America

Typeset in Palatino

Library of Congress Cataloging-in-Publication Data
Multiple Sklerose.   English.
Multiple sclerosis / edited by Jürg Kesselring.
p.   cm.
Includes bibliographical references and index.
ISBN 0-521-48018-3 (hardback)
1. Multiple sclerosis.   I. Kesselring, Jürg.
[DNLM: 1. Multiple Sclerosis.   WL 360 M9618m 1996a]
RC377.M83713   1996
616.8'34–dc20
DNLM/DLC
for Library of Congress   96-6151

A catalog record for this book is available from the British Library

ISBN 0 521 48018 3 hardback

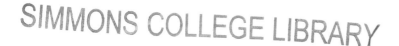

Contents

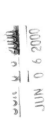

Foreword

In the past two decades we have witnessed a remarkable growth in our understanding of multiple sclerosis, and we are now on the threshold of an era in which effective treatment seems possible. Though the aetiology of the disease is not yet fully understood, evidence for an interaction between an environmental factor (perhaps viral) with a genetic susceptibility factor has grown. Four new studies just published (Ebers et al. 1996; Haines et al. 1996; Kuokkanen et al. 1996; Sawcer et al. 1996) have confirmed that the latter implicates several chromosomes; again, the HLA region of the 6th chromosome emerges as the most important.[†]

[†]Ebers GC, Kukay K, Bulman DE, Sadovnick AD, Rice G, Anderson C, Armstrong H, Cousin K, Bell RB, Hader W, Paty DW, Hashimoto S, Oger J, Duquette P, Warren S, Gray T, O'Connor P, Nath A, Auty A, Metz L, Francis G, Paulseth JE, Murray TJ, Pryse-Phillips W, Nelson R, Freedman M, Brunet D, Bouchard J-P, Hinds D, Risch N. A full genome search in multiple sclerosis. *Nature Genetics* 13 (1996): 472–476.

Haines JL, Ter-Minassian M, Bazyk A, Gusella JF, Kim DJ, Terwedow H, Pericak-Vance MA, Rimmler JB, Haynes CS, Roses AD, Lee A, Shaner B, Menold M, Seboun E, Fitoussi RP, Gartioux C, Reyes C, Ribierre F, Gyapay G, Weissenbach J, Ilauser SL, Goodkin DE, Lincoln R, Usuku K, Garcia-Merino A, Gatto N, Young S, Oksenberg JR. (The Multiple Sclerosis Genetics Group). A complete genomic screen for multiple sclerosis underscores a role for the major histocompatability complex. *Nature Genetics* 13 (1996): 469–471.

Kuokkanen S, Sundvall M, Terwilliger JD, Tienari PJ, Wikström J, Holmdahl R, Pettersson U, Peltonen L. A putative vulnerability locus to multiple sclerosis maps to 5p14-p12 in a region syntenic to the murine locus *Eae2*. *Nature Genetics* 13 (1996): 477–480.

Sawcer S, Jones HB, Feakes R, Gray J, Smaldon N, Chataway J, Robertson N, Clayton D, Goodfellow PN, Compston A. A genome screen in multiple sclerosis reveals susceptibility loci on chromosome 6p21 and 17q22. *Nature Genetics* 13 (1996): 464–468.

Much has been learned about cellular mechanisms involved in pathogenesis and repair, and the evolution of the lesion is now much better understood through the exploitation of magnetic resonance imaging (MRI) and spectroscopy. A secure early diagnosis can be made earlier in the course of the disease through the application of MRI, evoked potentials, and cerebrospinal fluid analysis.

Developments in MRI have produced powerful new tools for monitoring the effectiveness of treatment. As a result, putative therapeutic agents can be screened relatively quickly to see whether they have an influence on at least some aspects of the pathological process. One of the most encouraging developments has been the demonstration that a number of agents–most notably the beta-interferons–reduce the frequency of acute pathological activity, and that this can be reflected in a modest decrease in relapse rate. Convincing evidence for a useful effect on disability (surely the most important criterion for an effective treatment) is still awaited. But the progress over the past five years gives grounds for optimism.

In this timely book, the background to these advances is described; the areas of greater and lesser certainty are delineated and the prospects for future progress are laid out; and the practical management of the patient as well as of the disease are detailed. This is an exciting time for the study of multiple sclerosis, and Dr. Kesselring and his colleagues show why.

W. I. McDonald
National Hospital for Neurology and Neurosurgery
London, England

Contributors

Dr. Walter Fierz
Institute of Clinical Microbiology and Immunology
Frohburgstrasse 3
CH-9007 St Gallen
Switzerland

Professor Christian W. Hess
Head of the University Department of Neurology
Inselspital
CH-3010 Berne
Switzerland

Professor Ludwig Kappos
Leitender Arzt
Kantonsspital Basel
Petersgruben 4
CH-4031 Basel
Switzerland

Dr. Jürg Kesselring
Head of the Department of Neurorehabilitation
Rehabilitation Centre Valens
CH-7317 Valens
Switzerland

Professor Hans Lassmann
Institute of Neurology, University of Vienna
Schwarzspanierstrasse 17
A-1090 Wien
Austria

Dr. Jürgen Mertin
Medical Director
Josef-Wolf-Clinic for Neurorehabilitation
Krankenhausstrasse 12
D-93149 Nittenau
Germany

Abbreviations

ACTH	adrenocorticotrophic hormone
ADEM	acute disseminated encephalomyelitis
ADL	activities of daily living
AFP	α-fetoprotein
AIDS	acquired immunodeficiency syndrome
ALG	antilymphocytic globulin
4-AP	4-aminopyridine
AZA	azathioprine
BAEP	brainstem auditory evoked potential
CMCT	central motor conduction time
CNS	central nervous system
CoP-1	copolymer 1
CSF	cerebrospinal fluid
CSL	soluble cerebellar lectin
CyA	cyclosporin A
EAE	experimental autoimmune encephalomyelitis
EAN	experimental autoimmune neuritis
EDSS	expanded disability status scale
EFA	essential fatty acid
GABA	γ-aminobutyric acid
GFAP	glial fibrillary acidic protein
HIV	human immunodeficiency virus
Ia	immune-associated antigen
IEF	isoelectric focusing
IFMSS	The International Federation of Multiple Sclerosis Societies
IFN	interferon
Ig	immunoglobulin
IL	interleukin
INH	isoniazid
IR	inversion recovery
MAG	myelin-associated glycoprotein
MBP	myelin basic protein
MCV	mean cellular volume

MEP	motor evoked potential
MFT	myofunctional therapy
MHC	major histocompatibility complex
MOG	myelin oligodendrocyte glycoprotein
MRC	Medical Research Council
MRI	magnetic resonance imaging
NK	natural killer (cells)
PGE	prostaglandin
PI	progression index
PLP	proteolipid protein
PML	progressive multifocal leukoencephalopathy
PNF	proprioceptive neuromuscular facilitation
PUFA	polyunsaturated long-chain fatty acid
RFLP	restriction fragment length polymorphism
SE	spin echo
SEP	somatosensory evoked potential
SSPE	subacute sclerosing panencephalitis
STAT	signal transducers and activators of transcription
STIR	inversion recovery with short inversion time
TE	echo time
TGF	tumor growth factor
TH1	T-helper-1 cells
TNF	tumor necrosis factor
TR	repetition time
VEP	visual evoked potential

Multiple sclerosis

PART I

General aspects

1

Historical perspective

The past is always with us, never to be escaped; it alone is enduring; but amidst the changes and chances which succeed one another so rapidly in this life, we are apt to live too much for the present and too much for the future.

Sir William Osler, *Aequanimitas*, 1889

Multiple sclerosis is a very conspicuous disease which, when full blown, has signs which no experienced clinician should fail to recognize. Nevertheless, until the Middle Ages, there are no descriptions in medical texts of any disease which we would recognize and diagnose as MS today. A possible exception to this may be the history of Saint Lidwina von Schiedham (1380–1422), a nun from the Netherlands (Medaer 1979). Over the course of 37 years, she showed waxing and waning clinical manifestations of symptoms which could be attributed to disorders of various parts of the nervous system.

The diary and letters of Augustus Frederick d'Este (1794–1848), an illegitimate grandson of the English King George III and cousin to Queen Victoria, do provide a record of a case of MS. In 1822, at the age of 28, he suffered from sudden visual disturbances after having attended the funeral of a close relative: "Soon after . . . and without anything having been done to my eyes, they completely recovered their strength and distinctness of vision." Five years later, while in Florence, both his legs became paralyzed: "I remained in this extreme state of weakness for about 21 days, during which period I fell down about five times (never fainting) from my legs not being strong enough to carry my body." In the following years he writes of "very violent pains" and that "my making water is attend with difficulty." Two years later: "whilst in the act of getting out of bed a considerable portion of stool flowed from me, without my having been made aware of wanting to go to the closed stool." In a note made in 1830, we can detect a hint of impotence: "I formed a liaison with a young woman – I find my acts of connection a deficiency of a wholesome vigour . . ." Some 13 years later, during which time he had been searching for cures in various spas and with various physicians, he noticed some sensory disturbances: "Sitting produces a numbness all down the back part of my thighs and legs, and gives me a curious numb sensation in the lower region of the belly. When standing or walking I cannot keep my balance without a stick." Three months after this, he records a feeling of vertigo for the first time: "For the first time in my life I was attacked by giddiness in the head, sickness, and total abruption of strength in my limbs." In 1844 Sir Augustus needed a wheelchair, "with which a 'wind-cushion', price 10 shillings, was used." The last entry in his diary was written in 1846, 2 years before his death. His writing is clearly affected by ataxia, the previously fluent, orderly script disintegrating into single letters. He describes the use of an orthopedic aid and ends full of hope: ". . . and I walk without my left foot, which some time ago always turned over outwards at the ankle joint unless supported by a steel upright, showing any disposition so to do. Surely this is a decided improvement! Thanks be to the Almighty!" (Firth 1948; McDonald 1983).

There can be found in several biographies of poets of that time, for example Heinrich Heine (1797–1856) (Jellinek 1990), and Eduard Mörike (1804–1875) (H.J. Grüsser, personal communication 1987), various signs and symptoms of disease which, in retrospect, suggest a diagnosis of MS.

Despite the paucity of historical examples, we may assume that the disease did not exist with the same signs, and certainly not with the same frequency, as it does today.

Jean Cruveilhier (1791–1873) is usually assumed to be the first to have described MS. This assumption (discussed by de Jong 1970, and S. Poser 1986) is based on the first monograph on the disease, which was edited by Charcot's pupil Bourneville in 1869 (Bourneville and Guérard 1869). Cruveilhier was professor of pathological anatomy in Paris and, between the years 1829 and 1842, he published a beautiful atlas with the title *Anatomie pathologique du corps human* (Cruveilhier 1829–1842). In the second volume there is a description of four disease protocols and an illustration of "Maladies de la moelle épinière." The disease is described as "paraplégie par dégéneration grise des cordons de la moelle," and Cruveilhier uses expressions such as "en tâches" and "en îles" to describe the pathological processes. He draws attention to the firm consistency of these spots, and was not able to compare them to any tissue in the body known to him. In his opinion, this disease was, like rheumatism, the sequel to suppressed sweating.

At about the same time, Robert Carswell (1793–1857), later to become professor of pathology in London, was working as a student in Paris when he produced nearly 2000 watercolors and drawings of normal and pathological tissues which later formed the basis of his work *Pathological anatomy: illustrations of elementary forms of disease* which appeared in 1838. He describes what we would today call MS as "a peculiar disease state of the cord and pons Varolii, accompanied by atrophy of the discoloured portions." One of his figures mirrors one from Cruveilhier's atlas so closely that it is tempting to assume both authors had used the same preparation as a model.

However, careful research into the years of these publications shows that the relevant figures in Cruveilhier's atlas, which was produced in 40 "livraisons," cannot have appeared before 1841, whereas Carswell's work was finished and published in 1838. Thus, the first patient whose disease was diagnosed as MS was French, but the lesions which formed the basis of the disease were depicted for the first time by a Scotsman (Compston 1988).

The dispute as to who was the first to describe MS – Cruveilhier or Carswell – might be resolved by the atlas *The morbid anatomy of the human brain, illustrated by coloured engravings of the most frequent and important organic diseases to which that viscus is subject*, by Robert Hooper (1773–1835), which was published in 1828 in London by Longman, Rees, Orme, Brown and Green (Hooper 1828). Hooper was a pathologist and practicing physician in London and he based his atlas on his experiences, gained over 30 years, of more than 4000 autopsies which he had performed at the St Mary-le-bone Infirmary (McHenry 1969). He describes "Diseased structures, and unnatural appearances without tumefaction: Morbid firmness, hardness, or induration . . . is not uncommon in the substance of the brain . . . It is mostly accompanied by a dark hue . . . With this preternaturally great cohesion of its particles, the brains feels not merely firm, but morbidly hard, and the cut surface does not show the natural number of bloodvessels in the medullary substance, nor does it receive the impression of the finger readily: and when the finger is removed, it quickly rises to its level . . ." and later: "The delicate colour of the medullary substance frequently undergoes a change. I have seen it of palestone or albine colour . . ."

The first clinical descriptions of MS were by Frerichs in Göttingen, Germany, and appeared in the middle of the last century (Frerichs 1849). Frerichs' clinical diagnosis of "Hirnsclerose" was challenged until, in 1856, his pupil Valentiner reported pathological findings from patients who had died and pronounced his master's clinical diagnosis to be "so brilliantly confirmed by postmortem examination." He highlighted a symptom which was later often neglected: "Psychological disturbances of higher degrees accompany the degeneration of the brain almost regularly." Treatment was very limited: "Without sanguinic hope of success he ordered the use of iodine potassium."

Rindfleisch, in Zurich in 1863, first identified the pathological changes of the blood vessels: "their wall is enormously thickened by the aggregation of nuclei and cells in the adventitia." He considered "often recurrent or persistent irritations of the entire central organs" to be a primary event, and changes in the parenchyma to be secondary phenomena: "The neuroglia undergoes a series of metamorphoses in continuation of the formative irritations from the vessel walls to the neighbourhood. This process carries throughout the mark of scantiness."

A vascular theory of MS was adhered to for several decades (Putnam 1933). It was based on the observation that plaques develop mainly in the neighborhood of small veins in which, from time to time, organized thrombi can be found. This theory led to several therapeutic trials with vasoactive substances and anticoagulants, but with no success.

Leyden (1863) summarized the state of knowledge of that time as follows:

1. women are affected much more often than men (25:1),
2. the onset of the disease is usually between the 20th and 25th year,
3. there had been only a single hereditary case,
4. there are two main etiological factors: exposure to cold and wet, and trauma,
5. psychological events are important in triggering the disease.

Jean Marie Charcot (1825–1893) gave the first comprehensive description of MS, describing its clinical peculiarities in his famous lectures at the Salpêtrière in Paris (Charcot 1872–1873; McDonald 1993). He distinguished myotrophic lateral sclerosis from MS, and evaluated tremor not as a disease but as a symptom. He clearly distinguished intention tremor from tremor with Parkinson's disease. The "classical symptom triad" of nystagmus, intention tremor, and scanning speech which is named after him was not considered important by Charcot himself, and he stressed repeatedly that the lack of one, or even of all three, of these symptoms could not preclude the diagnosis. He also drew attention to benign cases of the disease (Charcot 1879). As a successor to Vulpian to the chair of pathology, and possibly in collaboration with him, he elaborated the histology of MS and produced drawings of myelin loss and preservation of axon cylinders, proliferation of glia, and perivascular phagocytes containing fatty deposits (Charcot 1868).

Charcot maintained that the cause of the disease was unknown. He assumed it to have some connection with acute infection, and described cases in which it had been preceded by infections such as typhus, smallpox, or cholera. He also mentioned an association with exposure to cold, and with emotional factors such as grief, shock or trauma.

In 1906, Marburg described an acute form of MS which is still named after him. He postulated a myelinolytic toxin as a causal factor. This toxin theory was supported for several decades and received particular attention in the work of Baasch (1966), who thought the disease was caused by a chronic mercury infection from amalgam fillings in the teeth. Despite his elegant arguments, his conclusions were not confirmed.

The theory that MS is an infectious disease has had its supporters for more than a century, since Charcot and Pierre Marie (1884) (Larner 1986). In the 1930s, it gained new impetus following the observation that the histological picture of perivenous demyelination in postinfectious and postvaccination encephalomyelitis could not be distinguished from that seen in MS (Brain 1930).

On many occasions, specific organisms were isolated and considered as etiological factors. The search for viruses which could be responsible for MS is always accompanied by the same hope and confidence which, in the case of poliomyelitis, were rewarded by vaccination against poliomyelitis viruses. Various viral diseases in humans and animals may lead to changes in the central nervous system (CNS) which, histologically and otherwise, resemble MS. In viral disease, there may be focal inflammation as well as primary demyelination. The recognition of virus persistence in the CNS gave an important impetus to the search for a viral etiology for MS. Several chronic CNS diseases in animals (visna, scrapie, mink encephalopathy) and in humans (Creutzfeldt–Jakob disease, kuru) may be associated with transmissible agents. However, conventional viruses such as measles are also able to persist within the CNS under certain immunological conditions, such as in the case of subacute sclerosing panencephalitis (SSPE). Since the early 1960s, the measles virus has often been implicated in MS (Adams and Imagawa 1962) following the discovery on several occasions of elevated antibody titers against measles in some MS patients, and the detection of the measles viral genome in the brains of some people suffering from this disease (Haase et al. 1981). The fact that positive findings have not been found in all brains and body fluids examined does not exclude the possibility of an etiological connection. However, in the case of the measles hypothesis, definitive proof is lacking. If there were a causal relationship, vaccination against measles, which has been practiced for over 20 years in the U.S., should lead to a significant reduction in the incidence of MS in the near future. An association between MS and other viruses, such as rabies, parainfluenza, cytomegalovirus, corona, herpes simplex etc., has been suggested. Some of these have been dismissed as artifacts or laboratory infections, and further extensive research has failed to prove any connection with others.

A relationship between MS and particular forms of spirochetes (*Spirochaeta myelophthora*) which was postulated by Gabriel Steiner during more than 50 years of scientific work (Steiner 1931) could not be proved in numerous other studies. Nevertheless, this theory has recently received new impetus (Gay and Dick 1986) following the observation of MS-like pictures in encephalomyelitis caused by borrelia (see Chapter 11).

Similarly, a prematurely postulated causal relationship between MS and viruses of the group to which the human immunodeficiency virus (HIV) belongs (Koprowski et al. 1985) was refuted in numerous controlled studies.

The observation of perivenous infiltrates of lymphocytes stimulated great interest in the autoimmune theory of MS. It was possible in animal experiments to induce autoimmune disease following sensitization to myelin basic protein (MBP) (Rivers et al. 1933) – the so-called experimental allergic (autoimmune) encephalomyelitis which, in several respects, is similar to MS

(see Chapters 2 and 3). Interest in this has continued and has been stimulated by numerous further experiments.

Over the last century, interest in the various theories concerning the etiology of the disease has waxed and waned in a way which is reminiscent of the course of the clinical signs of the disease itself. In Chapter 5, an attempt is made to compile these theories into a hypothesis which takes account of all the relevant information.

It is interesting to read the old literature, and to compare what was understood about MS with the state of our knowledge today. Various conference volumes and review articles made history when they were published, and have been consulted by thousands of researchers over the years. They form the landmarks from which an overview may be gained of research past and present, and they contain many discussions which are worth reading, for example: the *Research Publications of the Association for Research in Nervous and Mental Diseases*, Volume 2 (1921) and Volume 28 (1950); *Annals of the New York Academy of Sciences*, Volume 122 (1965) and Volume 436 (1984); *Handbook of Clinical Neurology*, Volume 9 (1970) and Volume 47 (1986).

2

Pathology and experimental models

INTRODUCTION

Multiple sclerosis is one of the neurological diseases which were defined relatively early in the history of medicine. Descriptions of its macroscopic pathology first appeared during the 18th century, and a detailed summary of histological findings was given by Charcot (1868), whose basic study of MS can be regarded as the starting point for the intensive research into its clinical features, pathology, and pathogenesis which followed.

The clinical definition of MS includes a chronic relapsing or progressive disease course, and signs and symptoms which suggest the presence of multifocal lesions in the CNS. Neuroimaging, electrophysiology, and laboratory tests on the cerebrospinal fluid (CSF) may also help to establish the clinical diagnosis. In neuropathological terms, MS is defined as an inflammatory demyelinating disease of the CNS, which is characterized by chronic perivenous inflammation, multifocal plaquelike demyelination, and reactive glial scar formation. It is obvious that this neuropathological definition not only includes the typical cases of chronic MS, but also atypical cases of acute or monophasic manifestations of this disease. In addition, on the basis of neuropathology, MS is only one member of a larger family of diseases, the so-called inflammatory demyelinating disorders (Hallervorden 1940; Adams and Kubik 1952). These diseases may have an acute or chronic course, they may affect both the central and the peripheral nervous systems, and they may also present as transitional forms between the more clearly defined disease entities (Marburg 1906; Hallervorden 1940; Adams and Kubik 1952; Krücke 1973). For example, combined forms of

acute disseminated or hemorrhagic encephalomyelitis with MS have been described (Krücke 1973). In some MS patients, the peripheral nervous system may be affected with inflammatory demyelination similar to that found in the lesions of the CNS (Marburg 1906; Jellinger 1969; Lassmann et al. 1981a; Lassmann 1983a).

Although such acute and transitional cases are somewhat atypical, and represent only a small minority of all MS cases, their rapid progression and disease activity make them especially suitable for studies on the mechanisms of inflammation and demyelination of this disease. Thus, most of the data presently available on the pathogenesis of MS are, in fact, derived from studies of these atypical cases. In time, it should become apparent to what extent pathogenic concepts derived from the study of acute MS cases are truly applicable to chronic manifestations of the disease.

THE PLAQUES

The essential lesions of MS are the confluent demyelinated plaques scattered throughout the brain and spinal cord (Fig. 2.1). The macroscopic and histological appearances of these lesions were described in detail at the beginning of this century (Marburg 1906; Siemerling and Raecke 1914; Dawson 1916; Hallervorden 1940). In chronic, inactive MS, the plaques appear macroscopically as pale-gray, sharply demarcated, round to polygonal, frequently confluent lesions. On the lesional border, fingerlike extensions which follow the distribution of small venules can be seen entering the plaque (Dawson 1916; Fig. 2.1). Due to the astroglial scar tissue formation, the tissue texture is more dense

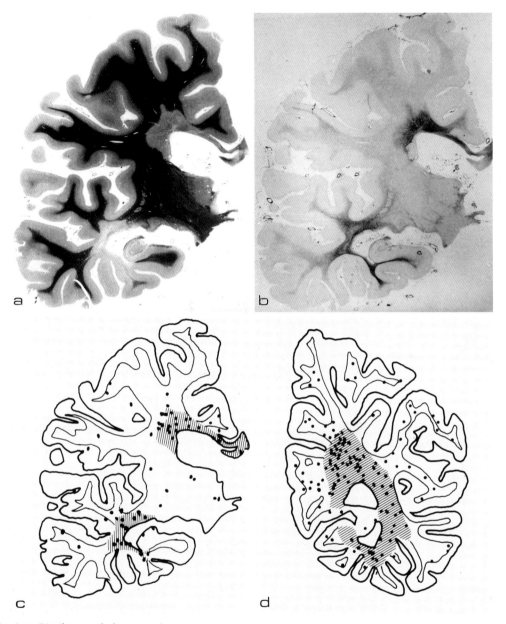

Fig. 2.1. Distribution of plaques in the CNS in active MS: large confluent demyelinated plaques with reactive gliosis in periventricular sites. (a) Luxol-fast blue myelin stain; (b) Kanzler stain for glia scar formation. × 1.) (c) Diagram of inflammation (points) and demyelinated areas (shaded) in the areas shown in (a). (d) A similar diagram of inflammation and demyelination in the occipital lobe of the same patient. Inflammatory infiltrates are not restricted to areas of demyelination, but are also present in high density in the surrounding "normal" white and gray matter.

in the plaques than in the surrounding tissue. Although plaques are located in both the white and gray matter of the brain, the color difference between myelinated and demyelinated tissue means that they are more clearly visible without the aid of a microscope in the white matter.

Histologically, the plaques are characterized by complete loss of myelin. In most of the lesions, oligodendrocytes are also lost, or are at least greatly reduced in number. In comparison to the myelin sheaths, axons are relatively well preserved in the lesions, although there is frequently some reduction of axonal density within the plaques. A typical feature of chronic inactive lesions is an intense glial scar formation (Fig. 2.1), characterized by an increased number of astrocytes and their cell processes, which are densely packed with glial filaments. These cells and their processes represent the majority of the cellular matrix between the demyelinated axons of the plaques. The myelin sheaths of nerve fibers which enter a plaque from the normal white matter terminate at a node of Ranvier, whereas the demyelinated axon can be traced into the demyelinated plaque, in what is known as segmental demyelination. Nerve fibers with atypically thin myelin sheaths and short internodal myelin segments are frequently found at the borders of inactive chronic plaques. These thin myelin sheaths seem to be the result of a limited degree of remyelination (see Fig. 2.5).

Besides demyelination, characteristic alterations of medium-sized or larger vessels are typical in inactive MS plaques. Light microscopy shows an intense perivascular fibrosis (Spielmeyer 1922). Under the electron microscope, the perivascular spaces appear to be dilated, and the perivascular glial limitans is separated from the vessel wall by septated connective tissue spaces which in many respects resemble small lymphatic vessels (Prineas 1979). It has not yet been determined whether these structures represent true lymphatic drainage sites (Prineas 1979), or simply connective tissue proliferation due to the chronic inflammatory process (Lassmann et al. 1981b).

Active MS plaques are different from inactive lesions in many respects. Macroscopically, active lesions are pink (salmon red) and less well demarcated than inactive ones. In addition, the active lesions have a soft consistency, possibly even softer than the surrounding normal brain tissue. Under the microscope, the characteristic feature of selective loss of the myelin sheath is visible. Although axons are relatively preserved in comparison to myelin, acute changes of axonal degeneration are frequent. The oligodendrocytes are difficult to evaluate, since in lesions with extensive inflammatory infiltration, differentiation between them and inflammatory cells is only possible with specific markers. However, as discussed below, the numbers

and structural features of oligodendrocytes within the lesions may vary in different MS patients. The tissue in active plaques appears spongy due to massive edema, and is heavily infiltrated by macrophages which are loaded with myelin degradation products (Fig. 2.2). In between, highly activated polymorphic and bizarre-looking astrocytes are present in the lesions, and these may sometimes give rise to diagnostic confusion with brain tumors.

Three main criteria are used to separate active from inactive lesions: the increased cell density, the ill-distinct plaque border, and the presence of macrophages with lipid debris. However, none of these three criteria is really reliable. Both the increased cell density due to inflammation, and the presence of macrophages with lipid debris may be present in lesions for a long time, possibly up to 6 months after the initiation of the lesion (Lumsden 1970). Similarly, the indistinct border of a demyelinated plaque frequently represents remyelination and not active demyelination (Prineas and Connell 1979; Lassmann 1983a). Thus, actively demyelinating lesions should be identified by the presence of initial myelin degradation products in the macrophages (Seitelberger 1969; Figs. 2.2 and 2.3).

Apart from the typical MS plaques described above, other lesions have been described in the literature.

Shadow plaques

Shadow plaques are mainly found in the brains of patients with either acute or chronic progressive MS (Lumsden 1970; Lassmann 1983a; Prineas 1986). They are similar to other chronic MS plaques in that they are sharply demarcated from the surrounding normal white matter. They are either found at the margin of large demyelinated plaques or are present as independent lesions (Fig. 2.4). Shadow plaques show a uniform reduction of myelin density due both to the presence of unusually thin myelin sheaths around the axons and to some reduction in axonal density. Like other chronic MS plaques, shadow plaques are characterized by dense astroglial scar formation. In rare instances, the early stages of shadow plaque formation may be associated with signs of ongoing lesional activity (Lassmann 1983a; Prineas 1986). For many years they were regarded as incompletely demyelinated lesions (Lumsden

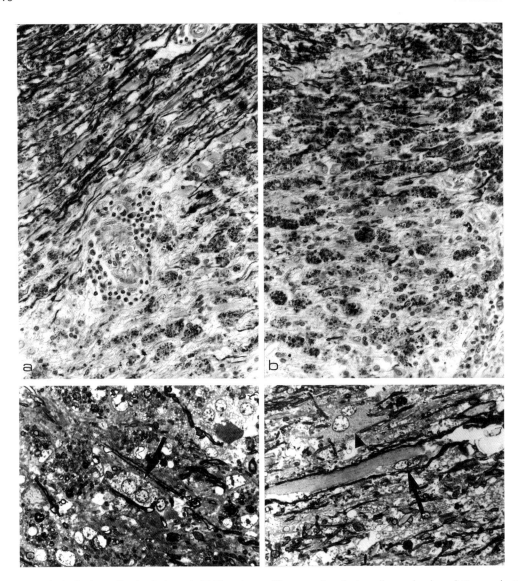

Fig. 2.2. Actively demyelinating lesions. (a,b) Chronic MS. The edge of an active lesion shows, in (a), a perivascular inflammatory reaction, with multiple macrophages with granular, MBP reactive degradation products in the demyelinated zone and between the preserved myelinated fibers at the plaque edge (a,b). (Immunocytochemistry for MBP; × 320.) (c) An actively demyelinating lesion in acute MS (Marburg's type). There are abundant small granular degradation products in the macrophages, and interfascicular oligodendrocytes (arrow) with cytoplasmic edema. (Toluidine blue; × 800.) (d) An actively demyelinating lesion in chronic MS. This shows infiltration of macrophages between axons and myelin (arrow), and extensive protoplasmic gliosis with multinucleated astrocytes (triangle). (Toluidine blue; × 800.)

Fig. 2.3. The borders of demyelinated plaques in different stages of demyelinating activity. (a) Acute MS. There is pronounced active myelin destruction and macrophages with early osmiophilic degradation products of variable size and structure (small granular inclusions appear adjacent to large, partly vesiculated degradation products). In the center of the plaque (lower portion of the figure), there is extensive protoplasmic gliosis and edema. (Toluidine blue; × 800.) (b) The edge of an actively demyelinating lesion in chronic MS. Adjacent to the normal white matter there are abundant macrophages with small granular degradation products (arrows). In the center of the plaque, pronounced fibrillary gliosis is apparent, together with some scattered macrophages with lipid inclusions (triangles). Protoplasmic gliosis is present in the surrounding white matter (thick

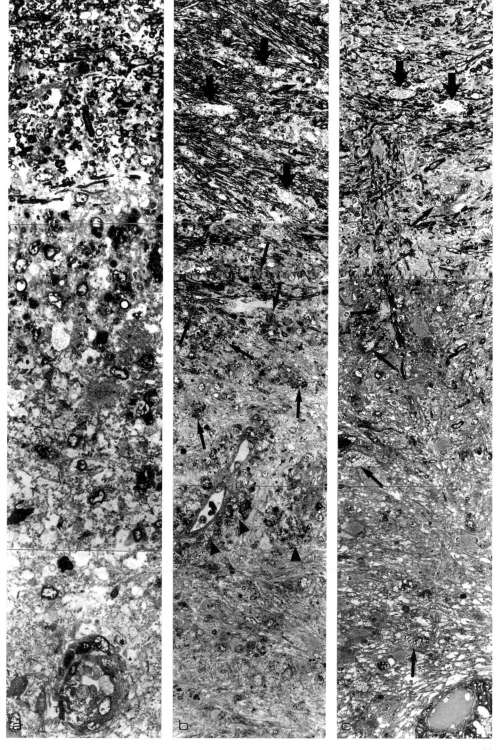

arrows). (Toluidine blue; × 800.) (c) A demyelinating plaque in chronic MS in a later stage of plaque formation than in (b). There are multiple macrophages with lipid inclusions (arrows), and extensive fibrillary gliosis in the lesions, as well as protoplasmic gliosis in the surrounding white matter (thick arrows). (× 600.)

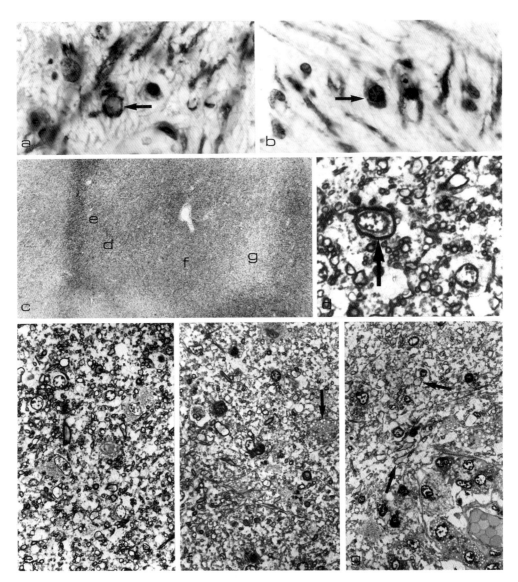

Fig. 2.4. Remyelination in MS lesions. (a) The edge of a lesion in acute MS. This shows thin MBP-positive myelin sheaths and an oligodendrocyte with cytoplasmic expression of MBP (arrow). (Immunocytochemistry for MBP; × 800.) (b) A demyelinated lesion in chronic MS. There are thin MBP-positive myelin sheaths, and an oligodendrocyte with cytoplasmic MBP reactivity (arrow). (Immunocytochemistry with anti-MBP serum; × 800.) (c) Chronic MS. A perivascular shadow plaque. The letters d, e, f, and g on the figure indicate the sites shown in detail in Figs. (d) to (g) respectively. (Toluidine blue; × 40.) (d) Edge of the shadow plaque with multiple thin myelin sheaths. One oligodendrocyte is surrounded by aberrant myelin (arrow). (Toluidine blue; × 1200.) (e) The edge of the shadow plaque with abundant, very thin myelin sheaths together with some normal myelinated fibers. There is extensive protoplasmic gliosis. (Toluidine blue; × 800.) (f) A more central portion of the shadow plaque with abundant small islets of thinly myelinated nerve fibers, and some macrophages with late myelin degradation products (arrow). (Toluidine blue; × 800.) (g) The central portion of the shadow plaque showing very few islets of thinly myelinated nerve fibers (arrow). (Toluidine blue; × 800.)

1970), and it only recently became evident that their thin myelin sheaths are due to remyelination rather than to incomplete demyelination (Lassmann 1983a; Prineas 1986).

Concentric plaques

Another rare lesion which is mainly found in cases of acute and subacute MS is the so-called concentric plaque. Concentric plaques can be the dominant lesions in concentric sclerosis (Balo 1928), but smaller ones may also be present in classical cases of acute or subacute MS. The lesions are generally located around a central blood vessel, and are characterized by alternating rings of myelinated and demyelinated tissue, giving them the appearance of onion bulbs. Their pathogenesis is still controversial, several different mechanisms having been suggested, including vascular factors (Courville 1970), secondary axonal degeneration, and topographical differences in the physicochemical properties of the extracellular matrix (Hallervorden and Spatz 1933). Recent studies suggest that the myelinated areas of concentric lesions may be formed by remyelination (Moore et al. 1985).

Destructive plaques

Destructuve plaques may sometimes be found in severe cases of acute or subacute MS. In these lesions, the axonal density is greatly reduced, and reactive axonal spheroids are frequent in the active stages. In more chronic lesions, the texture of the tissue is loose, and the extracellular space is dilated or filled with a dense astroglial matrix. In chronic MS, such destructive plaques frequently give rise to secondary tract degeneration in the brain and spinal cord.

Plaques with destruction of astrocytes

These are rare lesions in Caucasian MS patients, but have been found in MS patients in Japan (Itoyama et al. 1985). They are mainly located in the spinal cord. In the center of these large confluent plaques, astrocytes as well as myelin and oligodendrocytes are lost. Axons, however, remain preserved, and can later be remyelinated by Schwann cells derived from spinal roots. In the periphery of the lesions, a dense glial scar is found in which some demyelinated axons are remyelinated by oligodendrocytes.

Although these atypical lesions are rare, and mainly found in patients with acute and rapidly progressive MS, their existence suggests that the pathogenic mechanisms of plaque formation may be quite variable in different patients.

INFLAMMATION

The most remarkable alterations in the CNS of MS patients are the demyelinated plaques. It is therefore not surprising that for many years the significance of the accompanying inflammatory reaction was underestimated in the interpretation of the pathogenesis of the disease. Although early pathological descriptions of MS emphasized the presence of inflammatory infiltrates, the question of whether the inflammatory reaction was primary or secondary in nature was only recently addressed in detail in a large systematic study by Guseo and Jellinger (1975). They found inflammatory infiltrates in 60% of all cases investigated. Particularly intense inflammation was present in cases with active demyelination, no inflammatory infiltrates being found in some patients with longstanding inactive disease or in patients who had been treated with massive doses of immunosuppressive agents. Apart from these cases, very few were found in this series which presented with active demyelination in the absence of overt perivenous inflammatory infiltrates. Thus, until recently, controversy remained about whether the inflammatory reaction is a primary event, leading to demyelination, or a secondary response to the demyelinative process.

With the advance of modern immunology, pathogenic theories centered around the inflammatory reaction in the brain tissue. Active phases of the disease are frequently associated with characteristic fluctuations of T-lymphocyte subpopulations in the peripheral circulation (Bach et al. 1980). Neuroimaging studies in MS patients revealed that disease activity is associated with blood–brain barrier damage, which appears to be a result of the inflammatory reaction (Miller et al. 1988a). The most important evidence comes from experimental studies on autoimmune encephalomyelitis. As is discussed in detail below, in these models a T-cell-mediated inflammatory reaction can lead to inflammatory demyelinating lesions closely resembling those in MS.

With the availability of specific markers for leukocyte subpopulations, and with the improvement in immunocytochemical and electron microscopic techniques, it became clear that even when there were low numbers of inflammatory infiltrates, there was diffuse inflammatory infiltration of the tissue with T-lymphocytes and macrophages (Prineas and Wright 1978; Traugott 1984).

The perivascular inflammatory infiltrates are mainly composed of T-lymphocytes, which in actively demyelinating lesions also infiltrate the parenchyme of the CNS (Traugott et al. 1982; Nyland et al. 1982; Booss et al. 1983). However, the infiltration of the tissue with T-lymphocytes is not restricted to demyelinating lesions, but can also be found in the surrounding normal white matter (Booss et al. 1983; Traugott et al. 1983; Traugott 1984; Weiner et al. 1984). Although further characterization of lymphocyte subsets was attempted in several studies, the results are so far less clear. Some authors described a preponderance of CD4$^+$ (so-called helper/inducer) cells in active lesions and in the surrounding white matter, whereas CD8$^+$ (suppressor/cytotoxic) T-cells were concentrated in the inactive plaque center (Traugott 1984). Other authors emphasized a dominance of CD8$^+$ cells throughout the lesions, although the relative contribution of CD4$^+$ cells was still thought to be higher in active as compared to inactive lesions (Booss et al. 1983; Weiner et al. 1984).

Experimental studies on the immune surveillance of the nervous system (Wekerle et al. 1986; Lassmann et al. 1991), as well as the identification of autoreactive T-lymphocytes in the blood and CSF of MS patients (Olsson 1992), point toward a central role for T-cells in the induction of MS lesions. The selective recruitment and local proliferation of T-cells in the lesions should thus lead to an oligoclonal expansion of T-lymphoctyes in the plaques which can be detected by a restricted heterogeneity of T-cell receptor subtypes. In accordance with this concept, a restricted α/β T-cell receptor usage in MS plaques was described in a preliminary study (Oksenberg et al. 1990). However, these results were not confirmed in a large subsequent investigation (Wucherpfennig et al. 1992a), which found not only an unselective, polyclonal distribution of α/β T-cell recep-

tor subtypes, but also a different dominance of T-cell receptor subtypes in different brain lesions in a given MS patient. Thus, if autoreactive T-lymphocytes play a role in MS at all, it may be very difficult to detect them in established lesions as they may be masked by a high number of unspecific, secondary T-cells recruited to the established focus. This interpretation is in line with recent experimental data which showed that the pool of antigen-reactive T-cells in established lesions of autoimmune encephalomyelitis is small (Fallis et al. 1987).

However, the further characterization of inflammatory cells in MS lesions led to an unexpected finding. A surprisingly high proportion of T-lymphocytes with δ T-cell receptors was found within the plaques. Gamma/delta T-cells appear to form a first, and relatively unspecific, barrier against bacteria in mucous membranes (Kaufmann 1990). A considerable proportion of these cells is directed against stress proteins, which are highly conserved during evolution and present in nearly identical form in bacteria, animals, and humans. Stress proteins are synthesized in inflammatory lesions, and can be detected in inflammatory cells and glia cells in MS lesions (Selmaj et al. 1991a; Wucherpfennig et al. 1992b). In-vitro studies showed that the γ/δ cells which are directed against the stress proteins hsp 65 and 70 preferentially kill oligodendrocytes and the infiltration of MS lesions with γ/δ T-lymphocytes may therefore represent an amplification mechanism by which the tissue damage occurring during the course of an inflammatory reaction is potentiated by autoimmune reactions directed against endogenous stress proteins. The preferential cytotoxicity of this reaction against oligodendrocytes may partly be responsible for demyelination in MS plaques.

The majority of inflammatory cells in active MS lesions are activated macrophages (Traugott et al. 1983; Woodroofe et al. 1986) which are highly expressive for Fc-γ receptors and Class II histocompatibility antigens. In addition, located particularly in the perivascular spaces are plasma cells which mainly produce IgG and less IgM and IgA (Esiri 1977; Mussini et al. 1977; Budka et al. 1985). These plasma cells appear to be responsible for the intrathecal immunoglobulin synthesis which can be detected in the CSF and which is a characteristic feature of chronic MS.

An interesting aspect of the inflammatory reaction in MS is the distribution of cytokines in the lesions. Interleukin 1 (IL-1) was mainly found in areas of active demyelination. Cells with IL-2 receptors, as well as IL-2 itself, were found in the center of demyelinated plaques and in perivascular infiltrates (Hofman et al. 1986; Woodroofe et al. 1986). Interferon alpha (IFN-α) was found in macrophages, whereas IFN-γ was reported to be expressed in lymphocytes, astrocytes, and microglia (Traugott and Lebon 1988). Lymphotoxin was seen in T-lymphocytes and microglia, and tumor necrosis factor alpha (TNF-α) in macrophages and astrocytes (Selmaj et al. 1991b). However, these data have to be interpreted cautiously, since immunocytochemistry for cytokines is hampered by serious technical problems. More recently, mRNA for IL-1, IL-2, and IL-4 has been detected in active MS lesions by the polymerase chain reaction. Macrophages in the lesions also contained prostaglandin E (PGE) (Hofman et al. 1986). Overall, the data on cytokines in MS lesions are in agreement with the concept that a T-cell-mediated inflammatory reaction is essential in the pathogenesis of the lesions.

A key question in the pathogenesis of inflammatory demyelinating diseases is: how do inflammatory cells pass the blood–brain barrier and reach their target tissue? Specific antigen recognition at the luminal surface of brain endothelial cells appears to play only a marginal role in brain inflammation, if at all. In the normal CNS there is no expression of Class II histocompatibility antigens on the luminal surface of endothelial cells (Vass et al. 1986). In addition, the transport of autoantigens from the brain into the circulation through the blood–brain barrier appears to be even more restricted than the transport from the blood into the CNS tissue (Broadwell 1989). Activated T-lymphocytes can pass the normal blood–brain barrier in an antigen-independent manner (Wekerle et al. 1986; Hickey et al. 1991). More recent studies suggest that adhesion molecules are essential in the migration of leukocytes through the vessel wall (Shimizu et al. 1992). Adhesion of leukocytes on normal brain endothelial cells is poor; it can, however, be improved by exposure of endothelial cells to various cytokines (Male et al. 1990a; 1990b). Under normal conditions, cerebral endothelial cells express adhesion molecules such as ICAM 1, ICAM 2, LFA 3, CD44, and CD9 at low levels. In inflammatory lesions, the expression of these adhesion molecules is

increased, and new adhesion molecules are induced which are normally found only at specific sites of the vasculature (Sobel et al. 1990; Raine et al. 1990; Wilcox et al. 1990; Lassmann et al. 1991; Rössler et al. 1992). The interaction between VCAM, expressed on endothelial cells, and VLA 4, expressed on leukocytes, appears to play a special role in the recruitment of leukocytes to inflammatory brain lesions. A specific blockade of this interaction by monoclonal antibodies may prevent inflammation in autoimmune encephalitis (Yednock et al. 1992).

An important aspect of T-cell-mediated inflammation is the location at which antigen is recognized by T-lymphocytes in the lesions. T-lymphocytes recognize their antigen only when presented in the context of histocompatibility antigens. Whereas the expression of Class I histocompatibility antigens in the CNS is widespread, the expression of Class II antigens is more restricted (Vass et al. 1990). In MS lesions, Class II histocompatibility antigens are mainly found within the lesions and in their immediate vicinity (Woodroofe et al. 1986). The results of some light microscope studies suggest that these antigens may be present on the surface of astrocytes in the lesions (Traugott et al. 1985; Hofman et al. 1986; Woodroofe et al. 1986). This finding, together with observations on the presence of interferons (Traugott and Lebon 1988) and TNF-α (Selmaj et al. 1991b) in astrocytes, suggests that these cells may play an important role in the propagation of the lesions.

PATHOLOGY OF THE NERVOUS SYSTEM OUTSIDE THE PLAQUES

Although most of the studies on the pathology of MS concentrated on changes within the demyelinated plaques, it recently became clear that the normal white and gray matter outside the plaques is also affected. In biochemical studies, changes were found in the normal white matter with respect to the composition of myelin and an increase in the activity of proteolytic enzymes (Allen and McKeown 1979). These changes were partly interpreted as evidence of a generalized defect in myelin in MS patients.

However, microscopic demyelinated lesions are frequently present in macroscopically normal tissue. Such lesions alone can explain biochemical alterations in myelin in these areas.

Furthermore, the MS brain contains changes which are secondary to the presence of demyelinated plaques. These changes have been categorized as MS encephalopathy, and are mainly present in patients with longstanding severe disease (Jellinger 1969; Seitelberger 1973). They include secondary Wallerian degeneration due to axonal loss in plaques, chronic edema, and brain alterations induced by the poor general health of the patients, for example malnutrition, chronic infections, or uremia.

Wallerian degeneration in MS is due to axonal damage in demyelinated plaques which may be quite variable from case to case. In severe cases, it may lead to degeneration of long ascending and descending tracts as well as to a diffuse reduction in the volume of brain white matter. This may finally result in severe brain atrophy, with dilatation of the ventricles and the subarachnoid space.

An additional factor which may damage the nervous tissue outside the plaques appears to be the chronic inflammatory process itself (see Fig. 2.1). This leads to chronic disturbance of blood–brain barrier function, and to direct toxic effects of inflammatory mediators. Both a direct effect of certain cytokines as well as chronic edema can stimulate astrocytes, and thus result in scar formation.

DISTRIBUTION OF PLAQUES IN THE NERVOUS SYSTEM

A characteristic feature of MS pathology is the disseminated distribution of demyelinated lesions throughout the brain and spinal cord. Although plaques may appear at random in any areas of the CNS, certain predilection sites for plaque formation have been described (Steiner 1931; Hallervorden 1940; Fog 1950; Lumsden 1970; Oppenheimer 1978). In the brain, these sites include the periventricular white matter, especially at the lateral angle of the cerebral ventricles (see Fig. 2.1). Other areas with a high incidence of demyelinated lesions are the optic system (optic nerves and chiasm), the cerebellar peduncles, the cerebellar white matter, and the cortico–subcortical junction, particularly in cortical sulci. Within the spinal cord, the lesions are concentrated in the cervical portions, located mainly in the lateral columns (Fog 1950; Oppenheimer 1978).

The topographical distribution of plaques can be partly explained by the distribution of post-

capillary venules in the CNS. Since MS lesions in general arise around a central vein, the probability of an initial inflammatory focus is greater in areas with a high density of postcapillary drainage veins. In addition, however, the concentration of MS plaques at the inner or outer surfaces of the brain and spinal cord suggests that additional factors derived from the CSF may precipitate the lesions.

An additional indication that blood–brain barrier damage may facilitate the formation of plaques comes from observations that demyelination in MS may occur at sites of brain damage which are unrelated to the disease. Although a combination of MS with other brain diseases is rare (Jellinger 1969), demyelinated plaques can sometimes be found around small infarcts or vascular malformations.

A dogma of clinical neurology is that MS is a disease which is specific to the CNS. When lesions in the peripheral nervous system are found, the diagnosis of MS is questioned. This is justified in typical chronic MS, where pathological changes of the peripheral nervous system are mainly due to secondary axonal degeneration resulting from destructive spinal cord lesions or may reflect neuropathies in the course of metabolic disturbances or malnutrition (Hasson et al. 1958). In rare instances, however, primary demyelination can be found in the peripheral nervous system of chronic MS patients.

The situation is different in Marburg's type of acute MS. In this disease, primary inflammatory demyelination in the peripheral nervous system is common (Marburg 1906; Lassmann et al. 1981a; Lassmann 1983a). Although, due to the small number of cases described, a clear incidence figure cannot be given, it has to be considered that in Marburg's original description, all patients with acute MS showed peripheral nervous system involvement. Thus the presence of inflammatory demyelination in the peripheral nervous system does not rule out a diagnosis of MS.

DEVELOPMENT OF PLAQUES

In spite of many years of research, our understanding of the development of plaques in MS is still incomplete. There are several reasons for this.

Actively demyelinating lesions are rare in autopsy material from patients with chronic MS.

Thus most of the published data are taken from the study of active lesions from patients with acute, subacute, or atypical MS. It is not yet proven whether the pathogenesis of demyelination is the same in acute and chronic MS.

Furthermore, biochemical and immunological studies of active MS lesions are hampered by the difficulty of identifying such lesions macroscopically, and there are no biochemical markers available which allow the identification of the early stages of demyelination. Thus, the interpretation of the immunological findings in MS lesions is to a large extent based on analogy with experimental models of the disease, an approach which has not been proved to be justified.

There is little doubt that in inactive plaques of chronic MS, myelin and the large majority of oligodendrocytes are destroyed, whereas axons and nerve cells are relatively preserved. Such selective damage to the nervous tissue can be induced by several different mechanisms (Wisniewski 1977).

a. Primary damage of myelin sheaths may be followed by secondary degeneration of oligodendrocytes.
b. Myelin and oligodendrocytes may be damaged simultaneously in the course of plaque formation.
c. A primary cytolytic affection of oligodendrocytes may lead to secondary myelin destruction.

The clarification of these points is central to the understanding of the pathogenesis of MS.

Myelin

The alterations in myelin sheaths in active lesions were described in detail during the first decades of this century. In the plaques, myelin sheaths are selectively destroyed, and axons are relatively well preserved (Figs. 2.2 and 2.5). In actively demyelinating lesions, the myelin sheaths appear thin, with irregular pale-staining properties, or they may be transformed into small, granular degradation products (Marburg 1906; see also Figs. 2.2 and 2.3). In the early studies, an irregular destruction of the myelin sheath was described, which starts focally at any point in the internodium and then extends along the entire myelin segment (Marburg 1906). In addition, close contact between macrophages ("gitter cells") and the damaged myelin sheath, as well as the uptake of myelin fragments into macrophages were described early in the history of MS research (Babinski 1885). Further details of the patterns of demyelination were discovered using electron microscopic techniques.

Two different patterns of myelin destruction have been described. The first consists of an interaction of phagocytic cells with the myelin sheaths (Prineas and Connell 1978; Prineas 1986). These cells then take up small fragments of myelin. Contact between myelin and macrophages is frequently established through "coated pits," and myelin degradation products can then be found in macrophages in "coated vesicles." A similar pattern of phagocytosis is found in receptor-mediated uptake of macromolecules (Goldstein et al. 1979), and has also been described in the course of the phagocytosis of particulated immune complexes (Montesano et al. 1983; Mellman and Plutner 1984). This sequence of demyelination may thus suggest that myelin, opsonized by specific antibodies, is attacked by macrophages in the course of demyelination (Prineas 1986).

In less common instances, especially in cases where the inflammatory reaction is extensive and severe, an invasion of macrophages into myelin sheaths can be seen (Prineas and Raine 1976; Lassmann 1983a; 1983b), a mechanism which is similar to the "myelin stripping" observed in experimental autoimmune encephalomyelitis (see Fig. 2.2d). In addition, in acute cases with very severe inflammation, myelin sheaths may be transformed completely into vesicular material – "vesicular disruption of myelin" (Lassmann 1983a). It is not clear whether this vesicular transformation is a genuine pattern of demyelination or is mediated by autolysis of predamaged myelin sheaths. Furthermore, in some cases alterations in oligodendrocyte processes, described as "dying back oligodendrogliopathy" have been observed, that indicate a primary affection of oligodendrogenesis in the pathogenesis of demyelination (Rodriguez et al. 1993).

The myelin fragments which are taken up in macrophages are degraded within these cells to cholesterol esters and triglycerides (Seitelberger 1969). The earliest degradation products are small granular cytoplasmic inclusions in macrophages which have the same histochemical and immunocytochemical staining patterns as normal myelin (see Figs. 2.2 and 2.3). Under the

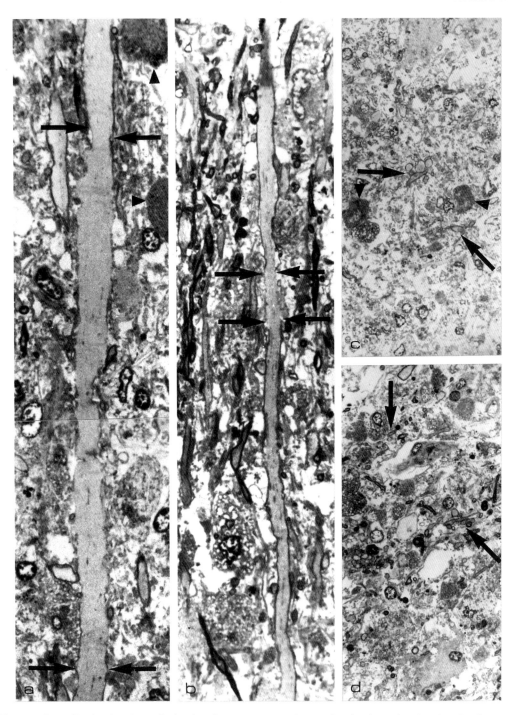

Fig. 2.5. Remyelination in MS. (a) The border of an actively demyelinating lesion in acute MS (Marburg's type). A longitudinal section through a demyelinated axon with two small segments of very thin myelin sheaths (arrows), and several axonal spheroids (triangle). (Toluidine blue; × 1500.) (b) An actively demyelinating lesion in chronic MS showing a remyelinated axon with very thin myelin sheaths and widened node of Ranvier (arrows). (Toluidine blue; × 1500.) (c,d) Central areas of an actively demyelinating lesion in acute MS with small clusters of remyelinated nerve fibers (arrows), and some axonal spheroids (triangles). (Toluidine blue; × 800.)

electron microscope, the degradation products can be seen to be built up by lamellated myelinlike inclusions. The initial chemical degradation of these inclusions can be visualized by the positive Marchi or OTAN reaction, which suggests an increase in hydrophobicity of the material compared to normal myelin (Hallpike and Adams 1969). The presence of these early myelin degradation products is at present the safest criterion for the identification of actively demyelinating plaques in MS (Lassmann 1983a; Prineas 1986). In later stages, the myelin degradation products are transformed into neutral lipid droplets (see Fig. 2.3) and some PAS-positive intracytoplasmic granules with a polymorphic ultrastructural appearance (Prineas 1975) which are removed from the tissue very slowly, and can be found within the lesions up to 6 months after plaque formation.

In actively demyelinating lesions, the macrophages are concentrated at sites where myelin sheaths are in the process of destruction (Seitelberger 1969; Prineas and Wright 1978; Hofman et al. 1986). In later stages, debris-containing phagocytes accumulate in the perivascular spaces (see Fig. 2.3). In spinal plaques which are touching the surface of the cord, debris-containing macrophages also drain into the CSF (Marburg 1906).

The vast majority of myelin degradation products are found in macrophages ("gitter cells"). In addition, however, debris may also be present in astrocytes in the form of small osmiophilic inclusions (Marburg 1906). Myelin degradation in astrocytes has been shown in vitro (Raine and Bornstein 1970b), in Wallerian degeneration, and in autoimmune encephalomyelitis (Lassmann 1983a). The conditions which stimulate astrocytes to become phagocytic cells in certain MS lesions are undefined.

Oligodendrocytes

Although in completely demyelinated, inactive plaques of chronic MS the population of oligodendrocytes is greatly reduced, or even completely lost (Prineas 1986), in the periphery of such lesions a variable number of oligodendrocytes is present which are engaged in the remyelination of nerve fibers (Prineas and Connell 1979; see also Fig. 2.5). It is, however, not clear whether these oligodendrocytes were preserved during the demyelinating process or whether they were recruited from a reserve pool of undifferentiated precursor cells.

In early ultrastructural studies, alterations in oligodendrocytes were described which mainly consisted of cellular edema, shrinkage of cytoplasm, condensation of the nuclei, and defects in cell membranes. However, it was difficult to differentiate these cells from the degenerating inflammatory cells which are frequently encountered in active MS lesions. Sometimes oligodendrocytes can be found embedded in the cytoplasm of other cells, in particular of astrocytes (Prineas 1986). However, in spite of complete demyelination, oligodendrocytes may be preserved either at the plaque edge (Raine et al. 1981) or even in the center of the lesions (Brück et al. 1994; see also Figs. 2.2 and 2.4).

Additional evidence which argues against a primary affection of oligodendrocytes comes from the comparison of MS lesions with those formed in disease with primary viral infection of oligodendrocytes. In progressive multifocal leukoencephalopathy (PML), the lesions are formed by the confluence of small demyelinated areas which correspond to the myelin territories of single oligodendrocytes. This gives the lesion a microscopic appearance reminiscent of moth-eaten tissues. Such lesions are fundamentally different from MS plaques, which are sharply demarcated from the normal white matter and are not associated with oligodendrocyte territories.

These data, taken together, indicate that at least in the majority of MS cases, the myelin sheath is the primary target of the destructive process, whereas oligodendrocytes may simultaneously or secondarily be affected in the course of myelin destruction. This interpretation is challenged by the observation of a disproportionately greater loss of myelin-associated glycoprotein (MAG) in comparison with other myelin proteins in MS lesions. Since MAG is mainly located in peripheral oligodendrocyte processes, these data were interpreted as an indication of primary oligodendrocyte dystrophy in MS lesions (Itoyama et al. 1980). Similar changes were also found in PML, which was taken as a model disease for primary virus-induced damage to oligodendrocytes, but were absent in the demyelinating lesions induced in the course of autoimmune encephalomyelitis. The experimental proof that oligodendroglia damage is a cause of the preferential loss of MAG is still missing. Furthermore, in experimental models of oligodendrocyte infection and virus-induced demyelination, a disproportionate loss of MAG was not found

(Vandevelde et al. 1983; Dal Canto and Barbano 1985). Similarly, the preferential loss of MAG was not present in MS plaques obtained from early autopsies with excellent tissue preservation (Prineas et al. 1984). Thus the extent to which minor myelin proteins such as MAG may be degraded more quickly than major myelin components in autopsy tissue has to remain unresolved.

With the availability of new markers and the development of new technologies, the fate of oligodendrocytes in MS lesions has again been addressed in recent studies. In some cases, evidence has been provided that oligodendrocytes may be completely destroyed in active lesions, but that new ones may be rapidly recruited from a pool of undifferentiated precursor cells (Prineas et al. 1989). The extent of remyelination appears to be partly determined by the availability of such precursors. In experimental systems, repeated demyelination and oligodendrocyte destruction within the same lesions may deplete this precursor pool and may lead to the establishment of persistently demyelinated plaques without remyelination (Ludwin 1980; Linington et al. 1992a). Other studies, however, led to different conclusions. The preservation of oligodendrocytes was described in early active lesions, and the cells were then lost at later stages in the formation of persistently demyelinated plaques (Selmaj et al. 1991a).

These somewhat conflicting results from different studies into the fate of oligodendrocytes in MS lesions may also be explained by an inherent variability in the development of plaques in different patients. In our own material, we found evidence for oligodendrocyte destruction together with a limited remyelination through precursor cells mainly in cases of chronic MS. In patients with very short disease duration, on the other hand, the majority of oligodendrocytes were preserved in the lesions, and rapid and complete remyelination was found throughout them (Lassmann 1983a; Brück et al. 1994; Ozawa et al. 1994). These data indicate that the mechanisms leading to demyelination may differ in patients with short- and long-standing disease duration (see also Chapter 5).

Astroglia

It is now well established that the alterations of astrocytes in MS lesions represent, at least in part, a secondary reaction to demyelination and tissue damage. In chronic MS lesions, astrocytes are moderately increased in number, and provide a network of processes which are densely packed with glial fibrils. These cell processes form a dense glial scar, in which demyelinated axons are embedded (see Fig. 2.3).

In active lesions, especially in cases of short disease duration, a protoplasmic glia reaction is mainly encountered (Field et al. 1962). The astrocytes appear as large, polymorphic cells with abundant cytoplasm, and may be multinucleated (see Fig. 2.2d). This pronounced astroglia reaction may sometimes imitate the pathology of a low-grade astrocytoma. However, the incidence of gliomas in MS patients is no higher than in members of a control population (Lumsden 1970).

Since alterations to the astrocytes similar to those described above can be found in a variety of other CNS diseases, they can be interpreted as a secondary reaction to tissue injury. There are, however, some aspects which may indicate an additional affection of astrocytes related to the immunological disease process. At the plaque edges of established lesions, the glia reaction may be found to extend a considerable distance into the surrounding normal white matter (see Fig. 2.3b, c), and may even be found in areas devoid of demyelination or secondary Wallerian degeneration (Allen and McKeown 1979). In addition, the increased activity of proteolytic enzymes found in the normal white matter of MS patients may be associated with increased lysosomal activation in astrocytes (Allen and McKeown 1979; Allen 1983). This general activation of astrocytes may be partly explained by the inflammatory reaction, since certain inflammatory cytokines may activate astrocytes (Fontana et al. 1980).

Another factor which points toward an immunological role of astrocytes in the lesions is the expression of histocompatibility antigens. T-cells recognize their antigens only when they are presented in the context of histocompatibility antigens (MHC antigens). Class I MHC antigens (HLA-A, B and C) are recognized by CD8[+] cells, whereas Class II MHC (HLA-D) positive cells present antigen to CD4[+] cells. Thus the presence of MHC antigen expression identifies cells as being capable of activating T-lymphocytes. Whereas Class I MHC antigens may be expressed by virtually all cells of the nervous system after stimulation with certain cytokines such as IFN-γ, the distribution of Class II MHC antigens is more restricted (Wong et al. 1984; Fontana et al. 1984).

In MS lesions, the expression of Class II antigens on astrocytes has been described in several studies (Traugott et al. 1985; Hofman et al. 1986; Woodroofe et al. 1986), performed on frozen sections. Class II MHC-positive astrocytes were identified by immunocytochemistry involving antibodies against glial fibrillary acidic protein (GFAP). Quantitative evaluation revealed that up to 50% of Class II positive cells at the border of actively demyelinating lesions may indeed represent astrocytes (Hofman et al. 1986). However, an unequivocal identification of Class II MHC expression on astrocytes is only possible using immune electron microscopic techniques, and convincing evidence on this topic is still not available. Furthermore, it appears that the contribution of microglia to Class II MHC expression was underestimated in these studies.

As has already been mentioned, in some MS cases, especially in Japanese patients, lesions can sometimes be found which are associated with the loss and derangement of astrocytes (Itoyama et al. 1985). Such plaques were found in the spinal cord, and were characterized by the loss of GFAP-positive cells and of myelin and oligodendrocytes. No information is yet available concerning the patterns of such tissue damage during the stage of active demyelination. However, similar lesions can be found in certain experimental models of autoimmune encephalomyelitis (Lassmann et al. 1980) in which the destruction of astrocytes is associated with extensive expression of Class II MHC antigens on virtually all cellular elements. In line with this observation, it has been shown in vitro that encephalitogenic, autoreactive T-lymphocytes may not only be activated by astrocytes, but may also destroy these cells in the course of antigen presentation (Sun and Wekerle 1986).

Axons and nerve cells

Whereas myelin sheaths and oligodendrocytes are destroyed in MS plaques, the axons and nerve cells remain preserved. However, as was pointed out in early studies on MS pathology (Marburg 1906), the sparing of axons is relative. A variable degree of axonal loss occurs in any chronic MS lesion. In actively demyelinating plaques, especially in severe cases of acute and subacute MS, acute axonal damage and reactive alterations in preserved axons, such as spheroids, are common findings (see Fig. 2.5a and c).

The consequences of axonal damage in the plaques may interfere with staging and pathogenic interpretation of the lesions. At the border of inactive demyelinated plaques, large globular myelin degradation products are frequently found which result from ongoing Wallerian degeneration, and which may simulate immunological activity in the lesions. Immunological studies on such lesions may lead to incorrect pathogenic conclusions. In addition, Wallerian degeneration at plaque edges may give rise to shadow plaque areas, which may make it difficult to evaluate the extent of remyelination.

As discussed above, axonal destruction in large plaques may lead to extensive secondary tract degeneration, especially prominent in the brainstem and spinal cord.

Nerve cell alterations have sometimes been described in MS lesions which mainly consist of "central chromatolysis," as a reaction to axonal damage, as well as increased accumulation of lipopigment. Overall, these changes appear to be secondary to the axonal damage. In single instances, acute destruction of nerve cells and neuronophagia have been described (Fraenkel and Jakob 1913). The relation of these changes to the underlying disease is not clear.

Remyelination

The first indication that remyelination may take place in MS came from Otto Marburg (1906), who described the appearance of extremely thin myelin sheaths in demyelinated plaques which were only visible following osmic acid impregnation. As one possible explanation for these changes, Marburg (1906) suggested they may represent an attempt at remyelination. These early observations were ignored during the following years.

In the early 1960s, the presence of remyelination was proven in certain experimental models (Bunge et al. 1961; Lampert 1965), and the characteristic morphological patterns of remyelinating nerve fibers have subsequently been defined (Blakemore 1976; Ludwin 1978). The alterations – the abnormally thin myelin sheaths, the shortened internodes, the presence of extremely short myelin segments, and the widening of the nodes of Ranvier – can also

be unequivocally identified in MS lesions (Suzuki et al. 1969; Prineas and Connell 1979;
Prineas 1986; see also Figs. 2.4 and 2.5). They
were found to be present in variable degree in
nearly all MS plaques at the border with the
normal white matter. In addition, similar
changes have been seen throughout entire
shadow plaques (Lassmann 1983a; Prineas
1986; see also Fig. 2.4). The first description of
shadow plaques came from Hermann Schlesinger (1909), who interpreted these changes as
incomplete demyelination. Recent studies,
however, suggest that even large confluent demyelinated plaques can eventually become
completely remyelinated (Lassmann 1983a;
Prineas 1986; Prineas et al. 1993a). Similarly, evidence for remyelination was found in the myelinated areas in a case of Balo's concentric sclerosis (Moore et al. 1985), but this finding was
not confirmed in a subsequent study on a larger
series of cases (Yao et al. 1994).

Controversy remains concerning the deriva-
tion of the oligodendrocytes which are responsible for remyelination in MS. A proportion of
oligodendrocytes may survive the active demyelinating episode, and may then be available
for remyelination (Lassmann 1983a). A significant proportion of mature oligodendrocytes can
be found in MS plaques at the earliest stages of
demyelination (Bruck et al. 1994). Furthermore,
myelin oligodendrocyte glycoprotein is abundantly expressed in oligodendrocytes in such
lesions. During development, this antigen appears very late in the course of myelination,
and is absent from undifferentiated oligodendrocyte precursors (Bruck et al. 1994). Alternatively, oligodendrocytes may be completely
destroyed, and remyelinating oligodendrocytes
may then be recruited by the proliferation of
cells at the lesional border or from undifferentiated precursors (Prineas 1986; Prineas et al.
1989). The recruitment of precursors and the
ability of mature oligodendrocytes to proliferate
are suggested from experimental models of demyelination (Ludwin 1978; 1980; 1984). Multiple demyelinating episodes in the same lesions,
which have recently been shown to occur in MS
(Prineas et al. 1993b), may then deplete the
pool of precursor cells which are available for
remyelination.

Recent evidence from our laboratory suggests that both mechanisms may be operating
in MS. The extent of oligodendrocyte destruction in the demyelinated plaques was found to

be very similar in different plaques from the
same patient, and was independent of lesional
activity. However, there was extreme variability in oligodendrocyte loss in different patients, ranging from nearly complete preservation to total loss (Brück et al. 1994; Ozawa et al.,
1994). Thus, depending on the patients studied, remyelination may occur either from preserved oligodendrocytes or through the recruitment of undifferentiated precursor cells.

It is thus generally agreed that remyelination
may occur in MS, although to what extent it
contributes to clinical recovery from the disease
remains unresolved. To address this point, several questions have to be answered.

a. What is the extent of remyelination in MS
   plaques?
b. Are there differences in the extent of remyelination in different MS patients?
c. What is the time course of remyelination?
d. Does remyelination in MS restore the electrophysiological functions of nerve fibers?

Although we are still far from definite answers to these questions, several interesting aspects have emerged during recent years.

The extent of remyelination in chronic MS
plaques in general is small; it is mostly restricted to a zone of less than 1 mm at the
plaque edge. As suggested from experimental
data, both the oligodendrocytes and their precursors appear to be lost completely in such lesions (Ludwin 1980). In addition, the extensive
glial scar formation appears to impede ingrowth of oligodendrocytes from the periphery
(Raine and Bornstein 1970a). Intrathecally produced demyelinating and myelination-inhibit-
ing antibodies may further impede the repair
process (Lassmann 1983a). In some cases,
mostly in acute but sometimes even in chronic
MS of long duration, large shadow plaques
may be present in high numbers, suggesting
that, under as yet undefined conditions, large
confluent plaques may be repaired.

Contrary to previous expectations, it turned
out that in acute, rapidly progressive MS, remyelination is more abundant than in the typical chronic disease variants (Lassmann 1983a).
In such acute cases, signs of remyelination may
be found adjacent to areas of active demyelination. Furthermore, shadow plaques are more
frequent in acute than in chronic MS (Lassmann 1983a; Prineas 1986).

The speed of remyelination also appears to

be different in acute and chronic MS (Lassmann 1983a). The finding that remyelination may frequently be found adjacent to active demyelination in the lesions of acute and subacute MS may be interpreted as evidence of recurrent demyelination in remyelinated areas (Prineas et al. 1993b). However, in experimental models of demyelination, it is not uncommon to find remyelination commencing within a few days of the onset of the demyelinating event. In contrast, in cases of chronic MS, remyelination, if present at all, is generally restricted to inactive plaques and is absent in actively demyelinating lesions. There, remyelination appears to start much later in the course of lesion evolution.

Although it has been shown in experimental models of demyelination that even incomplete remyelination may re-establish the electrophysiological function (Lidsky et al. 1980; Wisniewski et al. 1982), evidence for remyelination as a factor of functional repair in MS is still lacking.

A special form of remyelination is found in the spinal cord of MS patients. In these areas, ingrowth of Schwann cells into the demyelinated plaques may occur with subsequent remyelination with peripheral myelin (Feigin and Ogata 1971; Ghatak et al. 1974). Because of its different chemical and antigenic composition, this peripheral myelin is easily detected by histochemical and immunocytochemical techniques. Small islands of peripheral myelin are frequently found in the spinal MS plaques. Large confluent lesions which are completely remyelinated by Schwann cells are found in rare instances (Itoyama et al. 1985).

Experimental studies suggest that the ingrowth of Schwann cells with subsequent peripheral remyelination of central tracts is only possible when the astroglia population is severely impaired or destroyed during the active stage of demyelination (Blakemore 1976; Raine et al. 1978; Lassmann et al. 1980).

EXPERIMENTAL MODELS

Pathogenically oriented disease research into neurological disorders is difficult due to the limited accessibility of the nervous system tissue. Thus experimental models are especially important for our understanding of brain diseases. Indeed, many questions concerning the pathology and pathogenesis of MS in humans have only been addressed after similar phenomena have been described in experimental systems.

Depending on the questions asked, two different classes of experimental models have proved to be useful for MS research.

a. General models of the mechanisms of degeneration and regeneration in the nervous system, and of the mechanisms of demyelination and glial scar formation. Although these models might be quite different from MS itself, they have contributed considerably to our understanding of how myelin can be destroyed, how the brain tissue reacts to myelin destruction, and to what extent remyelination can occur.

b. Disease-specific models are designed to resemble closely the clinical course, the pathology, and the immunological features of MS. These models are thus suitable for the direct investigation of the pathogenesis of the disease, and for testing possible new therapeutic strategies.

The following discussion is restricted to the second class of experimental models.

Experimental autoimmune encephalomyelitis

In 1933, Rivers and his coworkers were able to show that the immunization of susceptible animals with brain tissue may induce an acute or chronic encephalomyelitis which, depending on the model studied, may be associated with extensive primary demyelination in the CNS. A disease which closely resembles acute MS was also observed in humans after autosensitization with CNS tissue (Seitelberger et al. 1958), or after immunization with rabies vaccine which contained remnants of brain tissue (Uchimura and Shiraki 1957). Depending on the immunized animal species and the model of sensitization, different courses of experimental autoimmune encephalomyelitis (EAE) can be observed.

The acute autoimmune encephalitis is the most simple and reproducible EAE model. Animals are sensitized with a single dose of CNS antigen together with adjuvant. The disease starts between the 8th and 15th day after immunization, and takes an acute monophasic course. Pathology is dominated by intense brain inflammation (Alvord 1970). Demyelination is only present in the late stages after disease onset (12 to 20 days after sensitization), and is restricted to small perivenous areas. During the following days, the inflammatory reaction subsides and the demyelinated fibers remyelinate completely. This disease pattern closely resembles that found in human acute disseminated leukoencephalomyelitis.

Hyperacute autoimmune encephalitis can be induced in specially sensitive animal strains with the use of a potent adjuvant such as pertussis toxin (Levine and Wenk 1965). The disease starts a few days earlier (7 to 9 days after sensitization), and in nearly all instances is fatal after a short time. Using neuropathological techniques, extensive inflammatory lesions are found throughout the brain and spinal cord. The inflammatory infiltrates are dominated by granulocytes associated with small perivenous hemorrhages and some demyelination (Levine et al. 1965; Lampert 1967). The pathological alterations resemble those found in acute hemorrhagic leukoencephalitis in humans.

Chronic models of autoimmune encephalomyelitis have been described in a variety of different animal species, such as mice, rats, guinea-pigs, rabbits, and monkeys (Rivers et al. 1933; Stone and Lerner 1965; Wisniewski and Keith 1977; for reviews, see Lassmann 1983a; Raine 1986). Today, the most commonly studied models are chronic relapsing EAE in guinea-pigs, mice and rats.

Chronic relapsing EAE in Strain 13 and Hartley guinea-pigs is induced by sensitization of juvenile animals with a single high dose of brain tissue and adjuvant (Stone and Lerner 1965; Wisniewski and Keith 1977). The disease takes a chronic progressive or relapsing course, and actively demyelinating attacks of the disease can be found even 12 to 24 months after sensitization. The disease goes through different stages (Lassmann 1983a). The acute and subacute stages (10 to 40 days after immunization) reveal pathologic alterations similar to those found in acute EAE. The dominant alteration is the perivenous inflammatory reaction; demyelination is sparse and restricted to small perivascular areas. However, in the chronic stage (more than 40 days after sensitization), large confluent demyelinated plaques are found. In the early phases of the chronic stage, inflammation is still very pronounced. Only at very late stages (after more than 100 days) does the inflammatory reaction decrease in spite of ongoing demyelinating activity. Detailed neuropathological studies on this model showed that all the essential features of the pathology of MS are closely mimicked. Differences are found mainly in quantitative aspects, such as the size of the lesions, and the extent of remyelination (Lassmann 1983a; Raine 1986).

Chronic EAE in mice (Lublin et al. 1981) differs in several essential aspects from that in guinea-pigs. Similar to other chronic EAE models, the disease runs a chronic progressive or relapsing course. The inflammatory reaction clearly dominates the pathology in the nervous system (Brown et al. 1982). Selective primary demyelination is present in the lesions, but is restricted to very small areas, and only exceptionally leads to the formation of confluent plaques. Larger lesions are generally associated with pronounced additional damage of axons.

In rats, too, a chronic relapsing or progressive disease can be induced with appropriate immunization schedules (Lassmann et al. 1980; 1986; Lassmann 1983a; Feurer et al. 1985). The pathology in these models, however, differs considerably from that described above. In the CNS, the inflammatory reaction dominates the pathology in the chronic stage of the disease. Large demyelinated lesions are rare, and, if present, reveal in addition to demyelination considerable damage of axons and astrocytes. Similar lesions have been described in a subpopulation of Japanese MS patients (Itoyama et al. 1985). Besides these pathological changes in the CNS, extensive inflammatory demyelinating lesions may also be present in peripheral nerves and nerve roots.

Target antigens for autoimmunity in EAE

The models described above were all induced by sensitization with complete CNS tissue. A major focus of EAE research was thus to identify the components which are responsible for the induction of an encephalitogenic autoimmune response.

The earliest identified target antigen of the CNS was the MBP (Kies et al. 1960). In more recent studies, the different peptide epitopes of MBP which are recognized by autoreactive T-cells were defined, and it became clear that they vary between different animal species and strains (Alvord 1984). As yet, the sequence of encephalitogenic peptides for humans has not been identified.

Sensitization with MBP generally leads to

acute EAE, a monophasic inflammatory disease of the CNS with little demyelination (Alvord 1986). With special immunization schedules, and by selecting especially susceptible animal strains, a successful induction of chronic relapsing disease variants was achieved (Panitch and Ciccone 1981). However, demyelination is sparse, even in chronic models, and is not comparable to that induced in chronic EAE in guinea-pigs or found in MS.

Another myelin antigen with encephalitogenic properties is proteolipid protein (PLP) or lipophilin (Madrid et al. 1982; Cambi et al. 1983; Trotter et al. 1987). Sensitization with this antigen leads to pronounced inflammation in the CNS. Demyelination appears to be more pronounced than after sensitization with MBP.

With the use of the T-cell line technology, and with more detailed knowledge of the structures and amino acid sequences of other myelin proteins, the spectrum of possible encephalitogenic target antigens is enlarging. Not only can the exact T-cell epitopes be characterized in the known encephalitogenic antigens such as PLP and MBP (Linington et al. 1990; Wekerle et al. 1991; Trotter et al. 1991), but new encephalitogenic epitopes have also been detected in other myelin and nonmyelin antigens, such as myelin oligodendrocyte glycoprotein (MOG, Linington et al. 1993), MAG, GFAP, and S-100 protein (Kojima et al. 1994). Additional candidates for encephalitogenic antigens are gangliosides (Cohen et al. 1981), and as yet undefined proteins of endothelial cells (Tsukada et al. 1987). In addition, the high percentage of γ/δ T-lymphocytes in MS lesions (Selmaj et al. 1991a; Wucherpfennig et al 1992b) further suggests that endogenous stress proteins may be the target for a pathogenic T-cell response in the lesions.

Besides these encephalitogenic antigens of the nervous system, other elements have been defined which may be recognized by antibodies and which are able to induce demyelination either in vitro or in vivo after injection into the CNS compartment. These antigens include galactocerebroside (Dubois-Dalq et al. 1970), gangliosides GM1 and GM4 (Roth et al. 1985; Schwerer et al. 1986), and possibly also sulfatide, and MOG (Linington et al. 1984a; Linington et al. 1987). This goup of demyelination-associated antigens may also include an epitope of MAG which appears to be the target of autoantibodies in demyelinating polyneuropathies

associated with gammopathies (Latov et al. 1981). A general requirement of a molecule to be the target for antibody-mediated demyelination appears to be its expression on the outer surface of the myelin/oligodendrocyte complex.

When the number of the already known target antigens for autoimmune inflammation and demyelination is considered, it is not surprising that sensitization with whole CNS tissue leads to more complex disease patterns than immunization with single antigens. Furthermore, these data suggest that antigen-specific therapy may be very difficult for a disease such as MS.

Passive transfer models

The EAE models which are induced by active sensitization are unpredictable and difficult to standardize. Thus, investigations into pathogenesis and therapy are complex.

As shown in 1960 by Paterson, EAE can be transferred by the intravenous injection of lymphocytes derived from sensitized donors. Subsequent studies revealed that the disease transfer is accomplished by T-lymphocytes against MBP. A major breakthrough was achieved in experiments by Ben Nun et al. (1981), who were able to establish long-term MBP-reactive T-cell lines with encephalitogenic activity. Similar encephalitogenic T-cell lines have subsequently been raised in mice (Zamvil et al. 1985). Transfer of these line cells generally induces an inflammatory disease of the nervous system with little demyelination (Fig. 2.6a and b). Chronic relapsing disease variants can be induced by repeated injection of these line cells (Vandenbark et al. 1986). Furthermore, in SJL mice, a chronic relapsing disease course was observed even after a single transfer of encephalitogenic T-cells (Zamvil et al. 1985). Although primary and secondary demyelination has been described in these chronic models, clear data on the extent and mechanisms of demyelination are not available.

The lack of demyelination in these pure T-cell-induced diseases raised doubts regarding their suitability as a model for MS. Recently, however, we were able to show that an intravenous injection of monoclonal antibodies against MOG at the onset of T-cell-mediated inflammatory disease of the CNS massively potentiated the disease severity and induced widespread confluent demyelination in the CNS (Linington et al. 1987). The lesions found

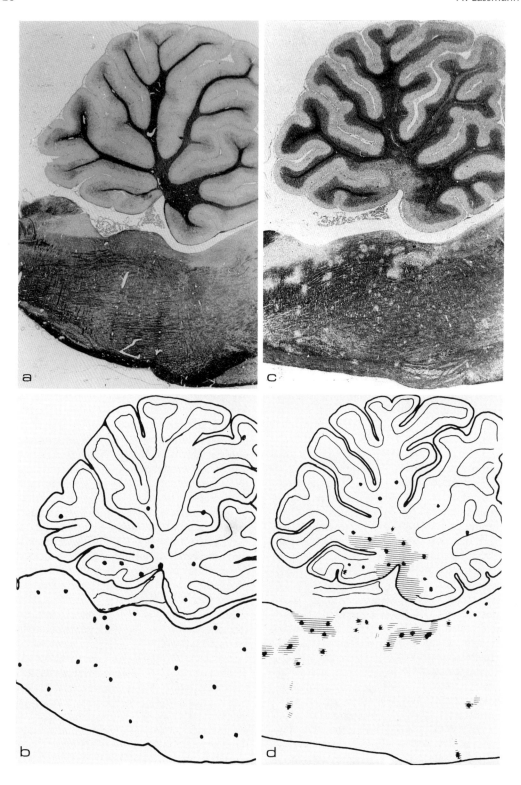

in this cotransfer model closely resemble those found in chronic EAE in guinea-pigs or in MS patients (Fig. 2.6c and d).

In general, the disease course in passive transfer models is monophasic. Even when there is extensive demyelination in the cotransfer experiments, the lesions become completely remyelinated and repaired within a few days following clinical recovery. However, repeated transfers of encephalitogenic T-lymphocytes with demyelinating antibodies result in a chronic relapsing disease pattern with large confluent, persistent demyelination (Linington et al. 1992a).

The close similarities of the lesions of chronic EAE and MS suggest that very similar immunological mechanisms are involved in the pathogenesis of demyelination and tissue damage. Thus, these models are especially valuable for the study of the development of inflammatory demyelinating lesions, and in particular for the evaluation of clinical diagnostic and therapeutic strategies. These data do not, however, prove that MS is an autoimmune disease in the proper sense. Very similar immunological mechanisms will be operating against a noncytopathic, persistent virus infection in the nervous system, and will lead to comparable structural features of the lesions.

Models of virus-induced demyelination

Although, as described above, the spectrum of MS pathology can easily be covered in models of autoimmune encephalomyelitis, it is difficult to explain the pathogenesis of MS solely on the basis of autoimmunity. First, it appears to be difficult to imagine how an autosensitization of such extreme severity may be induced in a normal human being in the absence of deliberate immunization. Second, unequivocal proof of a pathogenic autoimmune response in MS patients is still lacking.

A number of epidemiological studies suggest the involvement of an exogenous factor, possibly a virus infection, in the pathogenesis of MS.

Following the first descriptions of virus-induced inflammatory demyelinating disease in humans and experimental animals, a major focus of virology research was to develop animal models which more closely resembled the disease pattern of MS in clinical, neuropathological, and immunological terms.

Three major groups of virus-induced demyelinating diseases can be distinguished (Wisniewski 1977).

a. Direct cytotoxic infection of oligodendrocytes may damage the myelin-forming cells and lead to demyelination.
b. A permissive (noncytopathic) infection of oligodendrocytes may lead to the persistent expression of a virus-derived neoantigen within or on myelin-supporting cells. Such an antigen may be recognized in a similar way as an autoantigen in autoimmune encephalomyelitis.
c. A transient infection of oligodendrocytes or molecular mimicry may induce an immune response which is not only directed against the foreign pathogen, but simultaneously attacks the host. If this antigen is present in the CNS, an autoimmune encephalomyelitis will ensue.

Although these mechanisms are fundamentally different, it appears to be difficult to distinguish between them in established diseases of human or experimental virus-induced demyelinating diseases.

The most important models of virus-induced inflammatory demyelinating diseases are reviewed below. For further details on this subject, the reader is referred to more comprehensive reviews (Dal Canto and Rabinowitz 1982).

Theiler's virus encephalomyelitis

The murine Theiler's encephalomyelitis virus belongs to the class of Picornaviruses (Lipton and Friedman 1980). A large number of virus mutants have been investigated which induce acute, subacute, or chronic encephalitis. Espe-

Fig. 2.6. Inflammation and demyelination in EAE. (a,b) "Passive transfer" EAE induced by 10^5 MBP-reactive T-lymphocytes. The distribution of inflammatory infiltrates is indicated by the points in (b). There is no light microscopically detectable demyelination. (Luxol-fast blue staining for myelin; × 12.) (c,d) "Passive transfer" EAE induced with 10^5 MBP-reactive T-lymphocytes. At the onset of clinical disease, 5 mg purified mono-

clonal antibody against myelin oligodendroglia glycoprotein was injected intravenously. In addition to the inflammatory reaction, which is similar to that in (a) and (b), large confluent demyelinated plaques (shaded areas in d) are present, predominantly in periventricular sites. (Immunocytochemical visualization of proteolipid apoprotein; × 12.)

cially interesting is the chronic demyelinating encephalomyelitis induced by the DA strain of Theiler's virus (Lipton 1975). In an early phase, infection of neurons is the dominant event, leading to a panencephalitis of variable severity. In a second chronic phase of the disease, large confluent demyelinating lesions are found. Only very few viruses are present at this stage, located mainly in some axons and astrocytes (Dal Canto and Rabinowitz 1982). Other authors have also described the presence of virus in oligodendrocytes and their processes (Knobler et al. 1983). Early stages of demyelination are associated with "vesicular disruption" of myelin and myelin stripping (Dal Canto and Lipton 1975). During the whole course of the disease, the lesions closely resemble those found in chronic models of autoimmune encephalomyelitis. The disease can also be abrogated by immune suppression (Dal Canto and Rabinowitz 1982). The demyelinating process may also be inhibited by antibodies against Class II MHC molecules, suggesting that CD4$^+$ cells play a major role in the pathogenesis (Friedmann et al. 1987).

All these data suggest that immunological mechanisms play a central role in the pathogenesis of inflammation and tissue damage in this model. It is not yet clear whether the immune reaction is entirely directed against virus antigens or may also recognize autoantigens.

Canine distemper encephalomyelitis

Canine distemper encephalomyelitis is induced by a paramyxovirus which in many respects resembles measles virus (Hall et al. 1980). The disease in dogs starts 3 to 6 days after infection, with generalized virus spread, frequently associated with meningitis. In neuropathology, destructive lesions are found adjacent to selectively demyelinating plaques. Virus antigen is mainly found in astrocytes; a virus infection of oligodendrocytes has not been definitely proven (Raine 1976; Vandevelde and Kristensen 1977; Dal Canto and Rabinowitz 1982). In later stages of the disease, in particular in subacute or chronic disease variants, selective primary demyelination dominates. The selective demyelination may be due to direct virus-induced cytolytic damage of oligodendrocytes. However, in addition, damage of oligodendrocytes through macrophage toxins appears to be important (Vandevelde et al. 1982; Dal Canto and

Rabinowitz 1982; Bürge et al. 1989; Griot et al. 1989).

Coronavirus models

Infection of rodents with JHM virus (mouse hepatitis virus) leads to severe acute encephalomyelitis. Virus antigen is present in all cells of the nervous system, including the oligodendrocytes (Knobler et al. 1983). In more subacute disease patterns, infection of brain cells is more restricted, mainly affecting the oligodendrocytes and astrocytes. In these subacute forms, large confluent demyelinated plaques are common (Zimprich et al. 1991). The extent of demyelination correlates well with the extent of oligodendrocyte infection, and immunosuppression has little effect on the demyelinating activity. Thus, demyelination mainly appears to be a result of a direct virus-induced cytolytic effect.

In addition, however, at the time when subacute or chronic disease develops, T-lymphocytes can be isolated from the peripheral circulation which recognize MBP and are capable of transferring autoimmune encephalomyelitis to naive recipients (Watanabe et al. 1983). This observation indicated for the first time that a virus infection of the CNS may induce an autoimmune reaction which itself is capable of inducing and propagating the inflammatory disease. This observation offers a good explanation of how autoimmunity could be induced in a disease such as MS.

Other, less well-characterized, models of virus-induced demyelinating disease include visna and herpes simplex virus encephalomyelitis (Dal Canto and Rabinowitz 1982).

Until recently, MS was interpreted as being either a virus-induced or an autoimmune disease. Today, the data suggest that these two possibilities are by no means exclusive.

Models of inflammatory demyelination in the peripheral nervous system

Experimental autoimmune neuritis

As first described by Waksman and Adams (1955), sensitization with peripheral nervous system tissue leads to a disease which is similar to autoimmune encephalomyelitis, but which is restricted to the peripheral nervous system. Depending upon the mode of sensitization and the susceptibility of the animals, acute and chronic variants of the disease can be induced (Wisniewski et al. 1974; Pollard et al. 1975). Although in experimental autoimmune neuritis (EAN) the demyelination is more pronounced and selective in chronic than in acute models, even in the latter demyelination may be significant and widespread.

The major target antigens for the induction of EAN are the P2 protein (Brostoff et al. 1972), a basic protein similar to MBP in the CNS, and P0 protein, a glycoprotein similar in structure to adhesion molecules (Milner et al. 1987; Linington et al. 1992b). In some animal species, a disease similar to EAN has been induced by autosensitization with galactocerebroside (Saida et al. 1979) and gangliosides (Nagai et al. 1976).

Similar to EAE, peripheral autoimmune neuritis can be induced by the transfer of monospecific T-cell lines directed against P2 or P0 proteins (Linington et al. 1984b; 1992b). Contrary to the situation in the CNS, these EAN models are associated with significant demyelination. A possible explanation for the phenomenon may be that Schwann cells can express Class II MHC molecules and can present autoantigen to T-lymphocytes (Wekerle et al. 1986). Furthermore, Schwann cells may be destroyed by CD4$^+$ T-cells in the course of antigen presentation. However, as in the CNS, widespread confluent demyelination in the peripheral nervous system appears to be due to cooperation between a T-cell-mediated inflammatory response and demyelinating antibodies (Lassmann et al. 1986).

The value of experimental models for MS research

Experimental models are of critical importance for MS research. Nearly all clinical and immunological studies performed to date have been designed on the basis of experimental research on models of autoimmune or virus-induced demyelination. Similarly, the knowledge obtained from basic experimental neurobiological and immunological studies about inflammation as well as about demyelination and remyelination is essential for the interpretation of the structural alterations in MS plaques. This relates to all aspects of MS pathology, including inflammation, demyelination, remyelination, gliosis, and vascular alterations.

The MS models proper, autoimmune encephalomyelitis and virus-induced inflammatory demyelination, closely reflect the clinical features, pathology, and immunology of human inflammatory demyelinating diseases, including MS. They are thus suitable for the study of various aspects of the pathogenesis of the disease, the relevance of new diagnostic tools, as well as of new therapeutic strategies.

It has, however, to be emphasized that none of the models reflects all aspects of MS simultaneously. Thus, the most suitable model has to be selected for each aspect of MS pathology or pathogenesis. This implies that the questions being addressed have to be clearly defined at the outset of the studies, and the suitability of the model system has to be critically evaluated. Furthermore, when interpreting the results, the limits of the experimental strategies have to be taken into account, and the data gathered and the conclusions drawn must not be transferred to the human situation in an uncritical way. However, when these precautions are taken, experimental research will be the only way to unravel the pathogenesis of MS and to test new therapeutic strategies.

Acknowledgments

I thank Professor Dr. K. Jellinger and Professor Dr. H. Budka for supplying some of the material presented here. Helene Breitschopf, Angela Cervenka, Susanne Katzensteiner, and Marianne Leiszer are acknowledged for their expert technical assistance.

3

Genetics and immunology

INTRODUCTION

The immune system is well distributed throughout the whole body, its main sites of activity being in the bone marrow, thymus, lymph nodes, spleen, lung, and intestines. An important exception, however, is the CNS, which is normally isolated from the immune system. This special relationship between the CNS and the immune system (and its consequences) provides a key point in the understanding of the pathogenesis of MS, and its significance is discussed in this chapter. The key elements of the immune system are the lymphocytes and accessory cells, such as macrophages. These cells are armed with a highly complex arsenal of receptors and cellular hormones (cytokines) which enable them to communicate with their cellular environment and to protect the organism from intruders (Fig. 3.1).

First, we shall have a closer look at the receptors which help the cells of the immune system to recognize each other, other cells, and free molecules. The six most important types of receptors are: (1) the antigen receptors of the B-lymphocytes, known as antibodies, or immunoglobulins when they are in soluble form rather than cell bound; (2) the antigen receptors of the T-cells; (3) the Class I histocompatibility antigens; (4) the Class II histocompatibility antigens; (5) the cell surface markers of the T-cell subpopulation CD4; and (6) the cell surface markers of the T-cell subpopulation CD8. These recognition molecules all have a remarkably similar molecular structure (Fig. 3.2). They are all built from various domains of about 100 amino acids which are folded in a characteristic way and stabilized through an S-S bridge. Immunoglobulins, for example, are made up of 14 such domains, 5 in each of the two heavy chains, and 2 in each of the two light chains. The amino acid sequences of some of the domains show little variation, the so-called constant chains, and these are localized adjacent to the cell membrane in which the receptors are anchored. Other domains, further away from the cell membrane, are highly variable. They contain hypervariable regions which govern the specificity of recognition. From a genetic point of view, these molecules are members of a gene family which has evolved through multiplication and mutation from a common precursor. The functions of these receptors are strongly related and form the molecular basis of antigen recognition by the lymphocytes. This is the foundation of the extremely specific mode of action for which the immune system is known, with its ability to distinguish "self" from "foreign," and to react to antigen differences as small as single amino acid changes in a protein. However, another consequence of immune recognition is seen in the attack of organs in autoimmune disease.

THE HLA SYSTEM

The leading instruments in the orchestra of cellular and humoral elements of the immune system are the T-lymphocytes. They are assisted by antigen-presenting cells such as monocytes/macrophages, dendritic cells, and B-lymphocytes, etc., which present them with antigens from toxins, bacteria, viruses, or tumor cells, for recognition. In turn, the T-cells help the other immune cells, i.e., the macrophages, B-cells, and cytotoxic T-cells, to develop their effector functions of phagocytosis, antibody production, or cytotoxicity, in order to eliminate the antigen-bearing elements.

The above-mentioned recognition system of receptors which is the basis of these cell interactions will be discussed here in terms of a lock and key analogy. Antigen receptors expressed on T-cells as locks only recognize antigens if

Cellular and humoral elements of the immune system

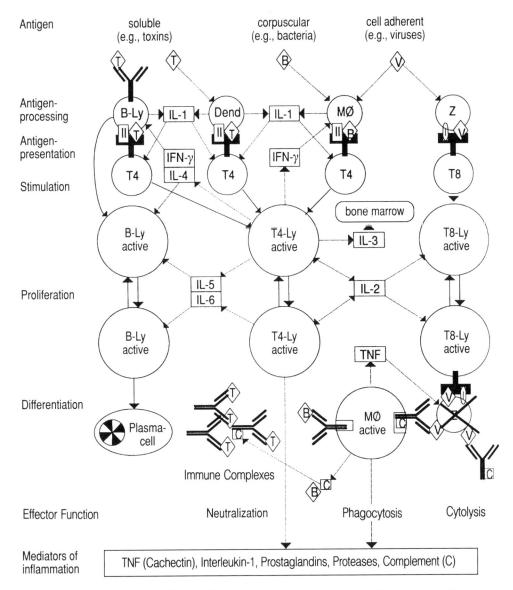

Fig. 3.1. Interaction of the basic cellular and humoral elements of the immune system. (ADCC, antibody-dependent cellular cytotoxicity; C, complement; CR, complement receptor; CTL, cytotoxic T-lymphocyte; Dend, dendritic cell; FcR, Fc receptor; IFN-γ, interferon gamma; IL, interleukin; Ly, lymphocyte; MO, monocyte/macrophage; TCR, T-cell receptor; TH, T-helper cell; TNF, tumor necrosis factor.)

they are presented by an individual key on the antigen-presenting cells. These key molecules are the transplantation antigens known as HLA antigens. As indicated by their name, these cell surface antigens were discovered during transplantation experiments in which T-cells were found to recognize "foreign keys" and reject the cells and tissues bearing them. These HLA molecules are genetically extremely polymorphic. As became apparent in transplantation immunology, everyone has their own individual set of HLA molecules. The special

Immunologic receptor-molecules of the immunoglobulin-gen-superfamily

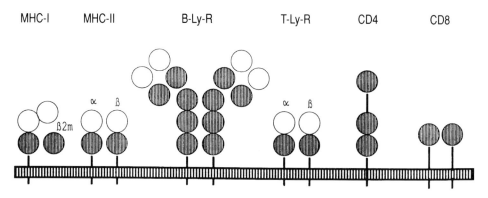

Fig. 3.2. Building plan of some basic immunological receptor molecules made up from closely related domains about 100 amino acids long.

characteristic of this lock and key system is that T-cells only recognize antigens which are offered by presenting cells on keys of the same HLA type, i.e., cells of the same individual. This phenomenon is called HLA restriction.

Research in another direction also led to the discovery of the same key molecules. Experiments with inbred mice and rats have shown that the ability to mount an immune reaction against a particular antigen is partly genetically determined. The genetic region for these immune response genes was found to be the same gene complex which codes for the transplantation antigens, the so-called major histocompatibility complex, termed HLA in humans (Fig. 3.3). Later, it turned out that within the MHC, the same genes and their products are responsible for both transplant rejection and immune response.

The main molecular mechanisms which control immune responses through the action of MHC genes have only recently been revealed. A fundamental aspect of them is that during antigen presentation, only short peptides, 5 to 15 amino acids long, rather than whole proteins are presented to the T-cells. These peptides (epitopes) are either synthesized in the presenting cells themselves (e.g., viral antigens) or produced through so-called antigen processing from ingested proteins by proteolysis in the lysosomes. Related to these two possibilities of peptide origin are two classes of MHC molecules which present the peptides to the T-cells.

Class I MHC molecules are made up from a polymorphic chain which is coded for in the gene loci HLA-A, HLA-B, or HLA-C. The chain is built from three of the domains mentioned above. A fourth domain is noncovalently linked to the chain, namely the invariant β2-microglobulin which is coded for outside the HLA complex on a different chromosome. Class I molecules serve as "keys" for a subpopulation of T-cells which carry the surface marker CD8 and whose main effector function is cytotoxicity. Class I molecules mainly present endogenously produced (for example viral) peptides, which explains their recognition by cytotoxic CD8 T-cells. The molecular structures of the Class I antigens have recently been elucidated by crystallography, and the remarkable picture which emerged was one of a pocket made up by the two polymorphic domains of the molecule in which a peptide of typically nine amino acids lies embedded. Since the HLA allele-specific amino acids are mainly directed toward the inside of the pocket, and therefore influence the peptide binding and consequently the recognition by the T-cells, the controlling effect of the HLA molecules on the immune response is at least partly explained. Class I molecules are expressed on practically all cells of the organism, except on those of the CNS parenchyma where their concentration is very low.

In contrast to the almost universal Class I expression, HLA molecules of Class II are only expressed on certain cell types which serve as accessory cells and which have an immediate immune function. They are not usually expressed on cells of the CNS parenchyma, which gives the CNS a privileged position in relation

Major histocompatibility complex (MHC) on chromosome 6

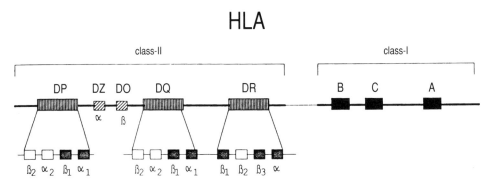

HLA

Fig. 3.3. Breakdown of the major histocompatibility complex (MHC) on chromosome 6. Empty boxes represent pseudo genes which are not expressed.

to the immune system. Class II molecules have also been called immune-associated (Ia) antigens because of their immune regulatory function. They are assembled from an α and a β polypeptide chain which are coded for in the gene loci HLA-DP, HLA-DQ, or HLA-DR (see Fig. 3.2). Each of the two chains coupled on the cell membrane is constructed from two domains, so that the overall structure, with four domains, looks similar to a Class I molecule, with its three domains plus the associated β2-microglobulin as the fourth domain. The crystallographic structure of the Class II molecules has now also been revealed, and it shows a similar molecular pocket made up from the two polymorphic domains of the α and β chains. The pouch, however, is open at both ends, and can therefore accommodate peptides which are 10 to 15 amino acids long. Peptides presented by Class II molecules come from exogenous proteins processed by the antigen-presenting cells.

Class II MHC molecules serve as keys for a subpopulation of T-lymphocytes which carry the surface marker molecule CD4, and have mainly a helper or inducer function, invigorating other immune cells such as macrophages, B-lymphocytes, and cytotoxic lymphocytes. CD4 T-cells are indispensable to the induction of an immune response, and consequently their partners, the Class II-expressing, antigen-presenting cells, also have a fundamental role in the initiation and control of an immune reaction. The expression of Class II (HLA-D) mole-

cules is strongly regulated. A lymphokine produced by activated T-lymphocytes, IFN-γ, induces enhanced expression of Class II molecules, even on certain cells which do not normally express HLA-D molecules. This is of great importance in the CNS parenchyma, where the lack of HLA-D molecules would otherwise prevent any contact with the immune system. Only after the disruption of this obstacle will HLA-D molecules be found in inflammatory lesions of the CNS, for example in the active MS plaque, and then not only on blood-borne macrophages, but also on cells of the CNS parenchyma. It would appear, from what is currently known, that the induction of HLA-D molecules and the activation of corresponding CD4 T-cells in the CNS are central in the pathogenesis of those diseases of the CNS which involve the immune system. Taking this into account, and in relation to the above-mentioned function of the HLA genes as immune response genes, the associations between HLA alleles and susceptibility to MS (discussed below) gain special significance.

Relation between the HLA system and MS

Associations between HLA types and susceptibility to MS are often different in different ethnic groups. The reasons for this are not yet clear. The following discussion relates only to the Caucasian population in whom susceptibility to MS is significantly associated with the HLA-DR2 haplotype (DRw15 subtype). The relative risk of developing MS in HLA-DR2-positive individuals is approximately four times higher than that for HLA-DR-negative individuals. Associations with Class I HLA alleles have been found for HLA-A3 and HLA-B7, but they are weaker and have not been confirmed in all studies. These associations are probably due to linkage disequilibrium within the HLA complex, since HLA-B7 is associated with HLA-DR2 in the general population. The association of HLA-DR2 with MS has to be compared with other idiopathic diseases with suspected involvement of the immune system. For example, the increase in relative risk for rheumatoid arthritis in HLA-DR4-positive individuals is about sixfold, that for diabetes mellitus Type I and HLA-DR3 and HLA-DR4 is about threefold to sixfold, respectively, and that for Hashimoto's thyroiditis and HLA-DR5 is about threefold. These are all disorders with a suspected pathogenesis similar to that of MS, i.e., in which T-lymphocytes play a central role in the inflammatory destruction of the affected tissue.

However, the association of HLA-DR2 with MS is not specific enough to be of importance for clinical diagnosis: the number of false-positive and false-negative cases is too large, since HLA-DR2 also occurs in about 20% of the healthy population, and 30% to 50% of MS patients are HLA-DR2 negative.

There are various reasons why the association of MS with HLA-DR2 is bound to be weak, although it is still of importance to our understanding of the pathogenesis of this disease.

Firstly, genetic analysis of the HLA complex is still incomplete. Progress in typing methods using the tools of molecular biology now allows for the analysis of genes which are not accessible with serological techniques, for example HLA-DQ and HLA-DP. Thus, various new HLA alleles have been defined with the analysis of the restriction fragment length polymorphism (RFLP) at the DNA level, and a significant association between MS and HLA-DQw6 has been found (Francis et al. 1991). The combination of DNA amplification techniques (PCR) and oligonucleotide probes allows for further analysis, particularly to examine whether specific segments of DNA which are common to various HLA alleles might correlate well with MS (Vartdal et al. 1989) – a possible relationship which could not be detected using classical methods. Furthermore, it is significant that the

Class II HLA molecules are assembled from an α and β chain, both of which are genetically polymorphic. Since, in principle, both chains combine freely, cis- and trans-combinations of α and β alleles might possibly be relevant (Spurkland et al. 1991). At present, the HLA Class II haplotype which is most frequently associated with MS is, in genomic terminology, DRB1*1501, DQA1*0102, DQB1*0602. In addition, new, immunologically important, polymorphic genes have recently been discovered in the region between HLA-DQ and HLA-DP. They code for proteins such as peptide transporters (TAP) which have important functions in the process of antigen presentation by accessory cells. A recent study, however, has not detected an association between such TAP2 alleles and MS; but a strong linkage disequilibrium was found between the allele TAP2*01 and the DRB1*1501, which belongs to the haplotype that confers a high risk for MS (Bennetts et al. 1995).

A second reason why a complete association between HLA alleles and MS is not to be expected comes from immunological studies. In many experimental immunological animal models, such as EAE, it has been found that apart from the MHC genes, other genes play a significant role in the control of the immune response and, more importantly, that only certain combinations of MHC alleles and non-MHC alleles correlate with a particular immune response. An example of this is the genetic system of the immunoglobulin allotypes (GM) in which the polymorphism of the genes which code for the γ chain of the antibodies is studied in relation to disease susceptibility. Although, depending on the study, there seems to be only a weak or no association between GM allotypes and MS, the combination of certain alleles of the GM system with certain alleles of the HLA system carries a higher risk for disease (Salier et al. 1986). Another example might involve the antigen receptor of the T-cells. This is because, with regard to the above-mentioned physiological function of the HLA antigens as restriction molecules for antigen presentation toward the T-cell receptor, it is reasonable to ask about the genetic polymorphism of the "key" but also about that of the "lock", i.e., the T-cell receptor. Since the analysis of the genes which code for the T-cell receptor is recent, the field is still open. Nevertheless, preliminary studies have shown certain associations with MS (reviewed by Oksenberg et al. 1993). However, it is to be expected that only the study of combinations of HLA alleles and T-cell receptor alleles will show increased correlation to MS, and to other diseases. Finally, it is possible that there are also other genes which influence immune responses.

A third reason for a weak association concerns the fact that, apart from genetic effects, unspecified environmental influences are also known to affect susceptibility to MS, which again suggests there is no absolute correlation with HLA types.

It is therefore significant that, despite all these reasons – incomplete analyses of the HLA complex, polygenic effects, and additional environmental influences – associations have been found between HLA-DR2 and MS. The significance of HLA molecules will be discussed in more detail below. It remains here to mention that it is important for future studies to look not only at susceptibility to disease, but also at the correlation between different forms of disease progress, clinical symptoms, and laboratory parameters. Even more important is that the therapeutic effects found in clinical trials should be compared in different patient groups.

FAMILY AND TWIN STUDIES

As mentioned above, the immune regulatory Class II HLA molecules (HLA-D) are coded for in several gene loci of the HLA complex. In addition, Class I molecules also play an immune regulatory role. This multiloci system is potentially able to influence disease susceptibility, and it is therefore reasonable to search for the spheres of influence of whole sets of allelic HLA loci, i.e., to study HLA haplotypes. Because of the genetic diversity in the population, such analyses have to involve family and twin studies where whole haplotypes are inherited. Moreover, only this kind of analysis can prove that genetic influences exist which can only be suspected from epidemiological data.

A simple method is to compare the HLA haplotypes of sibling pairs when both are affected by MS. In randomly selected control sibling pairs, the probabilities of identity in two, one or no haplotypes are 25%, 50%, and 25% respectively. In an analysis of 100 families with at least two diseased siblings, compiled from 10 family studies published between 1973 and 1981; the distributions of double, single, and negative

congruity for the HLA haplotypes were 37%, 50%, and 13% respectively (Stewart et al. 1981). This is significantly different from the theoretical expectation. A similar analysis has been done with cousin pairs. Here, one would expect a theoretical congruity in one haplotype of 25%. Yet, 10 (60%) of 17 MS-affected cousin pairs shared one HLA haplotype, significantly more than expected. A detailed genetic analysis has been performed using the data from 15 family studies between 1973 and 1981; including 192 families with at least two affected family members (Ho et al. 1982). As a result, a strong influence of a genetic determinant was found which is closely linked to HLA-DR2. However, a similar strong influence of a determinant not linked to HLA was also detected. This determinant, although familial, is not necessarily genetic in nature, but might represent a family-related environmental factor. This hypothesis, however, has recently been refuted in a study with adopted family members of MS patients, where no effect of shared family environment was found (Ebers et al. 1995). However, these findings still do not exclude the possibility of a synergistic interaction between genes and common environmental factors.

The classical method of searching for genetic influences on the susceptibility to disease is the study of twins. The finding of a higher concordance rate in monozygotic than in dizygotic twins with regard to the disease under scrutiny allows us to assume the existence of a genetic control, provided that environmental factors are similar in both groups. It is of fundamental importance, however, that there is no bias in the selection of the twin population. Unfortunately, because of the relative scarcity of twins, this condition can only rarely be fulfilled, since the search for diseased twin pairs in itself often creates selection bias. This therefore may be the reason why different concordance rates have been found in the twin studies published so far. Overall, it can be concluded that higher concordance rates for MS have been observed in monozygotic twins than in dizygotic twins. A more recent study in Denmark was able to avoid the selection problem by comparing the twin register which exists in that country with the available MS register (Heltberg 1986). The comparison revealed 50 twin pairs with at least one member affected by MS. Of 19 pairs which were monozygotic, 4 (21%) were concordant for MS, whereas of 31 dizygotic pairs, only 1 (3.2%) was concordant. However, these numbers are too small to be significant. Another recent study in Canada minimized the selection problem by systematically questioning more than 5000 MS patients who were registered in the Canadian MS clinics as to their twin status. After confirming the clinical diagnosis and twin status, 70 twin pairs were left. Of these, 27 pairs were monozygotic, and 7 of these (26%) were concordant for MS, whereas of 43 dizygotic pairs, only 1 (2.3%) was concordant (Ebers et al. 1986). A 7.5-year follow-up of this population of twins, whose mean age eventually exceeded 50 years, revealed an increase in the monozygotic concordance rate to 31%, and in the dizygotic concordance rate to 4.7% (Sadovnick et al. 1993). Taking into account another critical point in twin research, namely the fact that monozygotic twins probably have a higher congruity of their environment than dizygotic twins of different sexes, it is preferable to compare the concordance rates for dizygotic like-sexed twins. Summing the corresponding numbers of both studies results in a dizygotic like-sex concordance rate of 2 out of 47 (4.3%), versus a monozygotic concordance rate of 12 out of 45 (27%).

Taken together, family- and twin-based studies confirm the genetic control of the susceptibility to MS. The important question remains, however, of whether familial MS cases are representative of all MS patients, since only 5% to 10% of MS cases are familial. It is possible that this group is etiologically distinct. This hypothesis is supported by the observation that, in the study of Mackay and Myrianthopoulos (1966), 6 of 9 concordant twins showed a familial accumulation of MS, whereas this was only the case in 3 out of 30 discordant twin pairs, which corresponds to the expected frequency in the whole population. Although the epidemiological correlation with HLA-DR2 does not support the idea that only a minority of MS cases are genetically controlled, it is still remarkable that the correlation to HLA-DR2 is stronger in familial than in nonfamilial cases. Zander (1986) reported 24 HLA-DR2-positive patients among 33 familial MS cases (73%), as opposed to 70 HLA-DR2-positive patients in 136 nonfamilial cases (51%), and a frequency of HLA-DR2 in the general population of 25%.

It should again be emphasized that the genetic factor, which has now been confirmed by family- and twin-based studies, and which is closely linked to HLA-D, is predominantly of importance because HLA-D molecules play a key role in the induction and regulation of specific immune reactions.

IMMUNOLOGY OF THE CENTRAL NERVOUS SYSTEM

There are several reasons to include MS as an immunological disease. One argument comes from the association between MS and certain alleles of the MHC Class II genes which code for key molecules of T-cell activation (discussed above). The second justification is based on the occurrence of activated T-lymphocytes together with the expression of HLA-D molecules in fresh MS plaques as well as the production of immunoglobulins, i.e., antibodies, in the CNS. The third reason is most strongly supported by evidence from experimental animal models of MS. Taken together, these are sufficient reasons to give some consideration to the physiology of the immune system in the CNS, bearing in mind particularly its privileged role with regard to the immune system.

First, we should have another look at the basic mechanisms of immune reactions. Apart from the specific receptor molecules discussed earlier, such as B-cell antigen receptors (antibodies), T-cell antigen receptors, the MHC molecules of Class I and Class II, and the CD4 and CD8 molecules, several cytokines and their receptors play a role in the interaction between the lymphocytes and their accessory cells (see Fig. 3.1). The activation of CD4 cells by MHC Class II-bearing antigen-presenting cells is dependent on the cytokine IL-1, which is produced by the antigen-presenting cells. Apart from its essential role in T-cell activation, IL-1 exhibits an extraordinary number of other activities, such as induction of acute phase proteins, fever and sleep, chemotaxis, cell adherence, and activation of endothelial cells, just to mention a few. Similar activities have been ascribed to TNF or cachectin, another cytokine produced by accessory cells.

The activation of T-cells leads to their transformation into metabolically highly active lymphoblasts with a high rate of proliferation. The cell division of the T-cells is again dependent on other cytokines, such as IL-2 and IL-4, which are produced by the activated T-cells themselves and which act in an autocrine fashion on the IL-2 and IL-4 receptors of the T-cells, leading to proliferation of CD4 and CD8 T-cells. At the same time, activating or inhibiting signals

Blood-brain barrier

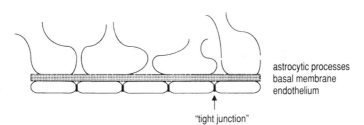

astrocytic processes
basal membrane
endothelium

↑
"tight junction"

Fig. 3.4. The blood-brain barrier is made up from, and functionally dependent on, the cerebral endothelial cell layer sealed with intercellular "tight junctions." Underneath is the basal membrane and a layer of tightly packed astrocytic foot processes.

go back to the antigen-presenting cells. Gamma interferon is a cytokine produced by activated T-cells which induces accessory cells to augment their synthesis and expression of MHC molecules. Other cytokines have an activating influence on B-lymphocytes (for example, IL-4, IL-5, IL-6, IL-10, and IL-13), and others stimulate bone marrow cells (for example, IL-3 and other colony-stimulating factors). CD4 T-cells are grouped into two populations according to their cytokine production profile: T-helper-1 (TH1) cells produce IL-2 and IFN-γ and mainly regulate the cell-mediated immune responses. T-helper-2 (TH2) cells produce the B-cell-activating cytokines such as IL-4 and mainly regulate the humoral immune responses. Apart from all these mostly activating cytokines, inhibiting factors are now also being studied, for example the family of tumor growth factor beta (TGF-β). A further humoral system which has been known for longer and whose function is on the effector side of the immune response is the complement system and the coagulation cascade.

Some of the above-mentioned cytokines also regulate the interaction of the immune system with the CNS, and will be referred to later in this chapter. An important fact to be emphasized again at this point is the central position of the CD4 T-cells and their counterparts, the MHC Class II-bearing accessory cells, in the interplay between the cellular and humoral elements of the immune system.

The blood-brain barrier

The pioneers of transplantation immunology recognized that the CNS is privileged from an immunological point of view. Experimental transplants into the CNS were only rejected when the recipient animal was previously sensitized by a skin transplant from the donor animal. A primary immune response in the CNS was apparently not possible, and there are various reasons for this. First, the CNS has no general lymphatic drainage which could transport antigens to the lymph nodes as in other organs. Second, in the CNS parenchyma, there is normally no expression of Class II MHC molecules (and only small amounts of Class I molecules), without which antigens cannot be recognized by T-lymphocytes. Third, and probably implicit in the previous points, the CNS is separated by the blood-brain barrier formed by endothelial cells which are firmly connected with each other by so-called tight junctions (Fig. 3.4). This barrier not only prevents the passive diffusion of higher molecular weight substances, but also to a large extent the passage of lymphocytes from the bloodstream to the CNS. Considering these obstacles, it is surprising that immune reactions take place at all in the CNS. However, there seem to exist regulatory mechanisms which allow for, and even promote under certain circumstances, interactions between the cells of the CNS and the immune system. Yet these regulations of the barrier obviously have to be restrictive, since each immune reaction also brings about a certain amount of tissue destruction which could be disastrous in the CNS with its very limited regenerating capacity.

A decisive inducing activity for changes in the blood-brain barrier seems to originate from activated T-lymphocytes. Experiments in vitro have shown that activated T-cells, similar to metastasizing tumor cells, have the capacity to

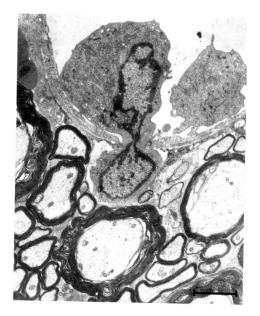

Fig. 3.5. Electronmicrograph from a rat spinal cord 4 days after injection of encephalitogenic T-lymphocytes. An inflammatory cell is migrating through the blood vessel wall.

penetrate a confluent layer of endothelial cells and to dissolve the underlying basal membrane (Naparstek et al. 1984). Resting T-cells are not able to accomplish this. Experiments in vivo also show this phenomenon (Fig. 3.5). When freshly activated and radioactive labeled T-cells were intravenously injected into rats, small numbers of labeled cells could be detected after a few hours in the CNS parenchyma (Meyermann et al. 1987). When such T-cells recognize antigens of the CNS, in this case MBP, they are further activated and proliferate. This results in local disturbances of the blood-brain barrier, leading to perivascular edema and consequently to the entry of other leukocytes which form inflammatory infiltrates. As a consequence of this, the well-known paralytic symptoms of EAE develop. If the primarily infiltrating T-cells cannot recognize any antigens in the CNS because their specificity is aimed at some irrelevant antigen (such as, for example, ovalbumin), the blood-brain barrier remains intact, the T-lymphoblasts revert to small resting cells, and are no longer detectable in the CNS after a few days. The animals remain without symptoms. The capacity of activated T-cells to pass through the blood-brain barrier is confirmed by the experimental observation that during a gen-

eralized activation of the immune system in the course of a graft versus host disease, T-cells are found in the CNS parenchyma (Hickey and Kimura 1987). Such a nonspecific invasion of activated T-cells into the CNS might reactivate a previously evolved specific immune reaction. It has been shown that in rats with a recent history of EAE, a new encephalitic bout can be induced by such a graft versus host reaction.

To summarize, the T-cell-mediated inflammatory changes of the blood-brain barrier are dependent on two preconditions: (1) T-cells have to be preactivated outside the CNS; and (2) T-cells have to be specific for an antigen within the CNS. This explains the above-mentioned phenomenon that experimental transplants in the CNS are only rejected when the animal has previously been sensitized by a skin transplant, i.e., when specific T-cells have been activated outside the CNS. It also explains why in the EAE model discussed below, disease is only induced by the transfer of activated but not by resting MBP-specific T-cells. The seeming limitation of this principle for immune reactions in the CNS is not necessarily one of hindrance to the normal function of the immune system in the course of an infection. Since infectious agents have to pass through the organism to reach the CNS, there is ample opportunity for lymphocytes to be activated before the CNS becomes infected. Such activated T-cells would then have access to the CNS to fight against the intruder.

The mechanisms leading to inflammatory changes of the blood-brain barrier after induction by T-cells are not yet known in detail. It is very likely that changes to cells resident in the CNS induced by interaction with the invaded T-cells are of fundamental importance. Ways of communication between T-cells and cells of the CNS are discussed below.

Interaction of T-lymphocytes with cells of the central nervous system

The endothelial cells of the blood vessels in the CNS are potential partners for T-cells. In-vitro experiments have shown that, after treatment with IFN-γ, cultured endothelial cells from the CNS are capable of expressing MHC Class II molecules and presenting antigens to the T-cells (McCarron et al. 1985). In contrast to endothelial cells from the CNS of a normal mouse, those freshly isolated from the CNS of a mouse with acute EAE were able to present antigens even without pretreatment with IFN-γ (McCarron et al. 1986). Also, HLA-D molecules have been described on CNS endothelium in vivo, although only with the use of light microscopy, with which it is difficult to distinguish whether the immunocytochemically detected HLA-D molecules belong to enothelial cells or to subendothelial pericytes. Another unsolved question is whether antigens of the CNS would be able to appear on the luminal side of the endothelial cells to be presented to passing T-cells. A direct antigen-specific interaction of T-cells with endothelial cells would, of course, be able to control changes in the blood-brain barrier in a very restrictive way. Even when there is no specific interaction of T-cells and endothelium via T-cell receptor and MHC Class II molecules, there are many nonspecific ways in which interaction could occur by means of adherence molecules and their receptors on endothelial cells and lymphocytes. In-vitro experiments have shown that IFN-γ from activated T-cells, or IL-1 which might originate from astrocytes or microglial cells, induces the expression of such adherence molecules on endothelial cells, thereby enabling the leukocytes from the blood to pass through the blood-brain barrier.

Immediately beneath the endothelium and the underlying basal membrane is a layer of tightly packed astrocytic processes which forms the CNS side of the basal membrane (see Fig. 3.4). These astrocytic foot processes play an essential role in the formation and regulation of the blood-brain barrier produced by the endothelial cells (Beck et al. 1984; Janzer and Raff 1987). Astrocytes also have a well-known function in the regulation of the internal milieu of the CNS and in the transportation of molecules from and to the blood vessels. Therefore, astrocytes have access to antigens of the CNS and are well positioned potentially to interact with incoming T-cells. Indeed, in-vitro experiments have shown that astrocytes are able to present antigens to the T-cells and thereby to induce them to proliferate (Fig. 3.6, following p. 48; Fierz et al. 1985; Fierz and Fontana 1986). Although astrocytes are primarily Class II negative in vivo as well as in vitro, activated T-cells produce IFN-γ, which induces astrocytes to express MHC Class II molecules (Fig. 3.7, following p. 48). Such activated Class II-positive astrocytes are then able to present antigens, in association with the "key" molecules, to the

T-cell receptors. This antigen-specific interaction restimulates the T-cells on one side to form metabolically highly active and rapidly proliferating T-lymphoblasts; on the other side, the astrocytes change their morphology themselves by retracting their widely spread processes and detaching them from the surface of the culture dish (see Fig. 3.6c). Resting inactive T-cells do not produce IFN-γ and are consequently not able to communicate with astrocytes. In this context also, therefore, as in passing the endothelium, the state of activity of the T-cells is decisive in the initiation of the immune reaction. Interestingly though, it has been found that certain viruses (coronavirus) or bacterial products (lipopolysaccharides or synthetic muramyl-dipeptide) directly induce MHC Class II molecules on astrocytes, independent of T cells (Massa and ter Meulen 1987).

The mutual activation of perivascular astrocytes and intruding T-lymphocytes could well be a pivotal step in the initiation of immune responses in the CNS. The induced alterations of the astrocytes could influence the function of the blood-brain barrier, leading to edema. Activated astrocytes also produce cytokines such as IL-1 which could induce adherence molecules on the endothelial cells and chemotactically attract further leukocytes, leading to perivascular infiltration. In addition, astrocytic alterations could also affect oligodendrocytes and consequently the myelin sheaths. The potential for such a mechanism is also shown in canine distemper disease, where it was found in vitro that the astrocytes rather than the oligodendrocytes are infected by the distemper virus, nevertheless leading in vivo to demyelination (Zurbriggen et al. 1986). Similar findings have been made in demyelinating encephalomyelitis in rats which is caused by the mouse hepatitis virus, JHM (Massa et al. 1986). It is even conceivable that astrocytic alterations have a direct effect on nervous conduction. Disturbances of the homeostatic functions which regulate the milieu of ions and neurotransmitters, caused by the interaction of T-cells with astrocytes, could impair nervous transmission and conduction, leading to paralytic symptoms long before demyelination occurs.

Finally, activated astrocytes might also influence microglial cells since, as has been observed in vitro (Frei et al. 1987), they produce IL-3 that stimulates microglial cells to proliferate. Microglial cells themselves are able to interact with T-cells in an immune-specific way, as they are able to express MHC Class II molecules upon stimulation by IFN-γ and to present antigens to the T-cells.

In contrast to astrocytes and microglial cells, the other two cellular elements of the CNS, the oligodendrocytes and the neurons, seem to have no way of interacting antigen-specifically with the T-cells, at least for the induction phase of an immune response, since no expression of MHC Class II molecules has been shown for either cell type. Nevertheless, these cells can also be induced to express Class I molecules if treated with IFN-γ so that, at least on the effector side, antigen-specific contact of oligodendrocytes and neurons with CD8 T-lymphocytes is possible. However, so far it has not been possible to demonstrate in animal experiments or in vitro, T-cells which would have an antigen-specific cytotoxic effect on oligodendrocytes or neurons. Although, in vivo, many CD8 T-cells can be found within MS plaques, it is unclear what function they might fulfill.

The role of immune mechanisms in MS patients

The mechanisms described above which might play a role in the induction and regulation of immune reactions in the CNS were mainly discovered by in-vitro experiments, partly at the molecular level. However, it is still difficult to analyze which of the possible mechanisms are operational in vivo and, particularly, which of them are critical for processes such as plaque generation in MS. Some insights can be gained, though, from the study of the pathology of MS lesions (see also Chapter 2). With the help of immunological techniques, it was possible to examine the cellular infiltrates in MS lesions in more detail. This first led to the discovery of some B-lymphocytes and plasma cells which produce the oligoclonal immunoglobulins found in the CSF of MS patients. Later, however, it was realized that most of the infiltrating cells are T-lymphocytes and macrophages (Traugott et al. 1983). With regard to the role of activated T-cells postulated above, it is of importance that signs of T-cell activation such as expression of IL-2 and IL-2 receptors could be traced in the plaques (Bellamy et al. 1985; Hofmann et al. 1986). The expression of HLA Class II molecules is also a conspicuous alteration in the MS plaques. HLA-DR has been

found on T-cells, B-cells and macrophages, but also on endothelial cells within the whole CNS parenchyma and on astrocytes in the center of plaques (Traugott et al. 1985; Traugott 1987). It has to be emphasized that the attribution of HLA-DR to cellular elements in these studies has been assumed on the grounds of light microscopy, evidence which must be confirmed by electron microscopy. Overall, these findings from pathology specimens are compatible with the pathogenic mechanisms observed in vitro. They do not, however, allow for conclusions to be drawn about the operation and regulation of functional interactions in the MS lesions. For such insights, experiments are necessary in vivo, which, of course, can only be conducted in animal models of the disease.

Nevertheless, an unintentional "experiment" with MS patients has recently been performed which demonstrated the critical role of IFN-γ in the disease process (Panitch et al. 1987). In a therapeutic trial, 18 MS patients were treated twice per week with IFN-γ for 1 month. Seven of the patients developed bouts. This exacerbation rate of 0.39 (per patient per month) was significantly higher than the rate during the two previous years (0.12) and during the 6 to 12 months after treatment (0.10). In contrast, treatment with IFN-α or IFN-β reduces the exacerbation rate, and a recent trial using this medication for the first time shows a positive immunomodulatory treatment effect (The IFN-beta Multiple Sclerosis Study Group 1993). These observations with MS patients are in accordance with the hypothesis that the expression of MHC Class II molecules, which is augmented by IFN-γ but not by IFN-α or IFN-β, is central to the induction of new lesions in MS.

Insight gained from such in-vivo "experiments" is, of course, an exception, and in-vivo pathogenic mechanisms in humans have to be studied by looking at the natural course of the disease. A somewhat indirect clue comes from nature's "experiment" – pregnancy. It is well known that the immune system is somehow suppressed during pregnancy by mechanisms which are not yet fully understood. Amongst other factors, α-fetoprotein (AFP) is a possible suppressive agent. It has been shown in vitro that AFP inhibits the induction of MHC Class II molecules by IFN-γ. In the last trimester of pregnancy, the blood levels of AFP are particularly high. The exacerbation rate in pregnant MS patients during this phase is lower than at other times, rising again post partum. An analysis of 199 pregnancies in 66 female patients with MS in Israel showed an exacerbation rate of 0.04 in the last trimester, compared with a rate of 0.82 in the first 3 months post partum. Nonpregnant women at the same age with a comparable duration of MS had an exacerbation rate of 0.30 (Korn-Lubetzki et al. 1984). If the reduction of the exacerbation rate during pregnancy is due to immunosuppression, it should be possible to influence the course of disease by therapeutic immunosuppression. Whether this is the case is discussed in Chapter 15.

A further in-vivo clue as to the pathogenic mechanisms comes from the observation that exacerbations in MS are frequently triggered by viral infections (by viruses not etiologically involved in MS itself). In a prospective study of 170 MS patients and 134 controls over a period of 8 years, the exacerbation rate was three times higher during a viral infection than during other periods without viral infections (Sibley et al. 1985). This observation can be linked to the above-mentioned experimental phenomenon that during a graft versus host disease, activated T-cells enter the CNS and reactivate EAE in remission. It is well known that viral infections generate abundant numbers of activated T-cells in the blood which are then able to cross the blood-brain barrier and might activate resting lesions by IFN-γ.

Further insights into in-vivo immunological mechanisms are to be expected from laboratory examinations of MS patients and from animal models of the disease. Evidence from the study of immunological parameters in MS patients and some recent observations from in-vivo experiments with animal models are discussed in the following sections.

Alterations of immunological parameters in the peripheral blood and cerebrospinal fluid of MS patients

The diagnosis of MS was always mainly established on clinical grounds, with minimal support from laboratory examinations. As an instrument with which to evaluate the course of disease and the prognosis, the laboratory has been of little help as changes in MS-associated parameters correlate poorly with the clinical stage of the disease. The advent of modern immunological laboratory tests has unfortunately done little to change this situation. This might have various reasons. Possibly of most importance is that the clinical picture of MS has little correlation with its pathological substrate, the lesion in the CNS. This is understandable considering that, because of the complex structure of the CNS, neurological deficits largely depend on the localization and less so on the number and size of lesions. This fact, well known to pathologists, has been reemphasized by the advent of in-vivo analyses of MS lesions by X-ray computer tomography and magnetic resonance imaging. So-called silent lesions are not only frequent during the course of diagnosed MS, but also occur in "healthy" individuals. It has to be expected, therefore, that laboratory parameters may correlate better with magnetic resonance findings than with clinical symptoms. Although such laboratory parameters seem to have less clinical relevance, they are certainly of value in our understanding of the pathogenesis of MS, and even more so for a rapid evaluation of treatment effects in clinical trials. A summary of laboratory findings in MS is given in a workshop report on "Cellular and humoral components of cerebrospinal fluid in multiple sclerosis" (Lowenthal and Raus 1987).

Humoral parameters

The laboratory parameter that so far correlates best with MS is the occurrence of so-called oligoclonal bands in the CSF (Fig. 3.8). The term oligoclonal bands relates to the analysis of immunoglobulins (antibodies) with the help of isoelectric focusing (IEF). Using this method, proteins (in this case immunoglobulins from the CSF or serum) are separated according to their electrical charges. Since each B-cell clone and the plasma cells originating from it produce antibodies of different specificities and different electrical charges, the IEF results in a multitude of individual protein bands. In the normal serum, the number of bands is so large that it almost appears as a continuum of adjacently positioned immunoglobulins. During activation of the immune system, for example in the course of a viral infection, single B-cells can multiply so abundantly that single bands emerge in the IEF. The same phenomenon is observed in the CSF, with the difference that in the normal CSF only a small amount of immunoglobulin is present, and therefore, with local production of immunoglobulins by B-cells and plasma cells during the process of inflammation in the CNS,

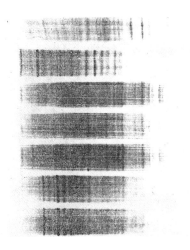

Fig. 3.8. Oligoclonal immunoglobulins from the CSF of an MS patient. Aliquots of 1 μl of native CSF were applied to an agarose gel and the proteins were separated by isoelectric focusing. After blotting on a nitrocellulose membrane, the immunoglobulins were identified by immunostaining with antibodies against human IgG.

IEF bands are conspicuous. Such bands produced in the CNS are only weakly or not at all visible in the serum, so that the finding of oligoclonal bands in the CSF in the absence of identical bands in the serum provides evidence of immunoglobulin production within the CNS. This complies with an augmentation of the immunoglobulin index [(Ig_{CSF}/Ig_{serum})/ (albumin$_{CSF}$/albumin$_{serum}$)] which gives a quantitative measure of immunoglobulin production in the CNS. However, the determination of oligoclonal bands is slightly more sensitive than the immunoglobulin index as bands are sometimes visible while the index is still normal. Local production of immunoglobulins in the CNS occurs in 80% to 90% of MS cases, but also in chronic infections of the CNS. The CNS-produced immunoglobulin is mainly IgG; raised levels of IgM and IgA are found less often in the CSF.

When immunoglobulin from post-mortem CNS material from an MS patient is looked at in terms of its banding pattern in the IEF, distinct patterns are found in individual plaques. This is in contrast to the finding in an immune response to a known antigen (subacute sclerosing panencephalitis), in which the same banding pattern was found in different plaques (Mattson et al. 1980). The banding pattern also varies from patient to patient. Astoundingly, within one patient the individual banding pattern

remains fairly constant over months or years. It can therefore be concluded that the immunoglobulin-producing B-cells either proliferate over a considerable length of time within the CNS, or that they have a long lifetime and are not constantly replaced by new cells. It has been suggested, therefore, that these B-cells might be nonmalignantly transformed and thereby escape normal regulatory controls, similar to a benign monoclonal gammopathy.

It would be interesting, of course, to know which antigens are recognized by these CNS-produced antibodies, but so far no clear picture has emerged. Quite frequently, one finds antibodies specific for common viruses such as measles or varicella, but they make up only a small part of the immunoglobulins in the CSF. Since they are not regularly observed, it is assumed that these antibodies stem from B-cells which reached the CNS randomly in a nonspecific way during the course of an inflammatory infiltration, and which continue to secrete the antibodies they have already produced in the blood. Antibodies to more or less well-defined antigens of the CNS tissue have also been described, but again no consistent relation to MS was found. Such antibodies are not pathognomonic for MS, but also occur in other demyelinating diseases. They might nevertheless play a pathogenic role in the effector phase of an inflammatory demyelination. In vitro, concentrated CSF of MS patients has been found to have a demyelinating activity, and in vivo, its local injection into the optic nerve of tadpoles induced demyelination. However, the chemical nature of this activity has not been identified. The possibility of a demyelinating action of antibodies is also supported by more recent animal experiments (see below). In addition, antibodies to MBP are found in the CSF of MS patients, but it is unlikely that they are demyelinating since MBP is localized intracellularly and is not expressed on the surface of the myelin sheaths. Nevertheless, in a clinical study, the amount of anti-MBP antibodies in the CSF correlated quite well with clinical progression and with exacerbation in patients with MS (Warren and Catz 1986). Part of these anti-MBP antibodies are bound in immune complexes which are frequently found in MS patients but which also contain other, not yet identified, antigens.

The occurrence of intrathecal immunoglobulin production, and particularly of immune complexes in MS, leads to the question of whether the complement system is also involved in the pathogenesis of the disease. Certainly, signs of intrathecal complement activation have been found, especially the terminal components C5 to C9 which form the membrane attack complex and are responsible for the cytolytic activity of complement (Morgan et al. 1984; Sanders et al. 1986). Complement activation could not only be induced by complexed antibodies, but also by broken myelin, as has been demonstrated in vitro (Vanguri et al. 1982; Cyong et al. 1982). Taken together, these factors seem to indicate that the complement system might convey an important effector function during demyelination.

Since the regulation of immune reactions within the CNS also involves the interaction of various cytokines, it is important to quantify them in the CSF. Of special interest seems to be the measurement of TNF-α in the CSF, which showed a relationship between the TNF-α levels and disease activity in MS patients (Sharief and Hentges 1991). The importance of this finding lies partly in the fact that the gene coding for TNF-α is located in the region between HLA-DR and HLA-B, and might therefore be partly responsible for the genetic association of HLA haplotypes and MS. It is of relevance in this context that in certain inbred strains of rats, the expression of TNF-α by astrocytes correlates with their susceptibilities to EAE induction (Chung et al. 1991), and that the potency of the ability of MBP-specific mouse T-cell lines to induce EAE correlates with their expression of TNF-α and TNF-β (Powell et al. 1990). Furthermore, a direct cytotoxic effect of TNF-α on oligodendrocytes has been described, as well as an activating effect on endothelial cells and the induction of astrocyte proliferation. The main sources of TNF are activated macrophages, but microglial cells, astrocytes, and T-cells are also able to produce it. In a recent clinical prognostic study, the in-vitro TNF production of blood leukocytes after short-term culture increased prior to relapses in MS patients (Chofflon et al. 1992).

A second macrophage product which can be measured in the CSF is neopterin. Neopterin is a general intermediate metabolic product which is extensively released by activated macrophages after they have been stimulated by IFN-γ. The biological significance of this neopterin release is not yet known, but since elevated serum neopterin levels are found in situations with activation of the cellular immune system, the measurement of neopterin levels has established itself as a diagnostic test with many applications, for example in monitoring viral infections, especially AIDS, and transplant rejection. In about half the number of MS patients with acute exacerbations or active progression, elevated CSF neopterin levels have been found compared to patients in remission (Fierz et al. 1987). However, this parameter is not specific for MS since elevated neopterin levels in the CSF are also found in other inflammatory diseases of the CNS.

Cellular parameters

As well as increased levels of immunoglobulins in the CSF of MS patients, 30% to 50% also have increased cell numbers. About 90% of these cells are lymphocytes, and about 90% of these are T-cells. There are also B-cells, monocytes/macrophages, and a few polymorphonuclear cells. The determination of the presence of CD4 and CD8 subpopulations of T-cells in the CSF was not particularly significant as the numbers more or less reflect the situation in the blood, which is discussed later. However, various reports demonstrated that a considerable proportion of the T-cells in the CSF of MS patients are activated. This was discovered using cell cycle analysis (Noronha et al. 1980), as well as by the detection of activation proteins on the T-cell surface (Bellamy et al. 1985; Hafler et al. 1985). Increased levels of activated T-cells have also been found in the blood of MS patients (Golaz et al. 1983), but reports of augmented spontaneous proliferation of blood lymphocytes in MS patients are controversial. In one study, it was noticed that peripheral blood T-cells from MS patients proliferated in vitro during IL-2 treatment for much longer than did T-cells from normal blood donors (DeFreitas et al. 1986). This prolonged proliferation was accompanied by an extended expression of IL-2 receptors on the T-cells. Evidence of a sustained T-cell proliferation in vivo comes from experiments which showed increased rates of somatic mutation in the peripheral blood T-cells of MS patients (Sriram 1994).

The cause of this state of activation of T-cells is not yet known. As with the oligoclonal bands, it was speculated that the T-cells might be non-malignantly transformed, particularly in the light of findings that MS patients have antibodies to certain proteins of HTLV-1. This human retrovirus transforms T-cells by inducing a pronounced and no regulated expression of IL-2 receptors, leading to the formation of T-cell lymphomas. Whereas such antibodies could not be found by various other groups, one study in Japan, where HTLV-1 is more common, also detected antibodies to HTLV-1 constituents in MS patients (Ohta et al. 1986). It is premature to postulate a role of possibly still unknown retroviruses in the etiology of MS, but the question of whether lymphotropic viruses are etiologically involved must be pursued further.

Another possible cause of the enhanced activation level among the T-cells could perhaps be found in the incompletely understood phenomenon that in a special in-vitro experimental setup, so-called suppressor activity of blood lymphocytes from MS patients seems to be diminished. Whatever the cause may be, the finding of activated T-cells in the CSF is of some importance with regard to the experimental pathogenic mechanisms discussed above, which led to the assumption that activated T-cells play a central role in triggering the disease process in MS.

Much was expected from the analysis of lymphocyte subpopulations in the peripheral blood when the techniques to measure them became available for routine diagnosis, particularly since some studies showed there to be a change in the CD4:CD8 ratios in MS patients which was dependent on the clinical course of the disease. However, these findings could not be corroborated in subsequent studies, and consequently this analysis has not found a place in the routine laboratory diagnosis of MS (Zabriskie et al. 1985). Various functional studies which described a reduced natural killer (NK) cell activity, i.e., an antigen-independent cytotoxicity of blood lymphocytes, in MS patients remain controversial, and the phenomenon needs further clarification.

As with the oligoclonal immunoglobulins, it would be helpful to know which antigens are being recognized by the T-lymphocytes in the CSF of MS patients, especially when they are activated. But here also the picture is still cloudy. Although techniques are now available to culture T-cells from the CSF and to clone them in vitro so that abundant cells are available for analyses, no disease-specific specificity of the T-cells against a particular antigen has emerged. Occasionally, T-cell clones can be

found which recognize some viral antigens, but presumably, like the virus-specific B-cells or immunoglobulins in the CNS, these represent T-cells present in the blood from earlier viral infections which have randomly intruded into the CNS during an inflammatory infiltration (Fleischer et al. 1984).

There has recently been intensive effort in many laboratories to characterize T-cell clones, grown mainly from the peripheral blood and partly from the CSF of MS patients and controls, which are directed against MBP, the main antigen of the animal model EAE. This effort has so far led to the following conclusions (reviewed by Martin et al. 1992). (1) MBP-specific T-cell clones have been regularly found in MS patients as well as in healthy controls, albeit in slightly larger numbers in the former. (2) The fine specificity of the clones is heterogeneously directed toward various epitopes of MBP. In one of the studies, with 13 patients and 10 controls, 215 T-cell lines recognized at least 26 different epitopes, with only slight differences between patients and controls (Meinl et al. 1993). However, a minority of patients showed a more restricted oligoclonal response which persisted over time, as has been observed with oligoclonal immunoglobulins. (3) The T-cell clones are mainly HLA-DR restricted, but the HLA-DR alleles involved are heterogeneous as well, even when the same epitopes of MBP are recognized. Again, there was no difference between MS patients and healthy controls. (4) The use of T-cell receptor genes by the clones is also heterogeneous, with regard to both epitope recognition and HLA restriction.

The cellular findings have so far been disappointing, and have to some extent made the prospect of an immune-specific therapy for MS less likely. On the other hand, only one antigen (MBP), possibly out of many other candidates, has been extensively studied in this way and, for practical reasons, T-cells have mainly been cloned from the peripheral blood rather than from the infiltrated MS plaques. A myelin antigen other than MBP which has been studied in this context is PLP, which was recognized by T-cell clones in a similar heterogeneous, non-disease-related fashion. However, a more recent investigation indicates that a quantitatively minor myelin protein, the oligodendrocyte glycoprotein (MOG), might be a more disease-specific target of cellular immune reactions in MS patients (Kerlero de Rosbo et al. 1993). This protein also seems to have some important role in the EAE model, as discussed below.

In summary, changes in immunological parameters, both humoral and cellular in nature, are certainly present in MS patients. The main alterations are found in the CSF, which confirms that the disease is restricted to the CNS. The nature of the changes can best be characterized as a chronically exacerbating non-specific state of activation of both the T-cell and the B-cell systems, as well as of the macrophages. Specific immune mechanisms against viruses or autoantigens are observed, but seem not to be strictly disease related. Some observations point in the direction of a nonmalignant transformation of B-cells and T-cells, leading to oligoclonal proliferation, but there is no clear evidence for this.

Immunological aspects of animal models

There are two kinds of animal models for human disease: (1) spontaneous disorders in laboratory animals which sometimes come very close to the human affliction but which can only be poorly manipulated and which pose problems similar to those of human disease for pathogenic studies; and (2) experimentally induced disorders which can easily be manipulated but which very often have associated experimental artifacts, and only partly mirror the human disease. For the study of MS, practically no spontaneous animal models are so far available. Experimental models of MS, on the other hand, are among the oldest and best studied immunological models. Two types of experimental disorders are mainly studied, namely autoimmune and viral-induced models. In both, the immune system seems to play a major pathogenic role. The following section does not include discussion of all animal models of MS individually, but is a synopsis of some of the most recent aspects of immunology.

Autoimmune models

The classical principle in experimentally inducing an autoimmune disease is to immunize the laboratory animal with organ extracts in complete Freund's adjuvant. Experimental autoimmune encephalitis is induced by immunizing animals with homogenized CNS material or with purified components thereof. The main disadvantage of this technique is the almost unlimited persistence of the antigen at the site of immunization, due to the persistence of the adjuvant. It follows that the disease evolves in the constant presence of an antigen deposit which continues to stimulate the immune system at a site distant from the target organ, in this case the CNS. This situation is therefore artificial since there is no evidence to suggest that immunogenic CNS antigens are present outside the CNS in MS. It is also difficult to study immunoregulatory mechanisms with this technique because of the persistent stimulation by the antigen deposit.

Therefore, attempts were made some time ago to separate the immunization phase of EAE from the effector phase by transferring the pathogenic principle from the diseased animal to a healthy recipient. When this procedure is successful, it is possible to examine the pathogenic principle, and this technique has been used to show that the disease can be transferred with T-lymphocytes, but not with serum. It then became possible to grow these T-cells as lines and clones in vitro, and to select them with regard to their antigen specificity. In this way, the capacity of the T-cells to be encephalitogenic in the recipient animal was not only preserved but also enhanced. This has led to the final proof that T-cells represent the specific pathogenic principle in EAE (Ben-Nun et al. 1981).

Subsequent studies with these encephalitogenic T-cell lines and clones has revealed the following (reviewed by Wekerle and Fierz 1985; Martin et al. 1992).

- The disease-transferring T-cells are exclusively of the CD4 subtype. They are only encephalitogenic when they have the right specificity and have been freshly activated in vitro before transfer. This demonstrates the fundamental role of immune-specific activated CD4 cells in the induction of EAE.
- The encephalitogenic T-cells are specific for myelin proteins. The main antigen used is MBP or its peptides, but other T-cell lines have also been described which are, for example, specific for the apoprotein of PLP, DM-20. T-cells which are specific for antigens that are irrelevant to the CNS (for example ovalbumin) do not induce any EAE. This demonstrates that the recognition of CNS antigens is necessary for the induction of EAE.

- Because of the MHC restriction of the T-cells, transfer experiments are mainly conducted in inbred strains of mice and rats. In these genetically homogeneous animals, the same epitopes of MBP are always recognized. This allows for the construction of synthetic peptides which are not encephalitogenic themselves but which block the presentation of natural peptides of MBP. The in-vivo application of such peptides can inhibit the development of EAE. In certain inbred strains, the same T-cell receptor genes are regularly used by the T-cells to recognize the MBP peptides. This allows the evolution of EAE to be inhibited by in-vivo application of antibodies against these T-cell receptor types. Both facts together have given rise to hopes that MS could be treated with immune-specific therapies. Since, in contrast to inbred animals, the genetic background in MS is very heterogeneous, despite some genetic susceptibility to disease, and since the pathogenic antigens are not yet known in the human disease, the hopes for immune-specific intervention have not yet been fulfilled (see above).
- In the rat, the adoptive transfer of encephalitogenic T-cells elicits an acute EAE, with paralytic symptoms first apparent after 4 days, a disease climax at day 7 to 8, and complete recovery after 3 weeks. The severity of such induced EAE is dependent on the number of transferred cells. Minimal symptoms can be evoked with 10^4 cells; more than 10^6 cells are lethal. Normally, 100% of the injected animals become diseased. The short latency period, the cell-dose dependence, and the homogeneous course of disease in all recipient animals make cell transfer EAE a very suitable animal model.
- The pathology of the induced disease consists of an acute, focal, perivascular, lymphomonocytic infiltration of the CNS, with involvement of the meninges. In contrast to MS, no consistent demyelination is observed. This clearly demonstrates that inflammatory changes alone, without obvious demyelination, can lead to extensive paralysis, but it also means that the disorder only partly mimics the pathology of MS.
- The induction of EAE with T-cells can be inhibited by the following measures: (1) irradiation of the T-cells before injection, which hinders their proliferation; (2) treatment of the recipient animal with immunosuppressive

drugs such as cytostatics or cyclosporin A, which represses cytokine production; and (3) treatment of the recipient animal with antibodies against activated T-cells. This demonstrates that the capacity of the T-cells to proliferate and to produce cytokines in vivo is essential for the induction of EAE.
- Animals which recover from transfer of EAE show a certain resistance to further induction of EAE by classical immunization with MBP. Such an immunity can also be achieved by injection of activated T-cells made nonencephalitogenic by irradiation, which indicates that such T-cells can be used to vaccinate against EAE. This demonstrates that T-cells induce immunological counter-regulations. The above-mentioned observation, that in inbred strains of animals only certain subtypes of T-cell receptors are used to recognize MBP, has led to the possibility of immunizing animals with specific synthetic peptides of the T-cell receptors involved, so that the treated animals acquire resistance to EAE.

The main difference between this cell transfer model and MS is the lack of demyelination and the acute, nonrelapsing and remitting course of the disease in the animal model. In contrast to this, in some EAE models induced by classical immunization, both demyelination and chronicity are observed. Whereas the chronicity is probably artificially caused by the persistent antigen deposit used for immunization, the demyelination could perhaps be explained in two ways. Firstly, in most of these models, whole CNS homogenate has to be used for immunization, which suggests that possibly antigens other than MBP are required for demyelination. Secondly, in the immunization model, both the cellular and the humoral parts of the immune system are involved, and it has been argued for some time that demyelination is mediated by antibodies. Yet, in the T-cell transfer model, antibodies do not seem to be involved.

Recently, however, it became possible to allow the cellular and humoral parts to be combined, under well-controlled conditions, in the transfer model. When, by using a small dose of T-cells to induce subclinical EAE, the animal is additionally treated in the early phase, at day 4 or 5, with a monoclonal antibody against MOG (Linington et al. 1984a), a massive EAE develops with extensive demyelination (Fig. 3.9; see also Chapter 2; Linington et al. 1988). Anti-

Synergy between autoimmune T-cells and antibodies

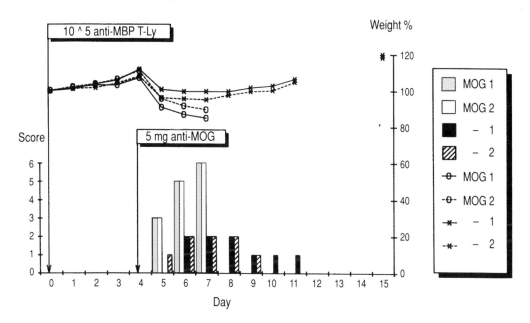

Fig. 3.9. Synergism between MBP-specific T-cells and antibodies against the myelin oligodendrocyte glycoprotein, MOG. Four Lewis rats were injected at day 0 with 10^5 MBP-specific T-cells; at day 4, two of the animals received in addition 5 mg of a monoclonal antibody to MOG. The MOG-treated animals showed a rapidly progressing demyelinating EAE, with a lethal outcome at day 8.

bodies against the same glycoprotein have also been found in the immunization model in the guinea-pig in correlation with the clinical course. Since these antibodies alone are not capable of inducing EAE, it is appropriate to speak of an actual synergy between T-cells and antibodies in this model. It is very likely that the T-cells are needed to open the blood-brain barrier and thus to allow the antibodies to reach the CNS. Furthermore, the T-cells are required to recruit macrophages which, together with the antibodies, are able to destroy the myelin. The EAE is not only enhanced by this mechanism, but also prolonged, since the repair by remyelination takes time. However, these animals also recover completely, and so far no relapses or chronic developments have been observed except when the animals are repeatedly treated with T-cells and antibodies (Linington et al. 1992a).

In summary, it is now possible to separate the cellular and humoral sides of the classical animal model, and to recombine the well-defined components under controlled conditions. Nevertheless, the question as to which mecha-

nisms lead to relapses and chronicity still remains unanswered.

With regard to the genetic influence on the susceptibility to MS (see p. 33), the genetics of EAE are discussed here. Since EAE models are studied in inbred strains of animals, and since only certain strains are susceptible to EAE, genetic questions can be particularly well addressed. A main genetic influence on the susceptibility to EAE comes from the MHC. Other genes outside the MHC also play a role. These non-MHC genes, however, have not yet been completely identified. The MHC genes control the specificity of the recognition of MBP by the T-cells since in different inbred strains of animals, different epitopes are recognized. Such disparities in the fine specificity of T-cells may be enough to alter the disease-inducing capacity of the T-cells (Beraud et al. 1986). The influence of MHC genes on the fine specificity of T-cells probably holds true also for other antigens, and is for the time being the best hypothesis to explain the influence of the HLA genes on the susceptibility to MS in humans. However, the effect of a particular HLA allele might not only encompass the specificities toward CNS antigens, but will probably also show up in antiviral immune responses which are not necessarily related to the etiology of MS. Hence, the altered immune response against measles viruses in MS patients, which has been observed both at the cellular level (Jacobson et al. 1985) and at the humoral level (Hankins and Black 1986), might be related to certain HLA haplotypes.

Viral models

In the viral animal models of MS, it also became increasingly obvious that the immune system represents an essential pathogenic factor. In principle, it is possible to distinguish between a direct cytopathic effect of a virus and the direct and indirect effects of the immune system which, on the one hand, strives to eliminate the virus by destroying the virus-infected cells, and, on the other hand, evokes autoimmune reactions. The three mechanisms (viral, antiviral, and autoimmune), which all lead to tissue destruction, are variably expressed in different viral models, but in reality it is difficult to discern to what extent the individual components are involved. The pathogenic effect of the immune system can be estimated by comparing the course of disease in infected normal animals with that in infected animals which carry an experimentally suppressed immune system. The autoimmune component which is triggered by the virus can be demonstrated by transfer experiments. In the mouse hepatitis virus model (JHM) in the LEWIS rat, it was possible to identify in this way encephalitogenic MBP-specific T-cells in animals with viral encephalitis (Watanabe et al. 1983).

There are various ways to explain how a viral infection can trigger an autoimmune reaction. One hypothesis which has been revived by the modern techniques of molecular biology and computer technology states that in certain viral proteins, there are amino acid sequences which are similar to those in proteins of the CNS (for example, MBP or PLP), which might lead to immunological cross-reactions (Shaw et al. 1986). Knowing, however, that the specific antigen recognition of T-cells is able to distinguish single amino acid changes within an epitope, the idea of sequence similarities is not yet very persuasive. To support the hypothesis, it has not only to be shown that actual cross-reactions between T-cells specific for viral and autoantigens occur, but it also has to be demonstrated that such T-cells are pathogenic when transferred into a healthy animal. These experiments are mandatory, since the disease-inducing capacity of T-cells is dependent on the right epitope being recognized, so that not every cross-reaction is necessarily pathogenic.

Viral models, like autoimmune models, are also genetically controlled, and the influence of MHC and non-MHC genes is effective here. In the case of the murine encephalitis triggered by the Theiler virus, it was found that a non-MHC gene which affects the susceptibility to the disease is very closely linked with the genes which code for the β chain of the T-cell receptor (Melvold et al. 1987). This observation supports the theoretical expectation that in MS also, associations to HLA and to polymorphic variants of the T-cell receptor genes should be found.

To summarize, the main points are as follows. Animal models and MS coincide in many immunological respects – in immune pathology, immune genetics, and the functional indications for actively ongoing immune processes. But one essential point so far separates MS from all models: whereas immune reactions in all models are clearly directed against well-defined viral antigens or autoantigens, it is still unclear which antigens might be of prime importance in MS. The lack of an answer to this question is, of course, related to the fact that the etiology of MS is still unknown.

Fig. 3.6. Tissue culture of rat astrocytes (stained green by fluorescent antibodies against the intermediate filament protein, GFAP) and MBP-specific T-lymphocytes (red nuclear staining). (a) The randomly assorted T-lymphocytes adhere to the astrocytes after addition of the antigen MBP. The astrocytes present the MBP to the T-cells and thus stimulate them to blast formation and proliferation (b) This interaction is restricted to the protoplasmic type of astrocytes which are induced to become spherical and to detach from the surface. (c) The fibrous type of astrocytes do not interact with the T-cells.

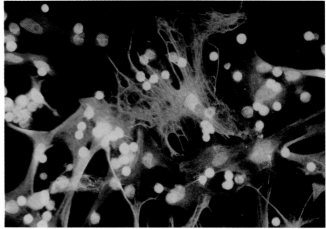

a

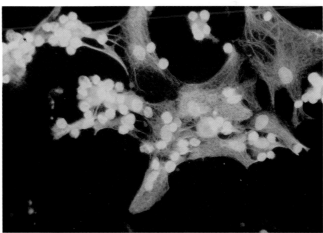

b

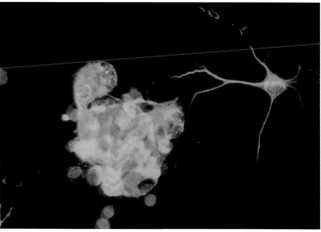

c

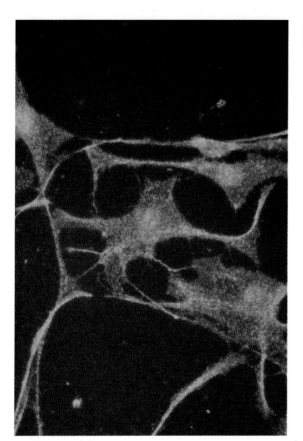

Fig. 3.7. Expression of MHC Class II molecules (red) on the surface of cultured rat astrocytes (green) after incubation with IFN-γ.

4

Epidemiology

INTRODUCTION

Studies into the prevalence of MS in Switzerland by Bing and collaborators (Bing and Reese 1926) rank among the pioneering works in epidemiology. Since then, two main types of epidemiological method have been used in the study of MS. First, numerous studies attempt to determine prevalence and incidence rates of the disease in different geographical regions as precisely as possible in order to find a pattern of disease distribution which would elucidate its etiological factors. Second, by comparing people affected by MS with healthy individuals in the same population, specific factors become apparent by which MS patients may be distinguished from nonaffected people. Factors are sought by these methods which cause or trigger manifestations of the disease. Such factors may either be related to genetic disposition or be environmental in nature. Theoretically, epidemiological studies should be able to answer the questions raised. However, they are burdened with methodological difficulties because the epidemiologist – in contrast to the experimenter in a laboratory – is not able to determine the experimental conditions under which the studies are carried out. It is therefore of the utmost importance that a rigorous methodology is respected in such studies (Kurtzke 1983b; Nelson et al. 1986; Martyn 1991; Beer and Kesselring 1994).

Precise criteria must first be determined by which the reliability of the clinical diagnosis can be verified. Because no single pathognomic test is available, the probability of the diagnosis must be checked against lists of criteria. These criteria now include clinical findings as well as data from electrophysiological and chemical examinations and imaging procedures (see Chapter 8). Only those cases which satisfy such well-defined diagnostic criteria should be included

in epidemiological studies. This prerequisite makes comparisons possible between studies in which similar diagnostic criteria have been applied. If they are applied rigorously, the diagnosis of MS is as accurate and reliable as, in other circumstances, is that of myocardial infarction (Ebers 1984). The diagnosis of MS made on these grounds is sufficiently accurate when compared with the pathological definition of the disease to enable reliable data to be gathered from epidemiological studies.

Within a defined population at a defined point in time, there exists a limited number of affected people. Most of them will show clinical symptoms of the disease (symptomatic cases); a certain number will be clinically asymptomatic, and any suspicion of the presence of the disease will be based on paraclinical examinations; and an undefined number may be affected by the disease without having any symptoms or signs at the time of examination (see Chapter 10). Studies on postmortem material are less relevant from an epidemiological point of view because such examinations are only rarely performed on diseased MS patients, although they would represent the most accurate means of diagnosis.

After determining the diagnostic accuracy, the rates of various parameters may be determined by which the prevalence of the disease may be ascertained in a particular area. Such rates are usually related to a population of 100,000 inhabitants.

Incidence rate

The incidence rate is defined as the number of new cases of a disease which appear within a defined period of time (usually one calendar year) within the population examined. The start of the defined period can be taken as the time at which the first symptoms occur or as the time of diagnosis. In a disease such as MS, the onset of which is so difficult to define clinically, it is impossible to obtain exact incidence rates. They would, however, be the only rates to indicate biologically significant fluctuations of disease frequency.

Mortality rate

The mortality rate determines the number of people who die of a disease within a defined period of time. It is also related to 100,000 inhabitants per year. Because MS is only rarely the primary cause of death, and therefore appears only rarely in statistics of causes of death, mortality rates play only a limited role in epidemiological studies of this disease. Statistics from the World Health Organization show, in most Western countries, a decrease in MS mortality of up to 25% over the last 30 years (Williams et al. 1991), whereas it seems to have remained constant in Northern and Eastern European countries (Lai et al. 1989).

Prevalence rate

The prevalence rate on a defined date (point prevalence rate) is the number of patients living on that date within the defined area, per 100,000 inhabitants in the area. Prevalence rates of MS are usually used in epidemiological studies of this disease. They depend on the incidence and duration of the disease, as well as on the availability of medical care, the accuracy of the studies, and the willingness of physicians to notify the epidemiologists of their cases. If incidence rate and mortality rate remain constant over time, and if no significant migration occurs, the prevalence rate is the product of the average incidence rate and the average disease duration. Because population groups differ in their age structure, it is more appropriate to define age-specific rates, i.e., rates according to age groups.

If a disease such as MS is relatively rare in an average population, its frequency cannot really be determined by direct questioning of all the inhabitants about the symptoms or signs of this disease. References from diagnosed cases must usually be accepted. It cannot be avoided that clinically relevant cases are not always found, and therefore even in the most accurate study, prevalence rates may only indicate the lower limit.

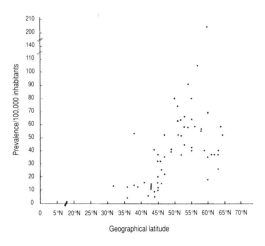

Fig. 4.1. Prevalence rates of MS per 100,000 inhabitants in relation to geographical latitude in Europe. (After Kurtzke 1983b.)

GEOGRAPHICAL DISTRIBUTION OF PREVALENCE

The results of studies on the frequency of MS, which have been obtained from over 200 prevalence studies in Europe which satisfy a well-defined quality demand (Kurtzke 1983b; Dean 1984), are summarized graphically in Fig. 4.1, in terms of the relationship between prevalence rates and geographical latitude. In Europe, the prevalence of MS rises with increasing geographical distance from the equator.

A high prevalence rate (more than 30 cases per 100,000 inhabitants) is found mainly between 44° and 64° latitude; a zone of medium prevalence (4–30 cases per 100,000 inhabitants) is found between 32° and 47° latitude. Near the equator, MS appears to be very rare. It is not certain whether prevalence increases continuously toward the poles, or whether "breaks" occur in which areas with high and low prevalence may be distinguished. These differences of prevalence rates in relation to geographical location cannot be explained as methodological artifacts, but seem to be a real biological phenomenon of the disease.

In the U.S., the observation of a North–South gradient of MS prevalence which was proposed by Limburg in the 1920s has been repeatedly confirmed in numerous later studies (Baum and Rothschild 1981; for a review see Kurtzke 1983b). A zone of high prevalence is found north of 37° latitude; the average prevalence rate is 60 per 100,000 inhabitants.

In Asia, prevalence rates of MS also appear to follow a North–South gradient. In comparison to similar geographical locations in Europe and America, prevalence rates in Asia (for example, in Japan) are lower by a factor of 10 (McDonald 1983a; 1986).

It is of interest that in Africa, only rare cases of defined MS have been reported. Even if one only considers the reports from hospitals, it seems reasonable to assume that MS is extremely rare in black Africa. Among whites in South Africa, the disease is as frequent as in the Mediterranean region, and corresponds to a medium-risk zone.

According to earlier studies, a zone of high prevalence is defined in Australia and New Zealand between 34° and 44° southern latitude; further toward the equator, MS is found, as in the northern hemisphere, with a medium frequency. More recent studies confirm this North–South gradient (Miller et al. 1990), and point to an average prevalence of 69 per 100,000 inhabitants (Miller et al. 1986). The disease is very rare among indigenous Maoris.

Overall, these data can be summarized as indicating that cases of MS are very rare in regions near the equator, their prevalence increasing toward the poles in both hemispheres.

GEOGRAPHICALLY WELL-DEFINED REGIONS

Because MS is relatively rare, it is recommended that more accurate epidemiological studies be carried out in populations which are not too large (less than 1 million inhabitants), and in geographically circumscribed regions (Dean 1984; Martyn 1991). This allows the examining epidemiologist personally to check the reliability of the diagnosis and the population statistics.

In southern Lower Saxony, a well-defined epidemiological area of about 0.25 million inhabitants has been studied systematically since 1968 with regard to cases of MS. Between 1969 and 1983, the prevalence rate increased from 51 to 89 cases per 100,000 inhabitants, whereas the incidence rate remained constant over the same period. This increase in prevalence rate can be explained in terms of a longer than average disease duration, and a longer life expectancy, which has been confirmed in several other studies concerning the course of the disease (see below). Another factor to explain this change in prevalence rates may also be the change in the age structure of the normal population (Martyn 1991).

The idea that high prevalence rates over a limited period of time within a defined region may be interpreted as a biologically relevant phenomenon in the sense of a true epidemic (Kurtzke 1983b) has not remained unchallenged (Lauer 1986). An accumulation of cases, such as has been observed on the Faeroe Islands (Kurtzke and Hyllested 1979; 1988) and in Iceland (Kurtzke 1980) since the Second World War, may only be interpreted as an increase in prevalence rate if equally reliable data are available for the time period before and after the apparent "epidemic" (Poser et al. 1992). On the Faeroe Islands, no single case of MS appears to have been identified before the year 1942, whereas in the years up to 1960, 24 definite cases were recorded. In subsequent years, only a single case was diagnosed, in 1970.

In the Orkney and Shetland Islands off the Scottish coast, careful studies revealed the highest prevalence rates (Poskanzer et al. 1980): 309 and 194 cases per 100,000 inhabitants. A more recent statistical analysis on these islands (Cook et al. 1985) demonstrated a reduction in the incidence rate. This reduction is interpreted as due to a diminished efficacy of a putative pathogenic factor from the environment, since it is assumed that the genetic background of the population examined has not changed (Swingler and Compston 1986).

In Great Britain, an overview of all prevalence and incidence studies carried out during this century (Swingler and Compston 1986; Phadke 1987) demonstrates again a North–South gradient of the prevalence of MS. There are, however, some regions which do not follow this rule (Orkneys: 258; North-East Scotland: 155; Wales: 113; East Anglia: 130 (Mumford et al. 1992); Northern England and Northern Ireland: 76–79; Southern England: 63 – all figures per 100,000 inhabitants). As far as comparisons are applicable in terms of variation of methodology, there is a linear relationship between the prevalence of MS and the distribution of the genetic marker DR2. This may be taken as an argument for the role of genetic influences on disease development (Spielman and Nathanson 1982).

The most recent studies from North America concerning MS are based on the registry of the Mayo Clinic in Olmstedt County, which is one of the most accurate sources of material for epidemiological examination. The data point to a prevalence of 160 in Rochester and 173 in Minnesota, per 100,000 inhabitants (Wynn et al. 1990).

In general, epidemiological studies into MS prevalence carried out later show a higher prevalence for the same region than earlier ones (Beer and Kesselring 1994). This may be due to increased life expectancy of the affected people, and to better ascertainment of the relevant cases in the second study. Furthermore, it may be assumed that physicians working in a circumscribed area become more aware of the disease after the first epidemiological study, and are more willing to refer their cases.

According to more recent studies of the prevalence of MS in Switzerland (Beer and Kesselring 1988; 1994; Groebke-Lorenz et al. 1992), carried out in various regions (Basel City and Canton Berne), there seems to be a minimal prevalence rate of 110 cases per 100,000 inhabitants. Compared to earlier prevalence studies in Switzerland (Bing and Reese 1926; Georgi et al. 1961b), this indicates a doubling of prevalence rates every 30 years – 1922: 20.3; 1956: 55.4; 1986: 110.4. The increase between 1922 and 1956 may be explained by methodological factors, whereas in more recent studies an increase in life expectancy of MS patients may be responsible. Since the prevalence rate is the product of incidence and disease duration, it increases in proportion to the average disease duration if incidence rate remains constant. In three earlier American studies (Ipsen 1950; Carter et al. 1950; Lazarte 1950), an average disease duration of 13 to 17 years was found, whereas in more recent studies an average disease duration of 25 (Phadke 1987) to 30 years (Frey 1986) has been reported. If disease duration doubles within the same time period as the prevalence rate, it may be inferred that the incidence rate within the same time period has remained constant. This may also be inferred from estimates of incidence rates based on a comparison of mortality rates and prevalence (Confavreux et al. 1980; Beer and Kesselring 1994). Most studies, although of different methodologies, indicate an incidence rate of between 3 and 5 per 100,000 inhabitants per year.

Even in such small regions as the Swiss Canton Berne (fewer than 1 million inhabitants), regional differences may be found which are statistically significant but very difficult to interpret. In large cities (more than 50,000 inhabitants) an average prevalence was found of 136.3 cases per 100,000 inhabitants; in smaller towns (with between 10,000 and 50,000 inhabitants) 137.7 cases; and in villages (with fewer than 10,000 inhabitants) 97.3 cases per 100,000 inhabitants. This difference was reported by Georgi et al. in 1961b. According to our study, prevalence is much higher in communities lying above 1000 meters above sea level (128.4 cases per 100,000 inhabitants) when compared to the average value in the Canton. The significance of this finding is not clear.

MIGRATION

If we accept that different prevalence rates in various geographical areas reflect a true biological phenomenon of MS, and that they express the risk of developing the disease within an area, it is of particular interest to examine whether the statistical risk of developing the disease changes if a population group migrates from an area with a high MS risk to an area with a low risk, or vice versa. Such studies have become possible now that migrations of populations occur over large distances.

Based on the pioneering work of Dean and collaborators (Dean and Kurtzke 1971; Dean et al. 1976), such migration studies have been carried out primarily in South Africa, Israel, and in an area of Greater London, England. Unfortunately, they are based on a rather small number of cases, but their results may be summarized as follows.

If the risk of developing MS is determined independently from the age at which migration occurred, it corresponds largely to the risk of the country of origin (Kurtzke 1983b). If the age at the time of migration is taken into account, and migration occurs during adult life, the risk remains that of the country of origin. On the other hand, the risk of the host country is acquired if migration occurs before the age of 15 years. This observation has been interpreted as meaning that the pathogenic factor relevant to the development of MS must be effective before the age of 15 (see Chapter 5). At least, it may be assumed that the time before puberty is the critical period during which geographical location is relevant for the determination of disease probability (Fishman 1982). Certainly, the risk of developing the disease is determined at least several years before the appearance of its clini-

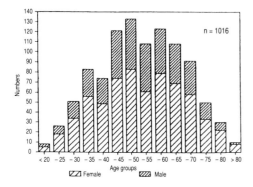

Fig. 4.2. Distribution of MS according to age group.

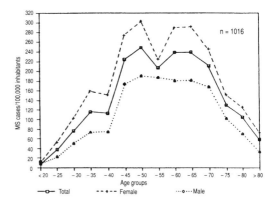

Fig. 4.3. Prevalence of MS per 100,000 inhabitants in relation to age and gender.

cal manifestations. To infer more from migration studies would be mere speculation.

DISTRIBUTION ACCORDING TO AGE, SEX, FAMILY, AND RACE

Comparison with numerous other studies indicates that our prevalence studies have produced representative data (Beer and Kesselring 1988; 1994). A total of 1016 MS patients were involved who satisfied the criteria proposed by C. M. Poser et al. (1983) for probable or definite MS risk. Based on these data, some further aspects of MS epidemiology can be given.

- The mean age of all patients was 50.7 (+/− 14.7) years. There was no difference with regard to gender. The mean disease duration at the time of examination was 17.4 (+/− 12.1) years.
- The distribution according to different age groups is shown in Fig. 4.2: 47.6% of the MS population are between 40 and 60 years old; 0.7% are below 20 years; and 1% are above 80 years.
- Age-specific prevalence rates according to gender are shown in Fig. 4.3: the highest age-specific prevalence is found in the age group between 45 and 50 years (302.7 per 100,000 inhabitants).
- Gender distribution: of 1016 patients, 63.9% were female, and 36.1% were male, corresponding to a ratio of 1.8:1 (female:male). A

similar sex ratio is found in most of the more recent studies, whereas in earlier reviews (Brain 1930), a predominance of males was reported. Whether a change in sex preponderance has occurred over the years cannot be ascertained in retrospect.

- Sex-specific prevalence is 137.3 per 100,000 inhabitants for females, and 82.0 per 100,000 inhabitants for males, a difference which is highly significant.
- We found familial cases in our own study in 8.6%, whereas even higher percentages have been found by other authors (Ebers 1983: 12.5%; Sadovnick et al. 1988: 17.5%; Wikström et al. 1984: 29%). The risk decreases within a family with increasing degree of relationship from the infected person. Relative risk is 20 for siblings, 12 for parents and children, and 5 for cousins. We cannot see any reason to separate familial cases from sporadic ones as single clinical entities, as has been proposed.
- Differences according to race and ethnic groups: the literature may be summarized by saying that MS only rarely exists in Bantu, Eskimos, Hungarian gypsies, and Hutterites in Northern America (Kurtzke 1983b; Waksman and Reynolds 1984), and that it is 10 times less frequent in oriental races than in populations of Northern European or North American origin living in comparable geographical locations (McDonald 1986).

5

Pathogenesis

The preceding chapters provide an overview of the pathology of MS and its relationship to experimental models (Chapter 2), on genetic disposition and immunological changes (Chapter 3), and on some epidemiological characteristics of the disease and its geographical distribution (Chapter 4). The following is an attempt to develop the basis of a modern concept of disease mechanism, and, in particular, of the pathogenesis of the plaques which are fundamental to it. It is unavoidable that some aspects are hypothetical, since the true cause of the disease is not known. Out of the mosaic of knowledge, a picture of pathogenesis is emerging based on the best proven facts.

GENERAL PATHOGENESIS

The prevalence of MS varies widely in relation to geographical location and the ethnic background of the population examined. As discussed in Chapter 4, there is an increase in the prevalence of MS with increasing geographical distance from the equator in Europe and Northern America. This is not a methodological artifact, but reflects a true biological characteristic of the disease. A similar North–South gradient is found in Japan, although the prevalence rates there are lower by a factor of 10 than those at similar geographical latitudes in Europe and Northern America.

In some ethnic groups, such as Bantu, Eskimos, Hungarian gypsies and Hutterites in the U.S., MS appears to be extremely rare; whereas in certain geographical areas such as the Faeroe Islands and West Finland, accumulations of cases are described. The results of migration studies indicate that environmental factors are probably operative in MS pathogenesis, although any concept of the pathogenesis of MS has to take into account genetic factors as well. If a genetic influence on the disposition to the disease (MS susceptibility) is postulated (see below), the possibility of a genetically regulated protective influence must also be considered. More recent studies allow for differentiation between pathogenically heterogeneous disease courses. This is of prognostic importance, and has to be taken into account in therapeutic studies.

Genetic factors

Familial cases

Familial accumulations of definite MS cases over several generations are known, but it is obvious that they do not follow a simple Mendelian trait. Genetic examinations of affected families demonstrate this is not due to common environmental factors within a family (Francis et al. 1987). Such examinations point to an unusual combination of genetic factors which are responsible for susceptibility to environmental factors and the immunological reactions to them (Hartung et al. 1988). The risk of developing MS is 30 to 40 times higher for first-degree relatives than the average risk of 0.1% in the normal population (Sadovnick 1988; 1993).

Twin studies

Indications of a genetic influence on a disease may be gained from twin studies. In the context of MS, early studies of this type had the disadvantage that only twin pairs were described in which both twins were affected by the disease. This negative selection is excluded if MS patients are asked whether or not their twins are affected (Ebers et al. 1986). The incidence of 1:80 obtained by this method corresponds to that found in the normal population, which makes a negative selection influence unlikely. A concordance rate of 30% is found in monozygotic twins, and of 2.5% in dizygotic twins, which corresponds to the familial risk (Sadovnick et al. 1993). Pathological findings in CSF or in magnetic resonance imaging (MRI) of the brain in manifest MS occur more often in the nonaffected twins of MS patients than in the general population (McFarland et al. 1984).

HLA associations

There is a proven association between MS prevalence and certain HLA antigens which are coded for on chromosome 6 and are responsible for the control of immune regulation, but this does not occur everywhere to the same degree. The most strongly associated genetic marker (DR2) is found in a fifth of the normal caucasian population of Nothern Europe, whereas it is found in more than half of the MS patients in the same regions. On the Orkney and Shetland islands, which are the regions with the highest MS prevalence (more than 250/100,000 inhabitants), an association of the disease with DR2 is not demonstrable because this genetic marker is also widely distributed in the normal population (Compston 1982). In Europe, the prevalence of DR2 shows a North–South gradient similar to that of MS. DW2 (which is probably identical to DR2) appears to be very rare in the black African population, where MS also occurs only very rarely (McDonald 1986). Because the occurrence of DR2 is not correlated everywhere with an accumulation of the disease, and is not present, for example, in Arabs, Japanese and Israelis, an MS disposition gene may be postulated, but it cannot be identical to one of the HLA loci known so far (Compston et al. 1986). DR2 is neither necessary in all cases, nor sufficient as a single cause to induce the disease. Rather, it may indicate, together with other genetic markers, for example markers which code for the complement system and antibody structure (chromosome 14), an individual susceptible to developing the disease when induced by factors from the environment. There are indications that the course of the disease and its severity may be associated with a particular genetic constellation: A3, B7, and DR2 are found more often in women and in more benign cases; A1, B8, and DR3 more often in men with a more severe disease course (Hammond et al. 1988).

There is no doubt that the HLA molecules of Class I and II control the reciprocal recognition of cells of the immune system, although the exact mechanisms at the molecular level are not fully understood. The most important point for an understanding of pathogenesis is the fact that they not only initiate the immune reaction, but modulate it. If, as explained previously, the epidemiological data are interpreted as showing that infections in childhood are the initial event in the development of MS, then MS behaves similarly to most known autoimmune diseases: an external factor leads to tissue changes by which cell antigens are liberated and neutralized by an immune reaction. The factors which determine the site of such an immune reaction, wherever it persists, have not been sufficiently clarified, but certainly the HLA system plays a part. All diseases which are based on an autoimmune mechanism show a correlation to gene products which are coded for by the HLA complex. A strong association, as is found in MS, may be taken as an indication of an immune pathogenesis.

This means that an agent responsible for the initial event (a virus?) does not necessarily have to persist in order for the cascade of subsequent events to be sustained, and this also means that the initial event does not necessarily have to be induced by the same agent in all affected people. Furthermore, this concept may explain the fact that not all individuals who have experienced similar initial events will develop MS, because not all of them have the necessary genetic background. The same argument may be used to try to explain the very variable degree of the severity of the disease (see Chapter 10). These factors indicate that the immune system plays a decisive role in MS pathogenesis. A further argument is the well-known observation of increased intrathecal production of γ-globulins in the CSF (see Chapter 8). The plaque itself is basically formed by immunocompetent cells (see Chapter 2 and below), which are spread far into the macroscopically apparently normal white matter.

It is not certain whether the described changes of T-cell subpopulations in the peripheral blood and CSF of MS patients are an expression of the above-mentioned disturbances of immune regulation. The findings are still heterogeneous and not constantly reproducible. Naturally occurring circadian fluctuations of T-cell populations, and heterogeneity of reagents, may partly explain the different results found in different laboratories. The following observations are the best proven (Waksman and Reynolds 1984).

- Active blasts in blood and CSF.
- Elevation of helper/inducer T-cells in CSF at the onset of an exacerbation.
- Diminution of T-suppressor cells in the blood immediately before and during an exacerbation.
- Diminution of the activity of NK cells, and a corresponding diminution of IFN production in one third of MS patients.
- Activated monocytes in peripheral blood contain proteolytic enzymes and produce PGE2.

All these findings can probably be sufficiently explained by the fact that activated monocytes reach the CSF and plaques from the blood, and produce PGE2, which alters the surfaces of NK cells, and probably of T-cells, in such a way that they lose phenotypic markers or cease to express them. On the other hand, T-cell groups which disappear from the peripheral blood may be used to build new plaques. The diminution of suppressor activity may be understood as a corollary or consequence of an immune reaction which plays a role, although not completely understood, in the development of the plaques. It is not certain whether this is due to a phenotypic modulation or to active elimination from the blood compartment.

The following summary can therefore be given of the arguments for immune pathogenesis.

- Genetic predisposition: differences in races (+: Northern European origin (caucasians); −: Bantu, Indians, Eskimos, Maori etc.)
- HLA associations (DR2, B7, A3); genetic restriction on other chromosomes (for example chromosome 14).
- Induction of disease: susceptibility is increased after puberty, after viral infections, and after pregnancy.
- Immunocompetent cells within plaques.
- Intrathecal antibody production.
- Diminution of components of complement in CSF.
- Fluctuations of T-cell populations in blood and CSF.

Although most experimental work associated with MS is immunologically orientated because the immune system plays an important role in the pathogenesis of the disease, older concepts concerning disease development should not be excluded as they may valuably replenish the mosaic of hypotheses.

Environmental factors

The above-mentioned epidemiological studies on the Faeroe Islands and the migration studies from South Africa, Israel, and London, suggest that a "window of vulnerability" at the time of puberty might play a role in triggering MS. The clinical impression that MS patients have had their childhood diseases relatively late, or not at all, is supported by the finding of a significantly higher prevalence of MS in people who have had measles, mumps, or rubella infection between the ages of 12 and 15 (Alvord et al. 1987). A retrospective study on discordant monozygotic MS twins showed that the affected twin had much more frequently had simple infectious diseases during the first 15 years of life than the nonaffected twin (Currier and Eldridge 1982). Furthermore, the fact that the older siblings within a family are more frequently affected by MS (James 1984), and the fluctuations over years in the prevalence rates in inhabitants of islands (Cook et al. 1988) suggest that common widespread infections such as childhood diseases are probably relevant in the pathogenesis of MS (McDonald 1986; James 1988).

Concerning a possibly causal role in the development of MS, neurotropic viruses are examined mainly because they are able to persist within the CNS over years, and because they may produce some of the main characteristics of MS pathology: demyelination (for example, coronavirus or canine distemper virus in animals, papovavirus in humans), exacerbations and remissions (herpes simplex), or clinical manifestations only after a long incubation period (spongiform encephalopathy). None of them, however, has been shown to produce all the various characteristics of MS at the same time.

It has been known for a long time that an elevation of measles antibodies may occur in the CSF of MS patients (Adams and Imagawa 1962). This is, however, not specific, because it is found only in 60% of MS patients and may occur in other diseases such as lupus erythematosus. In the near future, it should be possible to demonstrate whether or not measles virus plays a role in the pathogenesis of MS as vaccination against measles has been performed routinely in the U.S. on large numbers of people for about 20 years.

Antibodies against numerous other viruses are found in the CSF in about two thirds of MS patients: herpes, influenza, parainfluenza, mumps, varicella, vaccinia, and others (Compston et al. 1986). However, it is not assumed that this is the result of an equally specific antibody reaction against a causal viral antigen such as is the case in the oligoclonal bands of SSPE, where antibodies are directed specifically against the responsible measles virus. Rather, it is postulated that an elevated antibody titer in the CSF of MS patients is a consequence of a disturbance of immune regulation (McFarlin and McFarland 1982; McDonald 1983a), or else it may represent "scars" following previous viral diseases.

On many occasions, an attempt has been made to detect virus particles in the brains of MS patients, but almost all inclusion bodies described may be interpreted as artifacts or as myelin breakdown products and unspecifically active changes within astrocytes (Allen 1981).

A viral genome, however, may remain active within the brain without virus particles themselves being morphologically detectable. Occasionally, genetic material of measles virus or herpes simplex may be detected in brains of MS patients by in-situ hybridization (Haase et al. 1981).

Up till now, it has not been possible to prove a causal relationship between an infectious agent and MS: no agent has been detected simultaneously by morphological and serological means. Nor has it been possible to transduce MS from patients to experimental animals by tissue or body fluids. Even in regions in which apparent epidemics of MS have been observed (Kurtzke and Hyllested 1979; Kurtzke et al. 1982), no single cases of familial occurrence were reported. The hypothesis of a transfectious, contagious infection is therefore improbable (C. M. Poser 1986). However, the possibility cannot be excluded, and it is even probable (see below) that infectious agents play a role as additional or triggering factors in predisposed individuals.

In summary, MS is interpreted as a late general reaction against infections which have occurred during a period of increased immunological vulnerability, rather than as a reaction against a specific agent (Alter 1981). In fact, none of the 14 claims which have so far been made that a single agent is responsible for MS has stood the proof of time.

Other possible environmental factors, such as accumulations of cases in the environment of a zinc factory (Stein et al. 1987), may be explained by an effect via the immune system (Schiffer et al. 1988). Numerous other environmental factors have been examined, such as nutrition habits, toxic influences, duration of sunshine, social status, etc., but it has not been possible to provide an adequate explanation of the cause of MS.

Factors triggering exacerbation

Multiple sclerosis patients frequently report events which they consider to be responsible in retrospect for triggering exacerbations. Systematic studies usually fail to prove such relationships unequivocally. Overall, in prospective studies (Sibley et al. 1985), significantly fewer infectious diseases have been found in MS patients than in a comparable population group. However, more than a quarter of exacerbations were found to have a temporal relationship with an infection, most frequently caused by adenoviruses (Lygner et al. 1988). Viruses may be operating either as primary immunogens or via the stimulation of an immune response or antigen presentation by cells within the CNS. A further argument for this latter assumption may be the fact that in a therapeutic trial with INF-γ, exacerbations were produced (Panitch et al. 1987), and the observation that INF-γ and TNF are increased immediately before the appearance of clinical manifestations of an exacerbation (Beck et al. 1988; Chofflon et al. 1992). Hormonal factors probably also play a role in triggering or preventing exacerbations. It is regularly observed (Korn-Lubetzki et al. 1984) that the exacerbation rate is lower in the last trimester of pregnancy in MS patients than at times without pregnancy. However, the exacerbation rate is increased in the first half-year, and particularly in the first 6 weeks, post partum. It is assumed that α-AFP, the concentration of which is particularly elevated in the last trimester of pregnancy, is acting directly by immunosuppression and by inhibiting the expression of MHC Class II molecules stimulated by INF-γ (see Chapter 3).

SPECIAL PATHOGENESIS OF PLAQUES

Blood–brain barrier

Clinical evidence

If observed over long periods of time, optic neuritis may be taken as a symptom of MS in three quarters of cases. In the acute stage, in a

quarter of cases, extravasation from the peripheral retinal vessels may be observed ophthal-
moscopically (periphlebitis retinae) (Engell
1986), or it may be demonstrated by fluorescence angiography (McDonald 1983a). This
finding is relevant to the pathogenesis of MS
because it indicates that an opening of the
blood–brain barrier and the blood–retina barrier, respectively, occurs even in areas where
neither oligodendrocytes nor myelin are present. This suggests that these signs of inflammation are not a secondary reaction against myelin
breakdown products. It may therefore be assumed that a vascular event plays an important
role very early in the pathogenic course.

Predilection sites of MS plaques are found in
mechanically stressed regions of the CNS: in
the optic nerves (under mechanical stress in all
movements of the eyes), along the lateral ventricles (pulsations of the choroid plexus), in the
cervical spinal cord (movements of the head),
and in the transition zone between thoracic and
lumbar spinal cord (movements of the back).
Experimentally, inflammatory/demyelination
foci are grouped in mechanically or chemically
altered regions: they are found along the tapping channel in stereotactic brain operations in
MS patients, or in mechanically or chemically
altered tissues in EAE. These findings are explained as a consequence of a transient opening
of the blood–brain barrier (review in C. M. Poser 1986; 1993).

MRI findings

Magnetic resonance imaging is very sensitive in
detecting changes of the white matter (see
Chapter 8), and may be used for repeated examinations of patients because it appears to
be completely harmless. The function of the
blood–brain barrier may be examined in vivo
by the intravenous application of the contrast
agent gadolinium DTPA in MRI. An enhancement of this contrast agent has been found in
almost all newly developed plaques identified
in serial examinations. This enhancement,
however, persists for only about 6 weeks (Miller et al. 1988a). Single cases are known in which
enhancement has been detected before signal
changes could be seen in the native scan on corresponding sites (Kermode et al. 1990). Enhancement of gadolinium DTPA in recently developed foci allows differentiation of forms of
the disease which appear clinically as one enti-

ty. In primary chronic progressive disease, only
very few new lesions are produced over 6
months, of which none is enhancing. Six times
more lesions, of which over 90% enhance, are
found over the same period of observation in
the same number of patients with secondary
progressive disease, i.e., those who had exacerbations and remissions earlier in the disease
course. It may therefore be assumed that there
are pathogenically heterogeneous forms of the
MS (Thompson et al. 1991). An increased water
content outside the plaques is found in the apparently normal white matter and in the cortex
of MS patients, as can be demonstrated by measuring relaxation times in MRI (Kesselring et al.
1989b). By comparing magnetic resonance parameters found in MS patients with those
found in experimental brain edema in cats
(Barnes et al. 1987; 1988), it may be assumed
that the MRI signal changes are due basically to
an increased water content in the acute as well
as in the chronic plaques.

Experimental findings

It is an important prerequisite for the interpretation of magnetic resonance images in MS
that the formalin-fixed brain should be examined on MRI. This allows a comparison between imaging and histological findings. The
signal changes in MRI correspond exactly to the
histologically defined plaques (Ormerod et al.
1987). The animal model of MS (EAE) may now
be examined using adapted MRI techniques
(Hawkins et al. 1990). As mentioned above,
EAE is an autoimmune disease against a myelin
component, such as MBP, which in many aspects resembles the human disease. Enhancement of the contrast agent gadolinium DTPA is
found only in areas in which postmortem histological signs of inflammation are detected. Enhancement persists, as in MS, for 5 days to 5
weeks. In EAE, the transport of the contrast
agent within vesicles across the endothelial
cells can be followed, and an increase in the
number of endothelial vesicles within acute
plaques has been described in MS as well
(Brown 1978). In the acute inflammatory focus
of EAE with an open blood–brain barrier, the
tight junctions between endothelial cells remain intact. The penetration of gadolinium
across the endothelial cells is an active metabolic process which may be blocked by metabolic
toxins such as dinitrophenol. If primary de-

myelination is produced by cuprizone, no inflammatory reaction is found, and there is no opening of the blood–brain barrier (Bakker and Ludwin 1987).

In summary, the opening of the blood–brain barrier occurs regularly and early, and persists for about 6 weeks in MS as well as in the animal model of EAE. This may be demonstrated in vivo by enhancement of the intravenously applied contrast agent gadolinium DTPA in MRI, as well as by the technique of positron emission tomography (Pozzilli et al. 1988). An increased permeability of the blood–brain barrier may be produced experimentally by trauma, and by toxic and chemical influences such as hypoglycemia and hyponatremia. In single cases, it has been observed that a new development of plaques may occur after viral infections such as varicella, measles, and rubella, and this also may be explained by a disturbance of the blood–brain barrier (for review see C. M. Poser 1986). In analogy to these experimental findings, it may be postulated that an alteration of the blood–brain barrier may also occur after other infectious diseases. The changes would then be the common denominator on which various pathological influences converge

This hypothesis is further supported epidemiologically when it is demonstrated in careful prospective studies that MS patients show an increased number of exacerbations in close temporal relationship with viral infections (Sibley et al. 1984; 1985). Due to the opening of the blood–brain barrier, the brain is more accessible for antigenic influences from the bloodstream, and antigenically active components of the CNS are exposed to the immune system: the CNS is no longer an immunologically privileged organ.

Having said this, a general hypothesis concerning some steps of the pathogenesis of MS may be summarized in the following way. Disposition to, as well as protective influences against MS are genetically determined, probably by genes in the region of the HLA complex or by others which are in close relationship to it. Indications that a single gene locus is responsible for disease disposition are lacking, and it appears more probable that an interaction of genes from various regions determines the disposition to the disease. Unspecified factors from the environment which are operative in childhood lead to a systemic disease in genetically predisposed people. This does not necessarily manifest itself in neurological terms, but produces a transient change of the blood–brain barrier. In this way, a first sensitization by antigens is possible. These may either be foreign antigens or autoantigens.

Pathogenesis of the inflammatory reaction

A hallmark of the pathology of MS is the inflammatory reaction, which is not confined to the plaques themselves, but affects large parts of the macroscopically normal-appearing tissue. The mechanisms which lead to inflammation in the nervous system can only be understood if the basis of the immune surveillance of the nervous system is clear.

Until a few years ago, the CNS was regarded as an immunologically privileged organ. This assumption was based on the observation that heterologous transplants which were rejected immediately in peripheral organs could be tolerated for some time in the brain or spinal cord. Two main factors were thought to be responsible for the privileged position of the nervous system in immune surveillance.

1. The blood–brain barrier impedes the penetration of cells from the immune system and of inflammatory mediators into the nervous system.
2. Elements of the nervous system do not express histocompatibility antigens. A specific antigen recognition is therefore not possible for T-lymphocytes in the CNS.

This concept of the nervous system as an immunologically privileged organ has been modified in recent years. In the normal nervous tissue, at any given time, a small number of hematogenous cells (especially lymphocytes and macrophages) are found which are continuously replaced by other cells migrating from the bloodstream (Hickey and Kimura 1988; Hickey et al. 1992). The barrier function of the blood–brain barrier is operative for immunoglobulins, inflammatory mediators, and for cells of the immune system in general, but not for activated T-lymphocytes (Wekerle et al. 1986a; Hickey et al. 1991). Furthermore, even in the normal nervous system, expression of histocompatibility antigens has been demonstrated within the meninges, in perivascular monocytes, and in some microglial cells (Vass and Lassmann 1990). Expression of MHC antigens is increased locally by various noxious stimuli, such as irritation by electric current, trauma, or lesions of peripheral nerves. This focal elevation of density of potential antigen-presenting cells determines these brain regions as predilection sites for the inflammatory reaction (Hickey 1991).

The following concept of immune surveillance of the nervous system was derived from these findings (Wekerle et al. 1986a; Lassmann et al. 1991b). If T-lymphocytes are activated in the peripheral immune system (i.e., in the context of an infection or an immune-stimulating therapy), some of these activated T-cells will penetrate into the nervous system. However, an inflammatory focus is initiated only if these T-cells find an antigen within the nervous system which is presented by antigen-presenting cells together with histocompatibility antigens. In this case, the T-cells will produce various cytokines (IL-2, INF-γ, TNF-α, lymphotoxin, and others). These cytokines activate endothelial cells, leading to an expression of adhesion molecules on the surface of the endothelial cells, and thereby to the recruitment of further hematogenous cells into the inflammatory lesion, and a breakdown of the blood–brain barrier. Furthermore, expression of MHC antigens and adhesion molecules is stimulated by locally produced cytokines. In this phase of inflammation, the nervous tissue is damaged by toxins from activated effector cells, and this leads to functional deficits and clinical symptomatology.

It is not yet clear how this inflammatory reaction is brought to an end within the nervous system. Some mechanisms considered include the specific inhibition of pathogenic T-cell populations by anti-idiotypic T-lymphocytes (Sun et al. 1988), local production of immunosuppressive cytokines such as TGF-β (Johns et al. 1991; Racke et al. 1991), or the production of glucocorticoids from the adrenal cortex (Mason 1991). In infectious diseases, the elimination of pathogenic agents is of decisive importance.

In contrast to other organs, the CNS contains no lymph vessels. Only in exceptional cases is a connection found to regional lymph nodes (Weller et al. 1992). For this reason, it is not yet clear how inflammatory cells leave the nervous system. However, more recent findings using the model of EAE indicate that T-lymphocytes do not leave the inflammatory focus but are destroyed by a preprogrammed cell death (apoptosis) (Pender et al. 1992).

Immunopathological findings in MS are compatible with the mechanisms described. T-cells and macrophages dominate within lesions, MHC and adhesion molecules are expressed on elements of the blood–brain barrier and on glia cells, and cytokines are locally produced in inflammatory cells and glia in activated demyelinating foci. The requirement for there to be peripheral T-cell activation before inflammation can be induced could explain the association of MS exacerbations with preceding viral infections (Sibley et al. 1984; 1985), as well as with immunostimulating INF-γ therapy (Panitch et al. 1987a; 1987b). Furthermore, the increased expression of MHC molecules following nonspecific tissue damage might explain why lesions are predominantly found in areas which are exposed to frequent traumatic stress (Oppenheimer 1987).

It is not clear, however, whether autoimmune reactions contribute to the pathogenesis of MS plaques. Autoreactive T-lymphocytes are not only found in the blood of MS patients, but also in healthy controls, although in MS, the incidence is higher by a factor of 100 (Olsson et al. 1990; Sun et al. 1991a; 1991b; Olsson 1992). However, no direct proof of the pathogenic relevance of an autoimmune reaction has so far been produced.

Pathogenesis of demyelination and tissue destruction

It may be inferred from the histological observation that axons remain largely intact, at least in recent plaques, that demyelination in MS depends on mechanisms acting directly on myelin or on oligodendrocytes. In principle, demyelinating foci in inflammatory/demyelinating diseases of the CNS may be explained by two different mechanisms.

1. A primary damage of oligodendrocytes with degeneration of the cells and secondary demyelination. In this case, the inflammatory reaction is not the cause of demyelination.
2. An immune reaction against one or several antigens of the myelin sheath. In this case, the immune reaction and the inflammation are the prerequisites of demyelination. Such a mechanism is not necessarily directed against autoantigens, but may be directed against foreign antigens (virus?), which are built into the membrane of oligodendrocytes or myelin.

There is also the possibility that antigens which trigger the immune reaction are not primarily located within the CNS. Experiments supporting this idea were performed on EAE induced in guinea-pigs sensitized by subcutaneous injection of tuberculin in complete Freund's adjuvant. After later injection of tubercle bacteria or tuberculin breakdown products into the CSF, a local inflammation in the brain, with disruption of the myelin lamellae and myelin breakdown by macrophages, may be induced (Wisniewski and Bloom 1975). Therefore, various antigens from outside the CNS may be responsible for part of the demyelinating process within CNS foci typically seen in MS. Such antigens may also be produced by infections within the organisms which do not themselves reach the CNS. In animal experiments, infection by coronavirus may lead to an allergic demyelination within the CNS when the virus itself is no longer detectable within the organism (Watanabe et al. 1983).

Proof of a viral infection of oligodendroglial cells in MS patients, or changes of oligodendroglial cells in the border region of foci or in the neighboring white matter, has not been produced in the studies done so far.

The possibility of primary damage of oligodendroglial cells is not completely excluded by these negative findings. More recent experimental studies, however, indicate that the second aspect of MS pathology, the inflammatory reaction, appears to be more important in terms of pathogenesis.

The first change in active MS plaques appears to be the penetration of activated T-lymphocytes from the bloodstream into the nervous tissue. This initial inflammatory reaction is associated with a focal breakdown of the blood–brain barrier and an influx of serum proteins into the lesion. Recent in-vitro studies demonstrated that oligodendroglial cells and myelin are particularly susceptible to macrophage toxins and complement factors. Selective destruction of myelin and/or oligodendroglia by the sparing of other components of the nervous system may be induced by cytokines (TNF-α, Selmaj and Raine 1988), oxygen radicals (Griot et al. 1989), and complement (Scolding et al. 1989). All the factors are produced in T-cell-mediated inflammatory reactions by activated macrophages, and reach the lesion across a disturbed blood–brain barrier. In such foci, demyelination predominates; it is, however, associated with considerable destruction of other elements of the

nervous system (axons, astrocytes). In this case, the immune reaction is not directed against myelin, and demyelination itself may be explained by the relatively selective vulnerability of myelin and oligodendroglial cells to toxins produced by macrophages. Such destructive lesions are observed particularly in the very acute forms of MS (Marburg 1906).

Apart from these nonspecific mechanisms of demyelination, some specific immunological phenomena seem to play a role. Gamma/delta T-lymphocytes, increased numbers of which are found within MS plaques, may initiate selective destruction by the specific recognition of stress proteins in oligodendroglial cells (Selmaj et al. 1991a).

A much more efficient mechanism of demyelination is induced by antibodies directed against epitopes on the extracellular surface of myelin sheaths and oligodendroglial cells. The most important target antigen of antibody-mediated demyelination is MOG (Linington et al. 1988). In the pathogenesis of demyelination in vivo, demyelinating antibodies act synergistically with encephalitogenic T-lymphocytes. The inflammatory reaction mediated by T-cells leads to an opening of the blood–brain barrier, and thereby allows antibodies and complement to penetrate into the nervous tissue. A large number of effector cells (mainly macrophages) are also activated. It is the role of antibodies to direct these activated effector mechanisms against myelin sheaths and oligodendrocytes.

In the context of a mild inflammatory reaction, the cooperation between T-lymphocytes and autoantibodies leads to widespread and very selective demyelination, with destruction of oligodendroglia. Such lesions are found predominantly and typically in forms of MS with a chronic course.

Factors may be found in the serum of MS patients which lead in cell cultures to swelling of myelin, disruption of lamellae, and stripping of the myelin sheaths from the axon. A more accurate examination of the serum proteins which lead to demyelination demonstrates that immunoglobulins are only partly responsible for these effects. The rest of the activity appears to depend on complement factors (Compston et al. 1991). For a long time, the search for demyelinating antibodies within the CSF was disappointing. However, a positive finding was not to be expected because demyelinating antibodies produced within the CSF would be absorbed immediately by the surrounding nervous tissue. In elegant experiments, Sun et al. (1991a) were able to demonstrate that in the CSF of 80% of patients with chronic MS, plasma cells are found which produce antibodies against MOG. These more recent findings are a strong argument for a decisive role of demyelinating antibodies in the pathogenesis of MS.

It is not clear which immune reaction against which target antigen initiates the primary disease process in MS. There are indications, however, that during the further chronic course of the disease, new T-cell-mediated and antibody-mediated autoimmune reactions against a large number of various antigens of the nervous system are induced. These autoimmune reactions appear to play an important role in the pathogenesis of demyelinating lesions in the chronic course of MS.

SUMMARY OF PATHOGENESIS

From what has been said, a few steps of MS pathogenesis may be summarized in a general hypothesis as follows (C. M. Poser 1986; 1993; McDonald and Barnes 1989; McDonald et al. 1992; McDonald 1993).

Disposition to, as well as protective influences against MS are genetically determined, probably by genes in the region of the HLA complex or in close relation to it. All specific factors from the environment which are operative in childhood lead, in genetically disposed individuals, to a systemic disease which does not necessarily become clinically manifest, but

which leads to a transient opening of the blood –brain barrier. By this means, a first sensitization occurs when antigens reach the CNS from the bloodstream. Such antigens may be foreign as well as from the same organism. In a later period of life, the blood–brain barrier is again made more permeable by nonspecific factors such as trauma, infections, hormonal or toxic influences. A secondary hypersensitivity reaction occurs which uses the previous sensitization as an "anamnestic adjuvant." The opening of the blood–brain barrier which is regularly demonstrated in early stages of the plaques, and which persists for about 6 weeks, is a prerequisite for the development of plaques, but it is not sufficient as the only explanation for it. Various triggering mechanisms are fundamental to the inflammatory reaction by immunocompetent cells and to the demyelinating process by macrophages and microglia. The assumption that MS is a continuous disease process over years, and that the clinical manifestations are only the tip of an iceberg, is supported by the observation of clinically silent but pathologically verified cases of MS (Georgi 1961; Phadke and Best 1983).

In the future, a better understanding of MS pathogenesis may be expected when the relationship between infectious diseases and MS is clarified, when antigens can be detected which lead to inflammation and/or demyelination, and when both these processes may be differentiated in vivo, for example in MRI. In all these directions of research, there is reason for hope.

6

Pathophysiology of impaired neural transmission

The symptoms of MS are determined not only by the localization of plaques, but also by changes in signal transmission. Electrophysiological methods are therefore established in the diagnosis of the disease.

ELECTROPHYSIOLOGY OF NORMAL NERVE FIBERS

A neuron is composed typically of a cell body with thin, branched processes, the dendrites, and an axon of variable length. Dendrites receive impulses from the axons of numerous other neurons by synaptic contact. A complex network is formed of neurons communicating with each other. Sensible unipolar neurons are an exception to this rule insofar as they do not have any dendrites. Their participation in the disease process of MS is by means of a long afferent axon in the peripheral nerve, and a long efferent axon in the dorsal column of the spinal cord. Central nerve fibers also consist of axons, as they do in the peripheral nerve, and may reach a length of up to 1 m in the CNS. The velocity of impulse conduction in nerve fibers or axons depends primarily on whether or not the fiber is myelinated. Unmyelinated fibers conduct very slowly, at about 1 m/s, whereas impulse conduction velocity in myelinated fibers depends on their total thickness. For a fiber thickness of 10–20 μm, the conduction velocity is about 50–120 m/s; for a fiber thickness of 5 μm, it is about 25 m/s. A myelinated nerve fiber consists of an axon cylinder and the myelin sheath. In the resting state, an electrolyte gradient (the resting membrane potential) is sustained over the outer membrane of the axon. The inner side of the axon has a negative electrical charge compared to the outer side.

Myelin envelops the axon over its entire length except at short intervals, the Ranvier nodes. Sodium channels mainly occur in the membrane at the sites of these myelin-free nodes, which, when transiently activated (opened), permit the passage of a short influx of sodium. This leads to an electromotor gradient which is opposed to the resting potential of the membrane and which builds up the action potential of impulse conduction (Fig. 6.1).

A single action potential lasts for about 1 ms, or slightly longer. It follows the all-or-none law, and is initiated as soon as the passive depolarization from the neighboring node reaches a certain threshold. In between the nodes, myelin acts as an electric insulator around the excitable membrane, and therefore the action potential of a node is only able to leave the axon at the next node. There, a new depolarization up to the critical threshold is produced, and thence an action potential. In myelinated fibers, the spread of action potentials thus becomes saltatory, and is much faster than the continuous impulse transmission in unmyelinated nerve fibers. After excitation, every excitable membrane loses its ability to be excitable for a certain period of time, known as the absolute refractory period. It also shows an elevated threshold for a certain length of time, known as the relative refractory period. This refractory period depends on rebuilding of the resting potential. Therefore, a nerve fiber is not able to conduct impulse volleys at high frequencies. In myelinated nerve fibers, the relative refractory period lasts two to three times as long as the action potential, about 3–6 ms. A second impulse arriving within the relative refractory period may be transmitted under optimal conditions. However, the safety margin for successful impulse

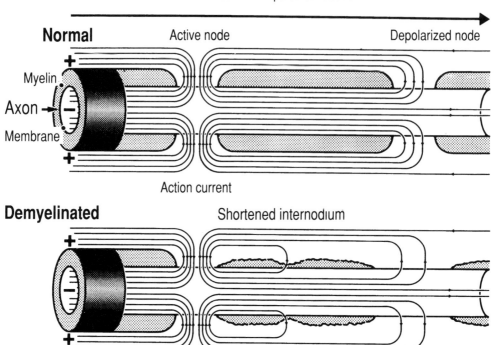

Fig. 6.1. Schematic depiction of saltatory impulse conduction in intact myelinated and partially demyelinated nerve fibers. At the active node, the action current flows as ion current across the opened sodium channels into the interior of the axon, and leads to passive electric depolarization at the next node. In demyelinated nerve fibers, less current reaches the depolarized node than in the intact fiber because of leakage. (Direction of impulse conduction from left to right. The length of the internodium (the section between two nodes) is shown relatively much too short for the sake of clarity.)

conduction is reduced for this second impulse, because even a slight loss of current over an internodium suffices to impede depolarization of the next node so that firing threshold is no longer reached. This means that the conduction of impulse volleys is particularly at risk if the electrical properties of nerve fibers are disturbed.

PATHOPHYSIOLOGY OF DEMYELINATED NERVE FIBERS

Electrophysiological properties

A characteristic morphological hallmark of the MS plaques is focal demyelination (see Chapter 2). This involves a more or less marked destruction of the myelin sheath whereby axons remain intact and Wallerian degeneration does not occur. The pathophysiology of the partially or totally demyelinated, or occasionally re-

myelinated, nerve fibers is not completely understood. However, a number of pathophysiological characteristics are known which facilitate the understanding of the signs and symptoms of MS.

If the myelin sheath is damaged, the resulting leakage of current and capacitance losses cause depolarization over the corresponding internodium to be impaired (see Fig. 6.1). It takes longer to reach the threshold on the next node, and therefore saltation of the excitation over the corresponding internodium is slowed. If demyelination is more marked, the excitation threshold is no longer reached, and impulse conduction is interrupted. The most severely damaged internodium is the weakest link in the chain of the nerve fiber, and determines the success of impulse conduction. Impulse conduction in completely demyelinated axons may be interrupted completely. It is restored, however, within a few days by the formation of new sodium channels in demyelinated internodia (Bostock and Sears 1978). Saltatory impulse conduction appears to occur occasionally even when myelin is lacking if sodium channels are distributed periodically, as in myelinated nerve fibers (Smith et al. 1982). Experimentally, spontaneous remyelination of central demyelinated nerve fibers has been demonstrated by which reliable impulse conduction may be restored (Smith et al. 1979). In the human CNS, corresponding proven facts are lacking. However, there are good indications that even in completely demyelinated nerve fibers in MS, a form of impulse conduction may be restored (Wisniewski et al. 1976), and that remyelination occurs (Prineas and Connell 1979; see also Chapter 2). In the latter case, internodia are shorter and the myelin sheath is thinner than originally. Therefore, conduction of reduced velocity is to be expected in remyelinated areas. Remyelination is again mainly due to oligodendrocytes or their precursor cells. Interestingly, it may be observed in transition zones to the peripheral nervous system, where it appears to be due to invasion of Schwann cells from the peripheral nervous system (Feigin and Ogata 1971).

Recent demyelination, even if it is only partial or limited to the paranodal area near the Ranvier nodes, may cause a reversible conduction block (Gilliatt 1982; Lafontaine et al. 1982). In the peripheral nerves, a conduction block of focal demyelination leads to the typical mechanism of neurapraxia which occurs, for example, in pressure lesions. Because axons retain their continuity and their trophic functions, there is little sign of atrophy, even months later and despite paresis. Several weeks after the removal of compression, normal impulse conduction is restored. It has been proven experimentally (McDonald and Sears 1970a), and by observations following tumor removal, that in central lesions as well, focal demyelination and local ischemia may produce a reversible conduction block. This leads to the assumption that findings from the peripheral nerves may be applicable to central lesions. In acute optic neuritis, partial restoration of vision as well as visual evoked potentials (VEPs) may occur after the acute visual loss and disappearance of the recorded potentials. This leads to the assumption that the mechanism of reversible conduction block is relevant in MS, and may play an important role during the recovery phase after a le-

sion. The diminution of impulse conduction velocity in demyelinated nerve fibers is particularly relevant in clinical neurophysiology. Prolonged latencies in evoked potentials are a diagnostic hallmark of MS, analogous to the slowed conduction velocity in peripheral nerves in demyelinating polyneuropathies (see Chapter 8).

Interestingly, even very marked prolongations of latencies in VEPs do not lead to very marked visual disturbances. They may only be detected by the Pulfrich phenomenon (von Pulfrich 1922; Frisen and Hoyt 1974). The arrival of a signal from one eye is interpreted within the cortex as faulty information about depth. In unilateral optic neuritis, a pendulum swinging on a straight line is perceived erroneously as circulating elliptically. The asynchronous arrival of somatosensory afferents from the skin due to the irregular slowing of impulses is responsible for the frequent paresthesia.

Clinically, it is probably more important that partially demyelinated peripheral and central nerve fibers have a prolonged refractory period. This impairs the property of conducting impulse volleys because the nerve fibers may not recover before further impulses follow a short time later (see above). Thus the maximal transmittable impulse frequency may be reduced drastically long before impulse conduction is interrupted (McDonald and Sears 1970b). When an impulse volley arrives, impulse conduction over a demyelinated area may be transiently blocked completely. Vibration sense is often reduced early in peripheral demyelinating polyneuropathies (diabetes mellitus) as well as in MS. This is probably due to an interruption of repetitive excitation in the first sensory neuron in the peripheral or central part of the dorsal columns. Normal functioning of motor control also relies on the capacity of corticospinal impulse volleys to be transmitted at relatively high frequency (Kernell and Wu 1967). This may be impaired in relatively minor demyelination.

Influence of temperature and calcium

It is of clinical importance that thermolability is increased in demyelinated nerve fibers. Normally, impulse conduction velocity increases linearly with increasing temperature because ion currents are accelerated as temperature rises. However, the impulse conduction of normal nerve fibers is blocked at a critical temperature of about 50°C when currents occur so quickly that the action potential becomes too short for the electrical energy to remain sufficient to excite the next node. Reduction of this critical blocking temperature is to be expected when myelin thickness, and therefore its insulating capacity, is reduced: if myelin thickness is reduced to one third and the length of the internodium remains constant, the critical temperature is reduced to about 40°C (Schauf and Davis 1974). Demyelinated nerves are much more sensitive in this respect as an increase of only 0.5°C may be enough to block impulse conduction (Davis and Jacobson 1971; Rasminsky 1973). Symptoms of MS characteristically become more marked with increasing body temperature, which may be explained by the properties of demyelinated nerves. The temperature effect is important because short-lived or fluctuating symptoms in MS are relatively common and should not be interpreted as exacerbations. Disturbances lasting only a few hours might be due to this so-called Uhthoff phenomenon (Uhthoff 1889; see also Chapter 7). Such symptoms may depend on body activity, fever, mental excitation, or exogenous temperature load.

It has been calculated that decreasing ion concentrations of calcium in the neighborhood of nerve fibers oppose the conduction block caused by increased temperature (Schauf and Davis 1974). This may explain the transient improvements of certain symptoms which can occur in MS patients following hyperventilation or treatment with sodium bicarbonate or EDTA (Davis et al. 1970).

Possible consequences of increased excitability

Excitability is abnormally increased in demyelinated segments of nerve fibers. This may lead to spontaneous discharges or discharges caused by mechanical stimulation (Rasminsky 1978; Smith and McDonald 1982; Nordin et al. 1984). A number of symptoms of MS might thus be explained: for example, paresthesia and facial myokymia may be due to spontaneous discharges of sensory or motor nerve fibers; Lhermitte's sign and phosphenes produced by eye movements (see Chapter 7) may be the consequence of mechanical stimulation of the dorsal column and optic nerves, respectively. In

Lhermitte's sign, such abnormal activity could be demonstrated by direct microneurography in humans (Nordin et al. 1984).

In experimental central demyelination, spontaneous activity may display the same rhythm of discharge as is characteristic of facial myokymia in MS, i.e., regularly recurring discharges in groups (Smith and McDonald 1982). Myokymias in the limbs consist of similar rhythmic discharges of motor units (Albers and Bastron 1981). Because similar lesions occur in peripheral chronic compression and in focal demyelination after irradiation, a similar mechanism is assumed. Painful tonic seizures in MS (Osterman and Westerberg 1975; see also Chapter 7) may also be explained by ectopic impulse generation. Such massive motor manifestations may not be caused by one single excitable nerve fiber. Defects of myelin may also facilitate ephaptic impulse transmission from one nerve fiber to another. Within a plaque, ectopic erroneous spontaneous activity may originate from a hyperexcitable fiber and may lead to widespread hyperactivity. Additionally, such motor phenomena may also be facilitated because of impaired inhibiting mechanisms.

Pathological ephaptic impulse transmission may also be a cause of paroxysmal neuralgia. In trigeminal neuralgia, for example, such transmission is postulated in the area of the proximal, focally demyelinated section of the nerve. It may occur from efferent motor nerve fibers onto afferent pain fibers. This could explain the triggering of paroxysms by minimal masticatory movements. Certain other paroxysmal symptoms which occur in many MS patients stereotypically and last only a few minutes (see Chapter 7) may also be explained on the basis of such ectopic impulse generation: paroxysmal ataxia, dysarthria, and akinetic attacks. It should also be considered that excessive or uninhibited activity in inhibitory central neuronal circuitry could explain paroxysmal negative symptoms. It must be stressed, however, that such considerations are still speculative, and the proper physiological role of ectopic activity and of ephaptic impulse transmission in MS is uncertain.

OTHER MECHANISMS OF IMPAIRED CONDUCTION

Although demyelinating lesions predominate in MS plaques, a certain amount of axonal loss and Wallerian degeneration occurs. This may reach a considerable degree in older plaques in advanced cases or in hyperacute inflammatory foci (see Chapter 2). Because axons in the CNS, in contrast to the peripheral nervous system, do not regenerate, the corresponding damage has to be considered as irreparable. This does not mean, however, that improvement of the symptoms would not be possible. As is known from patients with vascular lesions or after tumor excision, and from experimental work (Jacobson et al. 1979), redundancy and plasticity occur in the CNS to a degree which was probably previously underestimated. New synaptic contacts may develop by collateral sprouting of regenerating nerve fibers while others degenerate (Bernstein and Bernstein 1973), leading to a reorganization of the neuronal network. This allows adaptation to a new situation and partial replacement of lost functions, even in adults. Such morphological neuronal reorganization in the spinal cord might play a role in the development of spasticity (McCouch et al. 1958). Spasticity of the legs may then be considered, to a certain degree, to be a functionally useful adaptation (Murray and Goldberger 1974): the increased muscle tone may be necessary for standing and walking.

Concerning the dynamics of symptoms, the initial edema of the acute inflammatory focus is important because the tissue pressure and local ischemia may produce a transitory interruption of neuronal function. It is probably primarily intracellular edema. It was shown experimentally on the rabbit eye (Dalakas et al. 1980) that edematous astrocytes may produce reversible disturbance of function without demyelination. Some of the transient symptoms of an acute exacerbation might therefore be explained as due to edema, and the favorable effect of steroids on acute exacerbation is perhaps sufficiently explained by a more rapid resolution of edema.

As for certain inflammatory polyneuropathies, speculations have been published concerning a reversible neuroelectrical blockade of central impulse transmission by circulating agents such as antibodies in MS. Based on experiments with EAE and sera of MS patients, such a transmissible agent from the IgG fraction, blocking synaptic transmission, was postulated (Schauf et al. 1976). However, despite intense research in this field, a proven pathogenic role of such a factor in MS has not yet been demonstrated.

PART II

Clinical aspects

7

Symptomatology

A number of symptoms and signs are found in almost all cases of advanced MS. Among them are spastic paresis, ataxia of gait and the extremities, central visual loss, double vision, paresthesia, dysarthria, bladder and sexual disturbances, and fatigue. Although they are not specific for MS, they are so typical of the disease, particularly when occurring in combination, that they are accepted as clinical characteristics. However, it is not really helpful to consider combinations of a few individual symptoms as particularly characteristic. The combination of intention tremor, nystagmus, and scanning speech was identified by Charcot as the "classical triad"; pale optic discs, cerebellar ataxia, and pyrimidal signs were another combination identified by Marburg and Pette. If clinical diagnosis were limited to those cases in which these syndromes occur, a large number of MS cases verified at post mortem would be missed, or would only be diagnosed in the terminal stages.

Symptoms and signs which occur only rarely in definite cases of MS, such as aphasia, hemianopia, involuntary movements, marked muscular atrophy, or fasciculations, require specific and repeated differential diagnostic considerations.

There are also symptoms and signs which occur rarely in the MS population as a whole, but which are relatively typical for its diagnosis, even if they occur in single instances. Among them are Lhermitte's symptom, facial myokymias, painful tonic brainstem seizures and other paroxysmal phenomena, trigeminus neuralgia in young adults, and certain oculomotor disturbances such as internuclear ophthalmoplegia.

MOTOR ASPECTS

Pareses

Central pareses of the muscles of the extremities characterize the clinical picture in advanced cases of MS. However, motor deficiencies are responsible for the main complaints at the onset of the disease in over 50% of cases, particularly in primary progressive forms. Both legs are usually affected but weakness is only rarely marked to the same degree on both sides at disease onset. The next most frequent pattern of distribution after paraparesis is the affection of only one leg, and the next most frequent is hemiparesis. Rarely, only one arm is affected by central paresis in MS.

In advanced cases of MS, slight muscular atrophy is found, particularly in the hand muscles, an observation which was mainly emphasized in the older literature. It is not always easy to decide whether it is due to central lesions at the anterior horns of the spinal cord, to peripheral pressure palsies of the ulnar nerve in wheelchair patients, or of the median nerve in the hands of those who hold crutches, or whether it is due to inactivity in immobilized patients. It is certain that lesions of the peripheral motor neuron, particularly at the upper extremities, may be due to a plaque in the cervical spinal cord, and may produce fasciculations during an acute exacerbation (Garcin et al. 1962). Involvement of the peripheral nerves in the disease process of MS has been reported (Pollack et al. 1977; Lassmann et al. 1981a; Poser C 1993). However, lesions of the peripheral nervous system in MS always require a very careful search for other explanations. Marked muscular atrophies, and particularly fasciculations outside an acute exacerbation, should give rise to doubts as to the diagnosis.

The onset of central paresis varies considerably. Often, a feeling of fatigue in the legs or in the lumbar region can be seen in retrospect as an expression of incipient paresis. A feeling of feebleness is increased after exercise and after exposure to heat, more markedly so than in other etiologies. Pareses are slowly progressive over years, particularly if the disease onset is in the middle or older age group, and as a rule the initially affected extremity remains more markedly affected. Slowly progressive paraparesis and hemiparesis lead to differential diagnostic problems. If hemiparesis is due to MS, it is usually caused by a plaque in the lateral column of the upper cervical spinal cord, and therefore muscles of the face are rarely affected. Methods and values of additional examination, which are particularly important in such cases, are considered in Chapters 8 and 9. Sudden onset of hemiparesis or paraparesis has been reported in cases verified at post mortem; it is, however, very rare.

Spasticity and reflexes

For the clinician confronted with a patient with MS, it is of particular importance to determine signs of spasticity. Even more often than the above-mentioned paresis, these signs are largely responsible for the disability of affected individuals, and they are amenable to efficient treatment (see Chapter 13). During examination, one has to concentrate on clinically relevant phenomena, and to consider modern pathophysiological concepts of spasticity (Dimitrijevic and Nathan 1967a; 1967b; Conrad et al. 1984). Spasticity is defined as velocity-dependent increase of resistance, and is due to central disinhibition of the myotatic reflex arc.

In MS, the legs are usually more markedly affected by spasticity than the arms. Extensor spasticity of the legs, particularly of the quadriceps, may be advantageous for standing and walking as it may compensate for muscular weakness.

Gait in spastic patients is characterized by plantar flexion and supination/inversion. With increasing spasticity, gait becomes more difficult due to limitations of mobility of the joints and to simultaneous innervation of agonists and antagonists.

At the initial stage, flexor spasticity may lead to falls without warning; in later stages, it may make sitting and lying more difficult and the use of a wheelchair impossible. If this postural pattern of flexor spasticity becomes fixed as contractures, there is a danger of decubital ulcers developing, which themselves may increase spasticity. Preventive physiotherapy is of the utmost importance in this vicious circle. In advanced cases, extensor spasms may occur without a provoking pattern of posture or movement, even when lying at night, or particularly after rising in the morning. This type of spasm tends either not to be painful or to be less so than the flexor spasms which occur later in the disease course and which may be extremely painful.

Spasticity of leg adductors affects the sphincters of the bladder and bowel and makes nursing more difficult. It often develops during a phase of extensor spasticity, but it is not, however, diminished when flexor tone increases.

It is difficult to quantify spasticity more accurately than by clinical methods. Several methods have been challenged or are too time consuming for clinical practice. A useful possibility seems to be the polygraphic recording of muscle potentials by surface electrodes in the antagonistic muscles during a defined movement, for example by recording the activity in flexors and extensors during a circular movement on a bicycle. The activities of agonist and antagonist overlap in relation to the segment of the circle, and the degree of overlapping may be quantified as a measure of spasticity. An alternative way of measuring spasticity is to determine the velocity and acceleration/deceleration of defined angles on extremities over time, as used in gait analysis (Oesch and Kesselring 1995).

The reflex pattern in MS is often asymmetrical. Spastic increase of muscle tone is usually associated with increased reflexes and enlargement of the reflex zone. However, muscular reflexes may be diminished or absent. In very marked spasticity, limitation of joint mobility may impede visible reflex response. Diminution of reflexes may also be due to a plaque in the entry zone of the posterior root or in the posterior horn. It may then be considered as a sensory disturbance. Most commonly, the reflexes of the triceps brachii (C7), brachioradialis (C6), biceps brachii (C5), and triceps surae (S1) are diminished or absent.

When searching for multiple lesion sites, the phenomenon of reflex inversion may be of importance: reflexes of biceps brachii and/or brachioradialis may be absent, whereas the triceps reflex is increased on the same side. The elbow joint is thus extended when tapping the biceps tendon or the periosteum of the radius. This may be explained by a plaque in the anterior lateral column at level C5/6 which extinguishes myotatic reflex of the flexors, interrupts corticospinal fibers leading to the nuclei which innervate the triceps, and thereby inhibits its own reflex arc. The finding of an inverted triceps reflex is more indicative, but rarer: triceps jerk is absent while reflexes of the flexors, biceps and brachioradialis are increased. Such a finding alone proves the presence of two lesions, locally separated, one lying above C5/6 which disinhibits biceps jerk, and another one at level C7/8 which leads to the absence of the triceps jerk.

Absence of abdominal reflexes is often overvalued as a sign of impairment of the corticospinal tracts, as it can only be taken at face value in slim nulliparous patients without scars on the abdomen, and may be absent in 20% to 30% of healthy individuals.

The most important sign of a lesion in the pyramidal tract is still Babinski's phenomenon, in which stroking of the lateral part of the sole of the foot leads to tonic extension of the big toes, to fanlike spreading of the other toes, and, less markedly, to flexion of knee and hip. This sign cannot be simulated voluntarily, and it therefore allows reliable differentiation between organic and nonorganic pareses. Such differentiation often gives rise to uncertainty, especially in the early phases of MS. Babinski's phenomenon is positive in many MS patients, even without marked weakness.

SENSORY ASPECTS

Many MS patients complain of sensory disturbances; more than half have regularly done so in large series studied for long periods of time. At the onset of the disease, sensory disturbances are the most frequent complaints. Paresthesias are more common than hypesthesias (Sanders and Arts 1986). During examination, even the lightest touch of cotton is sensed, and the tip of a needle is registered as sharp, although perception in affected regions is described as "different": for example as "further away," "as if a second layer were below the skin," or "as if emery paper were on the feet." Such descriptions may lead to a diagnosis of hysteria, particularly in young women for whom no pathological findings are discovered on routine examination. A highly variable and often-changing distribution pattern of such paresthesias may be encountered. Particularly frequent is an onset in the fingertips, spreading over the arms, or from the toes and rising to the

gluteal or genital region. Before MRI was used, pathological anatomical explanations of such paresthesias were found only rarely. Clinicopathological correlation is difficult to determine in purely sensory symptoms, and such sensory disturbances occur relatively early in the course of the disease, and are therefore not examined at post mortem. Nevertheless, histological descriptions of plaques in sensory tracts are well known. They are found more often in the posterior columns than in the spinothalamic tracts. On MRI, plaques in the posterior columns may be clearly depicted (Kesselring et al. 1989a). However, somatosensory evoked potentials (SEPs) which are conducted via the posterior columns are often normal in such cases (see Chapter 8).

A clearly discernible sensory level at the trunk is rare in MS, and should give rise to further search for spinal cord compression.

Somewhat typical, but rare in MS, is the "deafferented hand of Oppenheim," which may lead to complete loss of use. A plaque in the posterior columns is the cause (Paty and Poser 1984). On examination, normal findings result from the testing of motor aspects and reflexes, and vibration sense is diminished or absent, two-point discrimination is enlarged (more than 5 mm on the fingertips, and more than 2 mm side difference), and joint position sense is absent. These findings help to discriminate acute loss of the use of a hand due to paroxysmal disturbance of motor function (paroxysmal akinesia, see p. 85) on clinical grounds alone.

If sensory disturbances are the only manifestation of an exacerbation, they tend to resolve within 1 or 2 months. Similar to motor manifestations, they may, however, be present chronically during the further course of the disease. Feelings are often then described such as "as if one were carrying an armour," "as if the skin were too narrow," or "a belt too tight." Many MS patients complain of an inner vibrating of the whole body; others describe a burning sensation or that the extremities feel cold or wet, without the cause of this being discovered on examination.

Interestingly, a diminution of vibration sense is almost always found in conjunction with a lesion of the pyramidal tract. This finding alone does not justify the postulation of a second lesion because it may be found in diseases confined entirely to the motor system, such as myotrophic lateral sclerosis or progressive spastic paraparesis.

The neck flexion sign described by Lhermitte et al. (1924) is so characteristic that it has been valued as pathognomonic for MS. However, the sensation is only subjective, and also occurs in other etiologies, such as cervical spine trauma, tumors of the cervical spinal cord, and malformations at the cranio–cervical junction (Kanchandani and Howe 1982). It may also be found in a quarter of cases of combined systemic degeneration (vitamin B12 deficiency) (Gautier-Smith 1973). It is uncertain whether it occurs in cervical myelopathy which is not accompanied by MS (Matthews 1991). Those affected describe an electric discharge spreading along the spine and occasionally into the extremities when flexing the neck. The sensation is unpleasant but not really painful, and therefore requires no treatment. A similar sensation may be provoked by laughing or coughing. This is not surprising in view of experimental investigations which demonstrate mechanical irritation in addition to ephaptic impulse conduction within the demyelinated plaque (Smith and McDonald 1982; see Chapter 6). Usually this disturbance disappears spontaneously over a few months. Often there is a certain habituation or fatiguability, and the sensation is provoked only a few times and then does not occur again for several hours.

Like most paroxysmal phenomena (see p. 85), the Lhermitte phenomenon seems to be more prevalent in Japanese patients, having been described in up to 42% of cases (Shibasaki et al. 1981), whereas its presence has been recorded in from 5% to 16% of patients in MS series in Western countries (Paty and Poser 1984).

In most textbooks on MS, pain is mentioned only briefly or not at all. In our experience, however, it is so frequent and distressing, and often treatable, that it deserves a special section (see p. 83).

COORDINATION

"Pure" cerebellar syndromes are rare in MS, and are almost unknown as an isolated initial symptom. However, objective signs of cerebellar deficiencies may be detected in a third of cases at initial examination (Matthews 1991). On the other hand, combinations of disturbances of coordination and motor deficiencies occur frequently during the course of the disease. If present to a marked degree in younger patients, they may indicate a somewhat poor prognosis (see Chapter 10).

Clinical examination of cerebellar functions is more difficult in patients with marked spastic pareses and disturbances of proprioception. Cerebellar involvement is marked by the lack of ability to measure spontaneously the temporal and spatial distances which is necessary for movement (dysmetria), disjointed movements due to lack of coordination of various muscle groups (dyssynergia), or disturbances or lack of change from agonistic to antagonistic movements (dysdiadochokinesia).

In MS, intention tremor is particularly frequent, and often very disabling. It was a sign in Charcot's classical triad of MS symptoms. It is characterized by movement of the extremities which is markedly increased in amplitude and intensity when a target is approached. In most severe cases, the affected individuals may become completely dependent as they are no longer able to feed or care for themselves. They may be able to hold a glass in their hand, but will spill its contents when they try to guide it to their mouth. This symptom is based on a lesion in the region of the dentate nucleus of the cerebellum and its connections. However, a slight increase in amplitude of movement when approaching a target may also be seen in other forms of tremor, and when MS is suspected, this sign alone does not prove cerebellar involvement and should not be taken as an indication of an additional lesion. Despite this, increasing tremor amplitude and intensity remains an important clinical characteristic in the differentiation of tremor forms which originate in the cerebellum from those which depend on other lesions in the extrapyramidal system.

Intention myoclonus may occur in the context of MS and may be particularly disabling. Every movement and even intention to move may cause uncontrollable movements of all extremities and of the trunk. It may be differentiated from true ballism on clinical grounds only by the fact that the movements are more stereotypical (Matthews 1991). In contradistinction to intention tremor, intention myoclonus may also affect body parts which are not involved in the intended movement itself. Lesions responsible for this are found pathologically in the circuit between red nucleus, oliva inferior, and dentate nucleus of the cerebellum, the so-called Mollaret's triangle (Hassler et al. 1975).

Dysarthria is an incoordination in the area of the speech musculature. Scanning speech is typical of MS and was part of Charcot's classical symptom triad: syllables and words are uttered irregularly, rapidly, and loudly, leading to an almost explosive character of speech. This sort of speech disturbance is characteristic of advanced cerebellar involvement.

Trunk ataxia leads to disturbance of equilibrium which renders gait more difficult. It may be little influenced by visual control. In MS, the most frequently occurring gait disturbance is a combination of spasticity and ataxia (spastic atactic gait), which occurs only rarely in other circumstances, such as in combined degeneration of the spinal cord.

Disturbances of ocular movements in MS include symmetrical horizontal directional nystagmus, which depends on lesions in the cerebellum and its efferents. Other forms of nystagmus, such as dissociated nystagmus of the abducting eye as part of internuclear ophthalmoplegia, are discussed elsewhere (see p. 77).

OPHTHALMOLOGICAL DISTURBANCES

Optic neuritis

It has been known for over a hundred years, since the classical work of Uhthoff (Uhthoff 1890), an ophthalmologist from Berlin, that MS plaques occur within the optic nerves. Assessment of their frequency in MS depends on diagnostic criteria and is variable. A study of more than 1200 MS patients which was specifically designed to address this question (Wikström et al. 1980), found involvement of optic nerves at disease onset in a third of cases (34.7%), and optic neuritis as an isolated initial symptom in 17% of cases. This should not be interpreted as indicating that disease onset should be defined unequivocally by optic neuritis, because in acute isolated optic neuritis prolonged latency in the nonaffected eye is found in a quarter of cases, indicating a subclinical involvement and dissemination of the disease process (Matthews et al. 1991).

Over the course of MS, optic nerve lesions are diagnosed in three quarters of cases (McDonald 1983b; McDonald and Barnes 1992). However, on postmorten examinations of chronic cases after long disease duration, involvement of the optic nerve is almost always found (Ulrich and Groebke-Lorenz 1983).

Clinically (Optic Neuritis Study Group 1991), optic neuritis manifests itself as anything from diminution of vision of variable degree, to complete visual loss. Normally, however, both eyes are affected with equal frequency. Generally, patients indicate very precisely the point at which they became aware of their visual disturbance. It begins rather suddenly, and is followed by further progressive worsening, usually lasting for 3 to 7 days, and rarely for longer than 14 days. The initial visual disturbance is described as blurring of vision, as a "veil or smokescreen," or as a "haze."

When measured objectively, the degree of visual loss may be very variable. Because of the tendency for improvement to occur spontaneously, this also depends on how long after the onset of symptoms the examination takes place. Most frequently, a reduction from counting fingers to 0.5 on Snellen charts is found within the first week after onset. On average, a linear relationship exists between visual loss and extension of demyelination when demyelination found at post mortem is compared to the last visual capacity measured during life (Ulrich and Groebke-Lorenz 1983). On the other hand, several exceptions to this rule have been reported: marked visual loss with only discrete demyelination, and, particularly interestingly, marked demyelination with normal vision as determined shortly before death (Wisniewski et al. 1976).

Restriction of visual fields usually takes the form of central or paracentral scotomata (Patterson and Heron 1980). The extension also depends on the stimulus used, and may reach far into the periphery of the visual field (Perkin and Rose 1979). In MS patients, subclinical deficits of visual field may be detected frequently by more refined methods of perimetry. This may be important for diagnosing a second lesion when dissemination of the disease process is suspected (Meienberg et al. 1982). Initially, patients can rarely see clearly, even in the periphery of the visual field, and even when objectively only a central deficit is found.

On fundoscopy soon after the onset of symptoms, the optic papilla appears normal in only about half of cases. On careful examination, blurred margins of the papilla are found in at least a quarter of cases, and striped hemorrhages close to the papilla are reported with variable frequency (up to 17%). Periphlebitis retinae, which may also be detected on fluorescence angiography (McDonald 1983b), is found in nearly a third of cases. It may be a mark of disease activity since the prevalence of regional sheathing is significantly higher in patients evaluated during an active phase than in those examined during a stationary phase (Tola et al. 1993).

Visual failure is usually associated with an afferent pupillary defect which is called Gunn's pupillary sign: the bright illumination of the normal eye leads to bilateral constriction of the pupils. When the light source is rapidly moved to the affected eye (within 1 second), the pupil is dilated initially and there is some delay before it constricts due to slowed afferents. Such a reaction may be detected in almost all cases of acute optic neuritis and in a high percentage after recovery of vision (Cox et al. 1981).

Acute optic neuritis almost always leads to a delay of latency of the VEPs, or no cortical responses may be reproduced at all (see Chapter 8). Difficulty in central fixation may be responsible for this if on examination the periphery of the visual field is not adequately stimulated.

Frequently, eye movements in optic neuritis are accompanied by pain which is located within the eye itself, supraorbitally, or as facial pain. It may be present only when pressure is exerted on the eye, or may last for several weeks. The pain usually reduces spontaneously or with steroid treatment before complete recovery of visual loss. This sort of pain may be present without other clinical signs of optic neuritis.

Lightning sensations, so-called phosphenes (Davis et al. 1976), may be perceived on saccadic eye movements and particularly during recovery. These are "positive" phenomena, with a pathophysiological basis similar to other paroxysmal symptoms in MS (see Chapter 6).

Good recovery of vision may be expected in 90% of cases after acute optic neuritis (McDonald 1983b; McDonald and Barnes 1992). The onset of recovery cannot usually be precisely determined. Vision recovers in 50% of cases 1 month after the onset of symptoms, and after a further month in all cases in which recovery is complete (Perkin and Rose 1979). Diminution of vision to 0.1 persists in 5% of patients after a single episode of optic neuritis. The extent of recovery cannot be predicted on the basis of the degree of initial visual loss.

Despite clinical recovery of vision, subclinical functional disturbances of the optic nerve may remain which may be detected with evoked potentials (Matthews et al. 1982), or by other special methods of examination. As has already been described by Uhthoff (1890), visual failure becomes worse with exercise and with rising body temperature. This may be used diagnostically when subclinical symptoms become apparent.

The Pulfrich phenomenon is found in at least half of patients with unilateral optic neuritis (Wist et al. 1978). A pendulum swinging in the frontal plane in front of the patient is perceived as moving elliptically because the visual impression reaches the cortex more slowly via the affected optic nerve than via the unaffected one.

The risk of recurrence of optic neuritis is reported to be between 20% and 31% (Compston et al. 1978). There is controversy as to whether a recurrence of ipsilateral optic neuritis is indicative of dissemination of the disease process in space and time and therefore justifies the diagnosis of MS (Ebers 1985; Kurtzke 1985; see also Chapter 8). For the patient, it is of particular importance to know the probability of an episode of optic neuritis leading to clinically definite MS.

In the literature, the percentage of cases of optic neuritis which develop into MS after observation for years or decades varies from 13% to 85%. Subclinical disseminated lesions, even in cases of clinically isolated optic neuritis (Ormerod et al. 1987; Morrissey et al. 1993), can be detected more often on paraclinical additional examination, and particularly using modern imaging procedures. Several authors go as far as to describe optic neuritis in each case as forme fruste of MS (Ebers 1985). Others calculate a risk on the basis of clinical studies of between 50% (Kurtzke 1985; Sandberg-Wollheim et al. 1990) and 80% (Compston et al. 1978; McDonald 1983b; Francis et al. 1987; Morrissey et al. 1993). This risk is influenced by several factors which in isolated optic neuritis may be taken as prognostic indicators of development into MS: genetic factors (fourfold increased risk in DR2–positive patients compared to DR2 negatives), recurrence (fourfold increased risk), and seasonal difference (threefold increased risk in optic neuritis in winter). If all these factors occur in a single patient, the risk of developing MS after optic neuritis is increased twelvefold compared to patients lacking these indicators (McDonald 1983b). If oligoclonal bands are present in the CSF of patients with isolated optic neuritis (in whom, however, we would not perform lumbar puncture), the probability of later dissemination appears to be higher (Moulin et al. 1983).

After simultaneous bilateral optic neuritis,

the risk of developing MS appears to be markedly lower compared to that after unilateral optic neuritis, and it is extremely low after an episode of bilateral optic neuritis in childhood (Parkin et al. 1984). Optic neuropathy occurring after the 50th year of age leads more rarely to MS because this diagnosis is rarer and its differential diagnosis is more extended in the higher age group (for example, ischemic papillitis).

Disseminated symptomatology manifests itself much more frequently within the first 4 to 5 years after an acute episode of optic neuritis (Ebers 1985; Hely et al. 1986), although single cases have been described following an interval of a decade.

In summary, long-term observations indicate that the risk of developing MS after an acute episode of unilateral optic neuritis can reach 80%. This risk is increased by factors such as DR2 positivity, recurrences, oligoclonal bands in CSF, and possibly by onset of visual disturbance during the winter months. Dissemination of the disease process is most commonly found within the first 4 to 5 years after acute optic neuritis.

Disturbances of ocular movements

Disturbances of ocular movements leading to double vision are found at disease onset in about one tenth of cases, and during the course of MS in at least one third (Reulen et al. 1983; Barnes and McDonald 1992). They become more marked with fatigue. In MS, they are rarely due to isolated deficiencies of cranial nerves, but usually to incoordination of eye movements, particularly in internuclear ophthalmoplegia. The basis of these disturbances is a lesion in the longitudinal medial fascicle which connects the nuclei of those cranial nerves which innervate the eye muscles. Clinically, they are characterized by inhibition of adduction on the side of the lesion, and dissociated nystagmus which is more marked on the abducting eye (Müri and Meienberg 1985; Thomke and Hopf 1992). The convergence reaction remains intact. In more discrete forms, only slowing of adduction saccades is found, which may be missed on clinical routine examination. It may be detected, however, in many cases by special oculographic methods, such as infrared oculography (Meienberg et al. 1986). Internuclear ophthalmoplegia may occur in other diseases, but it is so frequently caused by MS that this has to be viewed as the most prob-

able diagnosis until another one is proven. It used to be a clinical rule that MS leads to bilateral lesions of medial longitudinal bundles. On oculography, however, unequivocal unilateral lesions may be found (Müri and Meienberg 1985).

Very rarely, an isolated third nerve palsy may be an initial symptom of MS (Newman and Lessell 1990; Jellinek 1990).

Nystagmus formed part of Charcot's classical triad of MS symptoms (see Chapter 1), and is found in more than half of chronic MS cases. It is usually a symmetrical horizontal directional nystagmus with a rapid component to the lateral side. A similar nystagmus may also be seen in fatigue or if cooperation is difficult, and it should not be overvalued in MS nor accepted for diagnostic purposes as the sole indicator of an additional lesion. Acquired pendular nystagmus, frequently asymmetrical in both eyes and occasionally with rotary components, is usually seen in MS in conjunction with head tremor and with signs of trunk ataxia. It is due to lesions in the region of the cerebellar nuclei (Aschoff et al. 1974). Convergence nystagmus should be differentiated into congenital and acquired forms such as may occur in MS. Various forms of nystagmus may persist without clinical expression, and it is mainly of diagnostic value since no effective treatment is possible.

DISTURBANCES OF BLADDER FUNCTION

The problems caused by disturbances of bladder function are important for MS patients because they lead to considerable consequences in daily life. In the past, such disturbances were the main reason for the reduced life expectancy of MS patients. It is of the utmost importance that they are detected early, and that they are differentiated so that they may be treated appropriately (Fowler et al. 1992; Betts et al. 1993).

Between 50% and 80% of MS patients complain of bladder disturbances during the course of the disease; in 10% they form part of the initial symptomatology. Urodynamically relevant disturbances may be found in a much larger percentage – over 80% in the first 5 years after disease onset – even in early phases of the disease, when examined with refined urodynamic methods (Bemelmans et al. 1991). Adequate treatment is often necessary to prevent later complications (Fowler et al. 1992).

The most common causes of bladder disturbances in general are infections of the urinary

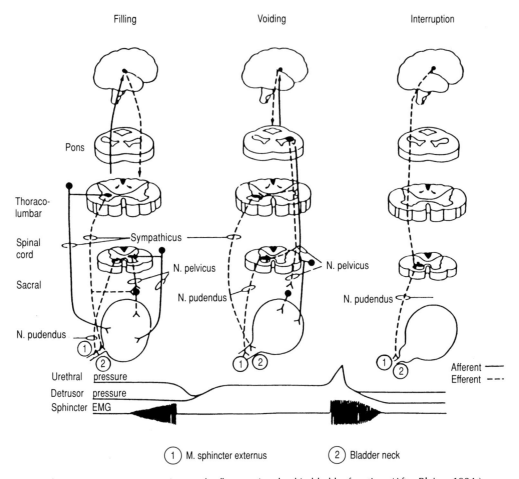

Fig. 7.1. The most important connections and reflex arcs involved in bladder function. (After Blaivas 1984.)

tract, and these must be sought in MS patients by urine examination. Urinary tract infections have to be excluded before neurogenic causes are examined further.

Modern therapeutic concepts are based on the analysis of the rather complex pathophysiology of neurogenic bladder disturbances which may be caused by MS (Blaivas and Barballias 1984). Physicians treating MS patients should be acquainted with them in order to organize appropriate examination and to initiate the most promising treatment.

It is not possible here to elaborate in detail on the physiology of filling and emptying of the bladder, but an overview is given which allows the type of disturbance to be determined and a suitable treatment to be decided upon.

The musculature of the bladder is organized and innervated such that normally about 350–500 ml of urine may be retained, and the bladder may be emptied completely under voluntary control. Continence in both sexes is controlled by smooth muscles at the bladder neck and at the proximal urethra. Micturition may be interrupted via the somatically innervated sphincter internus. Its activity alone is not usually sufficient to retain urine if proximal parasympathetically innervated muscles are not functioning.

The nerves and reflex arcs responsible for normal micturition are depicted in Fig. 7.1. They may be interrupted at various sites by MS lesions.

During the filling phase, extension of the bladder wall leads to discharges in the afferents of the pelvic nerve. After connection within the spinal cord, contraction of the striated external sphincter is mediated via the efferent somatic pudendal nerve. At the same time, afferent impulses are relayed via the sympathetic hypogastric nerve. These afferents are connected to sympathetic efferents within the thoracolumbar spinal cord by which detrusor contractions are inhibited and the tonus at the bladder neck is increased. The pressure within the urethra therefore remains higher than that of the detrusor, and thus filling of the bladder continues. During the emptying phase, afferent impulses are mediated via the pelvic nerve to the spinal cord where they ascend cranially and are relayed within the pontine micturition center. From there, other tracts descend which inhibit discharges of the pudendal nerve, leading to relaxation of the external striated sphincter. Activity within sympathetic efferents is inhibited by the same descending pathways in the spinal cord, leading to opening of the bladder neck. Relaxation of the external sphincter leads to a diminution of pressure within the urethra which is followed immediately by detrusor contraction and thus emptying of the bladder. In order to interrupt micturition, descending corticospinal pathways from the motor cortex leading to the pudendal nerve have to be intact. The sphincter internus is controlled via the pudendal nerve, allowing elevation of pressure within the urethra above that of the detrusor.

The so-called pontine micturition center is regulated via pathways from the frontal cortex, the thalamus and hypothalamus, basal ganglia, limbic system, and cerebellum. Voluntary control of bladder function is thereby effected. Furthermore, direct connections from the motor cortex to nuclei of the pudendal nerve within the sacral spinal cord (corticospinal tract?) allow voluntary control of the external striated sphincter of the urethra.

The most important reflex arc for bladder filling and retention of urine is formed from receptors within the bladder wall via the pelvic nerve to the sacral cord, and from there via the pudendal nerve to the external sphincter (sacral micturition center). Bladder filling is further controlled via a reflex arc of the sympathetic nervous system. Afferent sympathetic impulses from receptors within the bladder wall reach the thoracolumbar cord via the hypogastric nerve depending on the content of the bladder. Efferents allow tonic contraction of the proximal urethra via α-receptors. Excitation impulse is inhibited via another α-receptor transmission within the parasympathetic ganglion.

Detrusor activity is thereby inhibited, and pressure within the urethra remains higher than that within the bladder.

Bladder emptying is normally regulated via two connected circuits: on the one hand, a reflex arc is formed via the pelvic nerves (parasympathetically from and to the detrusor) and pudendal nerves (somatosensory and somatomotor from and to the striated external sphincter) to the sacral micturition center within the cord (S2–4). This reflex arc is controlled by another reflex arc which includes the aforementioned pontine micturition center: it contains afferents from parasympathetic receptors within the bladder wall via the lateral columns, and activity in the nuclei of the pelvic nerve (parasympathetic), hypogastric nerve (sympathetic), and pudendal nerve (somatosensory) within the sacral micturition center is controlled via descending efferents.

Disturbances of function of these complicated circuits may not be detected reliably enough on the basis of clinical history and neurological examination alone. However, therapy depends on adequate analysis of these functions. Combined urodynamic and electromyographic examination is therefore indicated if relevant bladder disturbances do not respond satisfactorily to trials of treatment (see Chapters 8 and 13).

Lesions above the pontine micturition center typically lead to destrusor hyperreflexia. Voluntary control over bladder emptying is no longer possible, although reflex arcs via the sacral and the pontine micturition center remain intact. The sequence of sphincter relaxation and detrusor contraction therefore may remain physiological, but voluntary control of this reflex is no longer possible. According to the type of lesion, the patient may perceive involuntary detrusor contractions as urinary urgency (i.e., an imperative drive to urinate); the time from the moment of perception of bladder filling to the moment of emptying is so short that uncontrolled micturition may occur if daily life is not organized to take account of this imperative demand. Occasionally, bladder emptying may be delayed by voluntary contractions of the external sphincter if direct connections between the motor cortex and sacral micturition center remain intact. Involuntary activity of detrusor alone does not prove a neurological cause because it may occur after pregnancy, as a result of obstruction, and idiopathically.

Typically, a lesion interrupting connections between pontine and sacral micturition centers leads to dyssynergia between detrusor and external sphincter. During involuntary detrusor activity, simultaneous contractions of the external sphincter occur, leading to occlusion of the bladder outlet with increasing pressure. Without treatment, the danger of vesico–ureteral reflux arises, which can lead to chronic kidney failure if it persists over a long period of time. Bladder disturbances in at least 50% of MS patients are due to detrusor–external sphincter dyssynergia (Goldstein et al. 1982). In 70%, they are associated with bilateral extensor plantar response (Goldstein et al. 1982; Awad et al. 1984).

Interruption of reflex arcs involving the sacral micturition center leads to areflexia of detrusor. This is rarely due to an isolated lesion within the conus medullaris in MS. Voluntary control of the external sphincter is no longer possible, and if the sympathetic pathways remain intact, occlusion of the proximal urethra leads to retention of urine. Sensibility in the saddle region is reduced, as is tonus of the anal sphincter, and bulbocavernous reflex is absent.

Isolated lesions of the sympathetic pathways concerned with micturition are almost unknown in MS.

Like all symptoms in MS, bladder disturbances may wax and wane during the course of the disease (Wheeler et al. 1983; Blaivas 1984). A repetition of combined urodymanic–electromyographic examinations may therefore be recommended if an appropriate therapeutic concept becomes ineffective or if new bladder symptoms arise.

From the clinical point of view, it is useful to differentiate the problems of bladder disturbances of MS patients due to failure to store and failure to empty (Blaivas 1984). Problems of filling and continence are most often accompanied by irritative symptoms such as frequent micturition, urgency of micturition, and incontinence or dysuria. They are usually due to hyperactivity of detrusor or insufficiency of the sphincter. Failure to empty, however, leads to obstructive symptoms such as retention of urine, reduced jet, and sensation of a filled bladder after micturition. These symptoms are caused by reduced activity of detrusor or obstructive lesions (including spasticity of the pelvic floor muscles). Rather than there being an immediate neurogenic cause, long-lasting blad-

der extension usually leads to reduction of detrusor activity. In many cases, bladder disturbances of MS patients are due to incoordination of detrusor and sphincter (the aforementioned detrusor–sphincter externus dyssynergia), which may lead to irritative as well as to obstructive disturbances.

When taking the clinical history of bladder disturbances, it is important to ask about earlier urinary tract infections, medical therapies, surgical interventions, and drinking habits. Bladder capacity is determined by ultrasound or catheterization after micturition. If there is more than 100 ml of residual urine, treatment is required as infectious complications are significantly more common than with residual urine of less than 100 ml. Based on the clinical history and neurological examinations, the three most important groups of bladder disturbances may be differentiated so that the treatment described in Chapter 13 may be indicated. However, if bladder disturbances in MS patients persist despite adequate treatment of the clinically suspected cause, further examinations may be indicated (see Chapter 8).

SEXUAL DISTURBANCES

Sexual problems are common in MS. If they are due to organic lesions, they are usually accompanied by disturbances of bladder function. Frequency figures vary widely in the literature because the subject is not considered equally important everywhere.

Loss of libido may occur in men and women. Erectile impotence is present in over half of men early in the disease course (Vas 1969). Sexual disturbances have been found in a careful investigation in over two thirds of patients with little motor disability (Minderhoud et al. 1984). In another study of unselected MS patients, 9 out of 10 men and three quarters of women indicated that their sex lives were unsatisfactory or that they had abandoned sexual activity completely (Lilius et al. 1976).

Patients with chronic organic disease often take it for granted that any disturbance of their sex life is due to the disease. The organic lesion itself is not usually the reason for such problems, but may be responsible in combination with psychogenic causes which are often present in such patients. For patients taking medication over years, its influence on potency has also to be considered. Penetration is only possible if erections last long enough, and this may be limited in MS patients as a result of organic causes. In such cases, bulbocavernous reflex is usually absent, and thermoregulation in the legs is reduced (Cartlidge 1972). If impotence is due to an organic cause, spontaneous erections are lacking in the morning, during dreaming, and during fantasy, etc. If psychogenic causes appear to be important, measuring tumescence of the penis during sleep (during REM phases) may be useful: it would be normal in psychogenic sexual disturbances.

In women, sexual activity is often impaired by loss of sensibility in the genital region and by spasticity of adductors (Lundberg 1981).

Sexual problems may arise for MS patients for several functional reasons, for example because of a fear of not satisfying, fatigue, or depression. The social contacts necessary to build up a partnership may also be reduced due to the disease, or to the fact that the patient has to organize his or her activities according to limitations set by bladder function. In existing relationships, it may be difficult for the nonaffected partner to change from the role of nurse to lover.

Although sexual problems in MS patients, whether due to organic or psychogenic causes, may, like all other symptoms of the disease, disappear, the fact that they have been present and may recur remains a psychological burden. In the partnership, psychological components are particularly important, even if organic causes of sexual problems are found. Therefore, therapeutic interventions have to take this into consideration.

PSYCHOLOGICAL DISTURBANCES

The emotional and relationship problems associated with MS have not always been fully appreciated by the medical profession, which has tended to concentrate on the physical aspects of this disease. Yet the psychological problems of MS often cause more suffering than physical effects. (Burnfield and Burnfield 1978).

Neuropsychological disturbances and psychiatric problems are common in MS (Schiffer and Slater 1985; Grant 1986; Rao 1986; Feinstein et al. 1993). It is difficult to differentiate which of the disturbances concerning affects and cognitive functioning are due to organic disease and which are psychological reactions to a disease which is always an enormous psychological burden, with its unpredictable course and potential to lead to severe disability and handicap.

Premorbid personality

It has been tried repeatedly, in retrospective investigations of patients already affected, to characterize a premorbid personality, and to determine characteristics of personality which dispose to the disease. Such investigations (Paulley 1976/7) claimed that the premorbid personality of MS patients should be characterized by hysterical aspects, as notes on "hysterical reactions" are frequently found in case reports of MS patients. Furthermore, such people were likely to have had difficulties in withdrawing from key figures during adolescence. In fact, MS may manifest itself in earlier phases of the disease by various symptoms which may be found in hysterical personalities: sensory disturbances, emotional instability, and particularly fatigue. If, from such observations, the inference is made that hysterical characteristics of personality may dispose to the development of MS, it only discloses a lack of ability to diagnose early manifestations of MS. "In its infancy multiple sclerosis used to be called hysteria" (Buzzard 1897; quoted in Schiffer and Slater 1985). Usually, the term "hysteria" is used imprecisely and includes conversion phenomena, dissociations, or only characteristics of individual personalities. Generally, it discloses more about the way physicians think about their patients than describing clinically relevant data (Grant 1986).

Cognitive functions

Reports of the frequency of disturbances of cognitive functions in MS patients are very variable, and depend on the methods used and on the type of patients examined. In about half of the patients in whom no mental disturbances are found on routine neurological examination, cognitive deficits may be detected during detailed neuropsychological examination (Rao 1986; Prosiegel and Michael 1993). Discrete or moderate impairment of cognitive functions may be found on neuropsychological testing, even in patients with disease of less than 2 years' duration (Lyon-Caën et al. 1986: 60%), without leading to disability in daily life. Patients with MS are more often distracted from tasks in which learning capabilities and memory are tested, although in the absence of distraction, learning capability remains intact. Visuospatial processes and memory appear to be more affected than verbal functions when compared to normal individuals and to patients with other neurological diseases (Grant et al. 1984; Carroll et al. 1984; Rao et al. 1984; Feinstein et al. 1993). The frequency and importance of such deficits increase during the course of the disease (Rao et al. 1984: 40%). They correlate with the extent of brain lesions as determined on MRI (Ron et al. 1991; Feinstein et al. 1993; Mattioni et al. 1993).

Systematic neuropsychological examinations of MS patients (for review see Grant 1986; Rao 1986; Prosiegel and Michael 1993; Wallace and Holmes 1993) disclose deficits mainly in tasks in which motor velocity, strength, and coordination are required. The deficits are less pronounced in tests requiring abstraction and conceptual thinking. After a longer duration of disease, disturbances of learning of verbal and nonverbal material are frequent. Disturbances of memory are found in a great number of MS patients in earlier phases of the disease (Grant et al. 1984; Good et al. 1992); in this group, according to performance in memory testing (Rao et al. 1984), changes of personality are often found, most markedly in the group with the lowest performance. More discrete disturbances of memory may, at least partly, be due to depression (Good et al. 1992).

Multiple sclerosis may occasionally lead to subcortical dementia. It is very rare in earlier phases of the disease, but later is often accompanied by severe physical disability (Surridge 1969).

Affective disorders

Clinical investigations into affective disorders in MS patients have mainly been carried out in recent years. Over decades, apparently, it was taken for granted that the mood of MS patients was typically euphoric, as described by many authors since Charcot (Cottrell and Wilson 1926). Euphoria describes a type of mood which is characterized by inappropriate/inadequate serenity (in view of the physical disability). Comparative investigations of patients with muscle diseases and similar physical disability demonstrated that euphoria in MS patients occurs only after long disease duration and with very marked neurological deficits, and is part of an "organic–psycho syndrome" caused by cortical MS lesions (Surridge 1969). Even in very severely disabled MS patients, this type of mood does not occur in more than 10%. Anosognosia (a lack of insight into the disease) may be a blessing for severely disabled patients and their caregivers. It is, however, as rare as euphoria in the early and middle phases of the disease (Grant 1986).

So-called affect incontinence (i.e., abruptly changing affective expressions which do not correspond to inner mood) may be very disabling for patients and those around them. Many patients describe a type of "internal disconnection" which does not allow them to express verbally or nonverbally affects which they feel interiorly. It corresponds to the pictures seen in pseudo bulbar palsy on a vascular basis, and is probably also due to an organic lesion.

Paroxysmal changes of mood, such as abrupt forced laughing or crying, may also occur in MS patients. Because of their similarity to other paroxysmal phenomena, and the lability of affects described above, we tend to consider these disturbances as due to organic lesions.

However, the most important affective disorder in MS patients is depression. It is characterized by an "inability to mourn," loss of hope, and pessimism, and is often associated with general loss of energy, sleep disturbances, weight loss, and lack of interest. Such episodes may precede neurological manifestations in MS. They may occur in most patients at some stage of their disease, and are occasionally considered a major symptom (Whitlock and Siskind 1980). In 20% to 25% of patients, depression may be so marked as to require treatment by a specialist (Schubert and Foliart 1993). The risk of suicide of MS patients, particularly in the earlier stages of the disease before and after the diagnosis, is markedly increased compared to that of the general population (Stenager et al. 1992). In the aforementioned psychiatric comparative study of MS patients and similarly disabled patients with muscle disease (Surridge 1969), depressive symptoms were equally frequent and were therefore interpreted as being a reaction to the disease. On the other hand, the observation that depressive episodes in MS patients are often associated with "endogenous signs," such as vegetative disturbances and diurnal changes of mood (Whitlock and Siskind 1980), is an argument for an organic basis.

Depressive disturbances in MS are so frequent and of such importance that they have to be analyzed and treated with particular care, sympathy, and persistence.

"Stress" and MS

It has been suggested repeatedly that psychological stress, be it due to sudden involuntary changes of life situation, traumatizing events, or difficult partnerships, might contribute to triggering exacerbations or even the disease itself. In earlier investigations (Pratt 1951), this influence has been denied. In more recent systematic investigations of events in the lives of MS patients which are outside the normal daily experience and which may lead to psychological stress, it was shown that 70% (Grant 1986) to 80% (Warren et al. 1982) of MS patients had experienced such events, compared to only 20% of controls. Frequently, these events occurred in close temporal relationship to exacerbations of the disease. However, it may not be inferred from these interesting observations that MS is a psychosomatic disease in the sense that its physical manifestations could be the immediate consequence of psychological disturbance. In the long-term management of MS patients, life situation and partnerships are of particular significance.

Because neuropsychological research in MS is a relatively new field of investigation, it is of particular importance that comparable test batteries are used for which normative data are available (Peyser et al. 1990; Prosiegel and Michael 1993; Wallace and Holmes 1993).

PAIN AND FATIGUE

For decades, MS was considered typically to be painless. Recent investigations, however, mainly initiated by those with the disease, demonstrate that pain is often a major problem which has to be taken seriously by relatives and caregivers. It may often be prevented or treated. Pain in MS is present in one third to one half of cases (Clifford and Trotter 1984; Vermote et al. 1986; Moulin et al. 1988) and may be considered by up to one third of patients to be the most disturbing symptom. The frequency of occurrence of pain is not related to the de-

gree of disability: it is more frequent in older people, when disease onset has occurred at a late age, in those with chronic progressive disease, and when there is spastic paresis and disturbances of coordination. It can be classified as follows.

1. Pain due to the disease process itself.
2. Pain which may be due to the consequences of the disease.
3. Pain due to disability and its associated problems.

1. Trigeminal neuralgia and painful tonic spasms are due to plaques lying within pain-conducting fiber tracts (see p. 73). More often, a persistent, not very intense pain in the extremities is described which is characterized as dull or stabbing and is often associated with a sensation of warmth. It is considered to be due to lesions in the dorsal columns (Paty and Poser 1984; Vermote et al. 1986). Very intense, so-called pseudoradicular pain of short duration may also occur in the extremities which does not follow the distribution pattern of anatomically defined regions.

2. Shooting spasms of the extremities are particularly marked in flexor spasticity of the legs (see p. 72) and are often extremely painful. Urinary infections due to bladder disturbances lead to pain in the urinary tract and may increase spasticity. Often, pain in the extremities and in the trunk is due to such infection-induced spasticity. The same mechanism may be involved in pain due to decubital ulcers. Although typically these occur in regions of reduced sensibility, they may increase spasticity considerably, particularly if infected. They can normally be avoided by careful nursing.

3. Pain due to disability or its effects may pose particular problems for MS patients. In most cases this type of pain can be prevented by adequate physiotherapy and comprehensive rehabilitation. Sixty percent of wheelchair patients complain of neck pain, and the comfort of those sitting in wheelchairs is not always considered carefully enough. The seats and back rests of wheelchairs sag after long-term use, and kyphosis of the thoracic spine, which is insufficiently supported by the weakened back musculature, is thereby increased. In order to compensate, patients extend their head and shoulders anteriorly, leading to painful muscular imbalance. Patients with MS often

show very marked degeneration of the joints caused by inappropriate loading of the cervical and thoracic spine, leading to complications affecting the peripheral nervous system. Too often, one can observe how wheelchair-bound patients have to adopt painful positions because others fail to communicate with them on eye level.

In chronic MS, painful osteoporosis (insufficient bone formation) may be due to inactivity or to irresponsible long-term prescription of steroid therapy which still occurs occasionally.

Lesions of the peripheral nerves are less dramatic, but are often overlooked and preventable. For example, lesions of the median nerve at the wrist can occur following the long-term use of canes, and of the ulnar nerve at the elbow in someone who uses an armrest on a wheelchair. On several occasions, we have seen lesions of the peroneal nerve below the head of the fibula caused by the belts of foot supports which have been too tightly applied to correct foot deformity.

A general feeling of fatigue and fatiguability is often considered the most disabling symptom in MS (Freal et al. 1984; Krupp et al. 1988). There is no easy pathophysiological explanation for this. It appears to be an organic phenomenon and should be differentiated from loss of energy due to depression (see p. 82). It may be exacerbated by exposure to heat, heavy meals or, according to the spontaneous reports of many patients, by smoking. It is improved at rest, less so by sleep. Fatigue in MS is probably not only due to increased muscular load, for example due to spasticity, bad posture, or increased respiratory exertion (Olgiati et al. 1986), but it is the subjective expression of those processes which form the basis of the disease. It is a symptom which is often misunderstood by partners, companions, and employers at the work place, as well as by physicians and caregivers. Fatigue and increased fatiguability are also the classical excuses of shirkers. The trust of patients must be gained in order to be able to make this important distinction. Although it is difficult to provide measurable clinical data, the similar experiences of many MS patients and the opinions of many experienced clinicians are valuable evidence that fatigue and increased fatiguability are important symptoms of MS which themselves may cause disability.

PAROXYSMAL PHENOMENA AND INVOLUNTARY MOVEMENTS

All manifestations of MS may occur only very briefly. They should be considered to be exacerbations if they last less than 24 to 48 hours (see Chapter 8). Apart from possible psychological stress factors (see p. 83), transient clinical symptoms are mainly due to Uhthoff's phenomenon: rising body temperature leads to amplification of clinical symptoms or the formation of new ones. Apart from such transient changes in the clinical picture in MS, paroxysmal clinical symptoms may occur, lasting only for seconds to minutes. Although they are somewhat rare relative to the whole spectrum of clinical symptoms of MS, they may be of particular importance to those affected, and should be recognized as they are amenable to symptomatic therapy.

Epileptic seizures

In the literature on clinical symptoms and signs of MS, there have been several reports of cerebral seizures since the first description by Leube in 1917. Indications of frequency vary widely: in the epileptological literature, we found up to 10% (Trouillas and Courjon 1972); in some neurological centers the average figure for epilepsy is 0.5%. Summarizing 20 publications since 1905 (Hopf et al. 1970) concerning MS patients, there are 207 cases with cerebral seizures, corresponding to 2.5%. This is in accordance with our own figure of 27 patients with epilepsy among 1016 MS patients (Beer and Kesselring 1988), and with another study from Finland (Kinnunen and Wikström 1986). If the age distribution of both diseases is taken into consideration, the coincidence cannot be by chance, and epileptic seizures appear to occur about 10 times more often than in the general population.

As far as types of epileptic seizures are concerned, two thirds are focal in nature, and in one third of cases, simultaneous central deficits (monopareses and hemipareses of sensory disturbance or sensory loss) are present on the same side.

It would appear that, on the one hand, plaques lying close to the cortex may induce seizures by mechanical and electrical irritation, and, on the other hand, lability of cerebral regulatory mechanisms accompanying an exacerbation may lead to manifestations of a constitutional disposition to seizures.

Paroxysmal phenomena of extracortical origin

Among motor paroxysmal phenomena, tonic brainstem seizures are of particular importance because they are often accompanied by severe pain. Typically, brief tonic muscle spasms occur, irradiating from one extremity to the other on the same side. They may be triggered by hyperventilation and vestibular stimuli (change of position). In larger series of MS patients, this symptom may be found in 4% (Matthews 1991). In the Japanese literature, its frequency is reported to be as high as 28%, and there are descriptions of manifestations on both sides (Shibasaki et al. 1981). The attacks may accumulate within a limited period of time and may then be considered as an exacerbation.

Based on histological examinations and computer tomography (Watson and Chiu 1979), the pathological-anatomical lesion is located in the brainstem.

Involuntary movements, as in Parkinson's syndrome or choreoathetosis, occur in MS exclusively paroxysmally. It is not unusual for patients to report brief choreiform athetoid movements and nontypical dystonia (Berger et al. 1984). The entire Parkinsonian syndrome of rigor, tremor, and akinesia is very rare in MS and there is probably no direct causal relationship (Sarkari 1968).

Apart from such positive paroxysmal phenomena, negative ones may lead to involuntary movement disorders in MS. Among them are paroxysmal dysarthria (Espir et al. 1966) and ataxia – episodes of blurred speech or inhibition of speech lasting only a few seconds to minutes (on average 15 seconds) – often accompanied by trunk ataxia, or incoordination of the extremities, or double vision. In paroxysmal loss of use (Matthews 1975; Osterman and Westerberg 1975; Castaigne et al. 1979), an extremity may not be used at all. A similar clinical picture occurs in kataplexy from the narcolepsy complex which on occasion may be shown to have a convincing causal relationship with MS (Grigoresco 1932; Schrader et al. 1980). In both conditions, there is a strong association to HLA DR2. Untreatable singultus (hoquet diabolique)

may be due to MS, as has been described in three impressive cases (McFarling and Susac 1979). Paroxysmal itching, as described in three women (Osterman 1976), appears to be somewhat less dramatic and is explained by the same mechanisms as the paroxysmal painful attacks.

Trigeminal neuralgia is much more frequent among MS patients than in the general population. In 1905 Oppenheim described, in his *Textbook of Nervous Diseases*, a case of syntropy, illustrating the postmortem finding of a demyelinating plaque in the entry zone of the trigeminal nerve into the pons. Symptomatic trigeminal neuralgia and idiopathic trigeminal neuralgia are not identical: MS patients are somewhat younger and often show sensory disturbances in the trigeminal region. There are probably also certain differences in the character of the pain since in one third of MS patients it may last a few seconds or longer. The course of the disease may be a little different in cases where it is accompanied by trigeminal neuralgia: onset is later, cranial nerve disturbances are more frequent as initial symptoms, pontine and cerebellar disturbances predominate, and in one third of cases pain also occurs at other sites.

Facial myokymia

Facial myokymia (Matthews 1966; Tenser 1976) is a conspicuous involuntary movement disorder occurring particularly, if not exclusively (Waybright et al. 1979), in MS. It involves a painless "waving" of facial muscles (Anderman et al. 1961). Patients complain of stiffness of one half of the face and that the affected side becomes distorted. There is ptosis and deepening nasolabial fold. Voluntary strength is not reduced, and active contractions of single facial muscles are followed by rapid fluttering in neighboring muscle groups which may not be apparent to an observer. On electromyography, characteristic groups of multiple units firing in their own constant rhythm are found (Matthews 1966).

FREQUENCY OF SYMPTOMS

Tables 7.1 and 7.2 summarize the frequency of symptoms occurring at the onset of the disease and over the entire course of MS in patients

Table 7.1 *Symptoms at disease onset, and percentages of patients experiencing them*

	(1)	(2)	(3)
Sensory disturbances	41.3	40	33
Visual disturbances (visual loss + disturbances of ocular movements)	36.9	34	30
Gait disturbances	31.8		18
Pareses	23.4	39	16 (approx.)
Vertigo	8.0	5	
Sphincter disturbances	5.5	5	
Fine motor disturbances	3.9		
Fatigue	1.6		
Epileptic seizures	0.7		
Psychic disturbances	0.6		

(1) Beer and Kesselring 1988, n = 688; (2) Matthews 1991; (3) Paty and Poser 1984, n = 461.

Table 7.2 *Symptoms during the course of the disease (%)*

	(1)	(2)
Remission	72	
exacerbating remitting		35
primary progressive		19
secondary progressive		47
Pyramidal lesions	99	> 80
Visual and oculomotor disturbances	85	ca. 80
Bladder disturbances	82	57
Brainstem and cerebellar disturbances		75
Dysarthria	55	20
Disturbances of equilibrium	80	
Sensory disturbances		83
Vibration sense	71	
Paresthesias	66	
Nystagmus	70	42
Gait ataxia	55	
Mental and cognitive deficits	45	

(1) 111 cases proven at autopsy (C.M. Poser et al. 1984); (2) 3248 patients with mean disease duration 10.8 years (S. Poser 1986).

whose disease was detected clinically or at post mortem. Percentages of the various symptoms have already been mentioned; often symptoms occur simultaneously at the onset of the disease. Such polysymptomatic onset occurs in 55% of cases, and in 50% of these is accompanied by paresis (Matthews 1991). Paresis as an isolated initial symptom occurs only in a quarter of cases. Cerebellar deficits occurring exclusively at disease onset are unknown. Individual cases may be marked by rare symptoms which are known to occur over the disease course, such as psychological disturbances, paroxysmal phenomena, fatigue etc. Despite very careful questioning of our patients, we were not able to detect a combination of symptoms which would allow for differentiation of the prodromal phase, as has occasionally been postulated.

8

Diagnosis

Le diagnostic de la sclérose en plaques est bien souvent l'objet de difficultés insurmontables.

Joseph Babinski, 1885

INTRODUCTION

The diagnosis of MS has far-reaching consequences in the lives of those affected and their relatives. It should therefore be made on the basis of rational and sound consideration. The description of the diagnosis by a leading MS researcher may well be accurate: "Multiple sclerosis is what a good clinician would call multiple sclerosis" (Kurtzke 1974). However, the physician who is confronted with a patient and his or her symptoms needs diagnostic criteria based on numerous reliable principles in order to establish a diagnosis. Rationally proven clinical diagnosis facilitates the discussion with patients and their relatives and allows for a more clearcut differential diagnosis. Various clinical studies – be they concerned with the course of the disease, with epidemiological problems, or with the use of therapeutic interventions – may be more easily compared if they incorporate a unified diagnostic terminology. A correct diagnosis may be made earlier if strict diagnostic criteria are applied (Izquierdo et al. 1985).

DIAGNOSTIC CRITERIA

The diagnostic criteria of MS have been in use for decades (Schumacher et al. 1965; McDonald and Halliday 1977). The diagnosis was usually based almost exclusively on the clinical history and on neurological examinations made during the course of the disease. The lists of diagnostic criteria were constructed mainly in order to compare clinical therapeutic studies. The probability of diagnosis was graded as "clinically definite," "probable," and "possible." How-

ever, first exacerbations and the early stages of the disease could not be diagnosed using these criteria. This is probably a serious disadvantage because the recognition of the early stages of the disease may be of particular importance in the search for exogenous etiologically relevant factors. Problems due to a lesion at a single location within the CNS, such as isolated optic neuritis or monotopic brainstem and spinal cord syndromes, may already be part of MS and are not embraced by these criteria. Insofar as such isolated symptoms may precede the disease or may be an early stage of it (McDonald 1983b; Ebers 1985; Ormerod et al. 1987), their correct diagnostic classification may be important for possible therapies, and certainly for a more comprehensive understanding of the whole clinical spectrum of the disease (Herndon and Rudick 1983).

The age limit placed on the onset of the disease (10 to 59 years) excluded a further, probably only minor, group of patients with a definite diagnosis as there are cases verified at post mortem in which the onset of the disease lies outside this age range (see Chapter 9).

The clinical diagnosis of MS always includes some uncertainty concerning the clinicopathological correlation. If additional data from laboratory examinations are included, the reliability of the diagnosis is markedly increased (Polman et al. 1985; Sanders et al. 1986a; Giesser et al. 1987). Prognostic indicators which are of greater interest to patients than the diagnosis itself are being searched for using special examinations such as electrophysiological measurements, biochemical analysis of CSF and serum, and imaging procedures (see Chapter 10). It is therefore appropriate to include such "paraclinical" parameters in newer diagnostic recommendations for MS (Poser et al. 1983, 1984).

In practice, it is best to adhere to a list of crite-

Table 8.1 *Diagnostic criteria in multiple sclerosis. Two groups of diagnostic reliability are differentiated: "definite" and "probable." In each of these groups, two subgroups are formed: "clinically supported" and "laboratory supported."*

Category	Exacerbation	Determination of lesions	Cerebrospinal fluid (oligoclonal bands)
		Clinically paraclinically	
Clinically definite			
1)	2	2	
2)	2	1 and 1	
Laboratory supported definite			
1)	2	1 or 1	+
2)	1	2	+
3)	1	1 and 1	+
Clinically probable			
1)	2	1	
2)	1	2	
3)	1	1 and 1	
Laboratory supported probable			
1)	2		+

ria designed for research protocols. The most widely used is the recommendation of the Poser Committee (Poser et al. 1983; 1984; Table 8.1), which is discussed later. A clear understanding has also to be gained of cases which are not diagnosed by these criteria (McDonald and Silberberg 1986; Matthews 1991). The practicing neurologist and physician are probably more often confronted by them than the clinician working in a hospital.

Relapse and remission

A symptom of neurological functional disturbance lasting longer than 24 hours and remitting after a certain period of time is considered to be an expression of a relapse, whether determined objectively as a physical sign or only as an anamnestic indication. A remission is a clear improvement of symptoms and signs lasting longer than 24 hours. It is significant only when it lasts at least 1 month.

Individual symptoms may occur in MS which last only a few seconds or minutes (see Chapter 7). Although they do not constitute a relapse on their own, they may be part of one if they accumulate over a period of days or weeks. In order to consider two relapses as being separate from one another, they should occur at least 4 weeks apart (Poser et al. 1983; 1984) or, more cautiously, 6 months apart (Ormerod et al. 1987). From our experience with acute disseminated encephalomyelitis (Kesselring et al. 1990), we consider this caution to be very important in avoiding confusion between MS and the monophasic disease ADEM (see Chapter 11). As a rule, for a definite diagnosis of MS to be made, two relapses should occur which are based on lesions at two different sites. This restriction should avoid the misinterpretation of monophasic diseases which have to be considered in the differential diagnosis. An exception to this rule are cases with at least two "typical" lesions and oligoclonal bands in the CSF, for which the diagnosis can be made during the first relapse. These cases will be more frequently identified when MRI (see p. 105) is more readily available. The danger then arises, however, that the diagnosis is made too readily without sufficient critical evaluation of the modern techniques.

Clinical evidence of lesions

Clinical evidence of lesions arises from pathological findings on neurological examination. Particular attention should be paid to those parts of the nervous system which are not suspected of being affected from the clinical history. Some examination procedures are not part of routine neurological examination, but they often yield pathological findings in MS, for example examination of color sense and luminance sensitivity (Foster et al. 1985), saccadic eye movements (Meienberg et al. 1986), Pulfrich's pendulum (Wist et al. 1978), or signs of periphlebitis retinae on fundoscopy (Engell

1986; Tola et al. 1993). Pathological findings not apparent during the examination can be accepted if they have been described earlier by a reliable examiner. For diagnosis, only those symptoms and signs should be considered which are characteristic of the disease. These include those based on the well-known predilection sites of MS plaques (see Chapters 2 and 7): optic neuritis, spasticity of the extremities, bladder disturbances, vertigo, oculomotor disturbances, etc. It goes without saying that MS is considered only when no other diagnostic explanation is present. Dementia, aphasia, epileptic seizures, affective disorders, and peripheral neurological deficits may be compatible with the diagnosis of MS, but they should not be considered alone as proof of its presence.

On rare occasions, symptoms present in a patient's case history may be considered as being of importance as objective signs if their description appears to be reliable and they are known to be relatively typical, for example optic neuritis or transient double vision, Lhermitte's symptom, and other paroxysmal phenomena (see Chapter 7).

Paraclinical evidence of a lesion

Paraclinical evidence of lesions is gained by procedures which are performed in addition to clinical neurological examination: electrophysiological investigations (see p. 90) and imaging procedures (see p. 105). With careful consideration of the indications and differential diagnosis, diagnostic certainty in MS is markedly improved by these investigations, and the length of time for which patients have to be observed in order to classify them with greater certainty is markedly shortened (McDonald and Silberberg 1986).

Separated lesions

In general, two lesions at different sites are required for a definite diagnosis of MS. It should not be possible to explain the various symptoms and neurological signs as being due to one lesion only. By convention, bilateral optic neuritis (Parkin et al. 1984) is considered to be due to a single lesion when both sides are affected at the same time (within 2 weeks); it is assumed to be due to multiple lesions if both sides are affected over a longer time interval. Since dissemination of the disease process does not nec-

essarily occur in cases of bilateral optic neuritis (Parkin et al. 1984; see Chapter 7), for diagnostic purposes this is not considered to be due to multiple lesions. Particular difficulties arise when clinically isolated monotopic lesions, such as isolated brainstem or spinal cord syndromes, and lesions at other sites within the CNS are detected by paraclinical investigations (Ormerod et al. 1987; Morrissey et al. 1993). In such instances, the process cannot be defined as multiphasic (see p. 128) as long as it cannot be determined unequivocally that the lesions are of different ages (Miller et al 1988a). According to diagnostic convention, a single clinical lesion may only be diagnosed as due to definite MS if oligocloncal bands are present in the CSF and if at least two separate relapses may be discerned from the case history.

Laboratory support

Only the diagnostic contribution of examination of the CSF is considered here, particularly the determination of immunological activity within the CNS: oligoclonal bands in electrophoresis of CSF (see p. 111). In cases of single clinical relapse and multiple lesions, and in cases of at least two relapses and only one lesion on clinical examination, the finding of oligoclonal bands in CSF determines the diagnosis of definite MS. The detection of myelin breakdown products in CSF may be interesting for determining disease activity, although it has little relevance to the diagnosis (A. J. Thompson et al. 1985).

Special cases

The Poser criteria set the age range of disease onset at 10 to 59 years. This limitation is justified for research purposes for which patients with other diseases need to be excluded. In daily practice, however, this age range would not be strictly adhered to since well-documented MS cases have been described in which disease onset was before the 10th and after the 60th year of life (Bauer and Hanefeld 1993; see Chapter 9).

Acute monotopic CNS lesions have to be considered in the differential diagnosis of MS (see Chapter 11). Cases in which clinical manifestations point to a single lesion which is already part of a disseminated disease process are of particular interest. Among them are isolated optic neuritis and isolated brainstem and spinal cord lesions. Multiple lesions outside the region in which they would explain the clinical symptoms are found in 50% to 70% of cases with these clinical pictures (Ormerod et al. 1987; Morrissey et al. 1993). This paraclinical finding on its own does not prove the diagnosis of MS: multiple lesions which cannot be distinguished from those seen in MS may occur in monophasic diseases such as acute disseminated encephalomyelitis (see Chapter 11).

If a diagnosis of definite MS is proven in serial examinations, new lesions are always detected.

Diagnostic difficulties often arise in chronic progresssive myelopathic syndromes in which no single relapse may be discerned. Cases of MS manifesting in such a way are not diagnosed by the aforementioned criteria. Oligoclonal bands in CSF and detection of clinically silent lesions by paraclinical investigations point to the diagnosis of MS (Kempster et al. 1987). In such cases it is often necessary to exclude a compressing lesion on the spinal cord by MRI or myelography.

NEUROPHYSIOLOGICAL INVESTIGATIONS
by C. W. Hess

Introduction

Numerous physiological methods have been recommended for the diagnosis of MS by which various functions of the CNS may be examined. Each of them may yield pathological findings in a proportion of patients. For several, mainly practical, reasons, only a limited number of laboratory examinations is widely used routinely. Introduction of a new method is hampered if the cost of new equipment exceeds the value of that already present in a clinical neurophysiological laboratory or in a neurological practice. On the other hand, the measurement of auditory and somatosensory evoked potentials has been widely used since the introduction of the technique of VEPs. In this case, the risk of misuse and diagnostic overvaluation of evoked potentials has to be guarded against. It is often forgotten that such technical examinations provide only a limited contribution, and they can never replace careful clinical examination. For the inexperienced examiner there is considerable danger of misinterpretation: the more ominous false-positive findings can occur more frequently than false-negatives ones. There is

significant individual variation and a broad band of normal values of single inter- and intra-parameters. This fact may often be overlooked, leading to misinterpretation and the description of a normal variant as pathological. For these reasons a neurophysiological laboratory should not cultivate too large a repertoire of routine examinations. Only in frequently used examinations can diagnostic certainty and reliability be acquired. An examination will provide a valuable diagnostic contribution if its indications are clear, it is performed carefully, and the results are evaluated critically. In general, a neurophysiological method of examination should be performed simply and rapidly, should not be invasive for the patient, and should be sensitive enough to detect clinically silent lesions. Furthermore, it is desirable that it produces specific results, a requirement which is difficult to fulfill with the methods currently available. Among evoked potentials, only a few standard examinations have been selected from a large number of stimulation and recording techniques. They are presented on the following pages.

Evoked brain potentials

The principle of afferent evoked brain potentials

In a strict sense, evoked potentials are measured by all electrophysiological methods which use a stimulus. By convention, however, the term is used only for electrophysiological investigations of the CNS. Afferent evoked potentials are made visible within the electrical activity of the brain by automatic averaging, a technique developed in the 1950s (Dawson 1951). Brain potentials evoked by various stimulus modalities are so small that they disappear in the far greater resting activity of the electroencephalogram. Electronic averaging devices allow a summation of electrical brain activity in relation to the repeated stimulus. The related responses become visible, and resting activity independent of the stimulus (biological background noise) is extinguished by summation; potentials occurring in constant temporal relationship to the stimulus are built up. Signal-to-noise relationship is improved by summing up more sweeps. The yield, however, is related to an exponentially increasing number of measurements. In practice, the number of sweeps to be measured is very limited. Large single artifacts, for example from adjoining muscles, comprise a possible source of error because they may be misinterpreted as stimulus-dependent potentials after a relatively small number of averages. It is important that the examiner observes the continuous build-up of signals and recognizes abruptly occurring artificial potentials. For the same reason, it is a rule in evoked potentials that each examination has to be repeated twice, and that only unequivocally reproducible potentials are accepted.

The quality of afferent evoked potentials depends mainly on minimizing artifacts. During recording, the patient should lie relaxed in order to avoid interference from muscle potentials. This is not always easy for anxious patients with pain. Therefore it is important that patients are as relaxed and as comfortable as possible, that they have an empty bladder, the room temperature is comfortable, and there is a calm atmosphere during examination. On some occasions, for example when examining small children, the use of a mild sedative such as diazepam may be justified. If all these factors are carefully considered, the stimulus responses will not be influenced to any relevant degree.

For the assessment of stimulus responses, reliable normative values are required which have been derived from a representative normal population by identical recording techniques. Normal values cannot be taken from the literature without examination because parameters of stimulation and recording vary from one laboratory to the next. Stimulus conditions are of particular importance in auditory and visual evoked potentials because amplitudes as well as latencies of the responses may be influenced to a significant degree. On the recording side, the same holds true for the filters used, whereas the precise characteristics of the amplifier in modern devices have no relevant influence in this respect. Each laboratory should determine its own normal limit by examining healthy individuals. Usually, normal values in evoked potentials are set to 2.5 standard deviations from the mean value. Further information concerning recording evoked potentials may be found in the literature (Halliday 1994).

Not all components of the evoked potentials arise within the cortex in the immediate vicinity of the electrode defined as the different one (Fig. 8.1). By electronic averaging, it is possible to record potentials originating relatively far away from the electrode. Therefore, subcortical

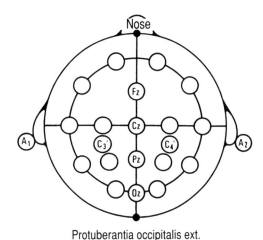

Protuberantia occipitalis ext.

Fig. 8.1. Electroencephalographic (EEG) recording points over the skull according to the "10–20 system." The recording sites most often used in evoked potentials are indicated.

regions and even sections of the spinal cord and of the brachial plexus are included. For recording of these distant and stationary potentials, the choice of the indifferent reference electrode is of decisive importance. Depending on the localization of the reference electrode, they become more clearly visible or even change polarity. Thus the directional relationship between the vector of the causative dipole and of the recording electrode pair is important. The terms different and indifferent electrodes, of course, are not appropriate for these distant potentials. In afferent evoked potentials, the definitions of different and indifferent are therefore arbitrary, and usually related only to "near" responses, for example to cortical potentials in scalp recordings. In recent years an international standard has been set amidst the enormous variability of recording techniques and nomenclatures. Continuing differences in parameters of stimulation and recording may partly be due to different diagnostic priorities and instrumentation. As usual in clinical electrophysiology, polarity is chosen such that negative potentials at the different electrode are recorded upwards. In brainstem auditory evoked potentials (BAEPs) it is convention to define the electrode near the ear as different, and the scalp electrode as indifferent. This is correct for the first cochlear component, and appears to be appropriate as long as one is not interested in the acoustically evoked late responses originating in the cortex.

In neurological routine diagnosis, the focus is on the early acoustically evoked potentials generated within the brainstem. Considering the various nomenclatures, it is recommended to use those which contain polarity and approximate normal latency: for example, P15 for a positive component with a mean latency of 15 ms. This system is used more generally in VEPs and in SEPs. An exception to this is BAEP, for which roman numerals are widely used.

The quality of information about evoked brain potentials may be improved by increasing the number of recording electrodes (see Fig. 8.1), which may also be expected to improve diagnostic yields. This involves a relatively greater instrument expense which probably does not pay off in routine diagnosis. Longer and more difficult preparations of recording would be required, and an enormous amount of data would have to be analyzed. Expensive brain mapping systems try to tackle this problem. Although commercially available systems appear very impressive in this respect, they do not bring decisive advantages compared to simple recordings with two to five channels. Therefore, on the following pages the systems of evoked potentials most commonly used in the routine diagnosis of MS are described.

Visual evoked potentials

Visual evoked potentials produced by checkerboard pattern reversal, as introduced by Halliday and collaborators in 1972, are sufficiently sensitive and do not cause distress to the patient. The examination, as described below, generally lasts a quarter of an hour; exceptionally, in difficult cases, it may take 40 minutes. It is well tolerated by patients and may be performed by a single examiner. The interpretation of the curve is relatively simple and the result is immediately available. A single amplifier channel and an averager, together with a stimulus generator and a stimulation field, for example a videomonitor or television set, are sufficient for routine examination (Fig. 8.2). The method is limited when there is lack of cooperation by the patient, be it voluntary or due to fatigue or generall ill-health.

Visual evoked potentials occupy the prime position among evoked potentials for other reasons too: they are able to detect the clinically silent second lesion (Kjaer 1982) which may be decisive for the diagnosis of MS. If a definitely

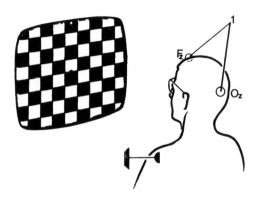

Fig. 8.2. Arrangement for stimulation and recording of VEPs. The retina is stimulated by inversion of the chessboard pattern produced on a television screen or videomonitor. This pattern reversal is repeated 64 to 128 times at a frequency of 0.5 Hz, and the EEG signal recorded from the occiput (with frontal reference) is averaged electronically at the same frequency.

pathological VEP is found in a patient with a recent spastic paresis of the extremities, further search for spinal cord compression is not of primary importance, and examination of CSF may suffice. In such a situation, pathological SEPs would not add much information. Pathological BAEPs would direct interest to the region of the brainstem as the most probable location of the lesion causing weakness. They would, however, not be able to prove the second lesion.

In VEPs, stimulation with pattern-reversal checkerboard is established for routine diagnosis of the visual system. If interest primarily concerns the optic nerve, each eye is stimulated separately. If, however, a retrochiasmatic lesion within the optic tract is being sought, binocular half-field stimulation is used (Fig. 8.3). In both situations, a median occipital recording (see Fig. 8.2) is generally sufficient, and the first large positive maximum P100 is measured (Fig. 8.4). Without changing the position of the recording electrode, the examination may be focused onto the prechiasmatic or retrochiasmatic part of the visual system by asking the patient either to fixate with one eye on the center of the stimulation field, or to fixate with both eyes on the left and right margins of the stimulation field, respectively. Only in exceptional cases are additional recording sites required if, for example, the main cortical component cannot be defined with certainty in complex configurations of the potential (Halliday 1994). The use of different types of stimulus is also recom-

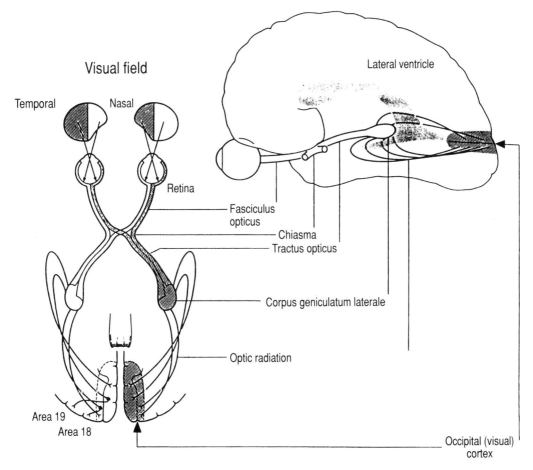

Visual field

Temporal Nasal

Lateral ventricle

Retina

Fasciculus
opticus

Chiasma

Tractus opticus

Corpus geniculatum laterale

Optic radiation

Area 19
Area 18

Occipital (visual)
cortex

Fig. 8.3. Schematic depiction of the visual system. When each eye is stimulated separately, the examination is focused on the optic nerves; with temporal and half-field stimulation of both eyes, it is focused on the optic tract and the optic radiation, respectively.

mended by asking the patient to fixate the center and the upper margins of the stimulation field (stimulation of the lower visual field), because the main positive component P100 is sometimes best seen with the one, sometimes with the other method. Although a stimulation field in a relatively small central area of the visual field is sufficient for generating pattern VEPs, a certain safety margin is recommended, for example a stimulation field of about 20 to 25 degrees of arc. Thus reliable responses are obtained even with imprecise fixation of the center. More peripheral parts of the visual field produce a slightly later and more or less marked positive component P135, which may render interpretation of response more difficult (so-called W-configuration, see below). Therefore, occasionally recording has to be repeated

with a reduced stimulation field in order to define P100 unequivocally.

To produce the largest possible amplitude of the evoked potential, the optimal dimension of the square of the checkerboard is about 15 to 30 minutes of arc. It is important, however, to use a larger pattern of about 1 degree of arc (50 to 70 minutes of arc) when searching for central, i.e., retrobulbar, lesions. A source of error of false-positive findings which is important for the neurologist is thus reduced because a pattern of this dimension produces potentials which are more resistant to anomalies of refraction and opaque media. Very fine patterns may be of interest to the ophthalmologist, for example for objective determination of refraction anomalies.

If oscillation frequency exceeds 8 Hz, a steady

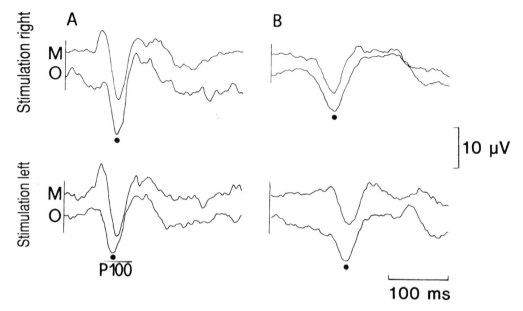

Fig. 8.4. Normal (A) and pathological (B) examples of VEPs. The upper curves (M) are derived when the patient is fixing the center of the stimulation field; the lower curve (0) when fixing the upper margin. Both eyes were stimulated separately by covering the unused one. The 42-year-old patient of curve B suffers from progressive paresis of the right leg and had never complained of visual disturbances. The latency of the positive component (P100) is found to be markedly pathological (130 ms) when stimulating the left eye, and normal (104 ms) when stimulating the right eye. In this case, VEPs indicate a diagnosis of "probable MS."

state potential is produced in which direct measurement of latency is not possible. Most commonly, a frequency of about 2 Hz is used. An average of 32 to 128 sweeps is necessary to produce a useful potential. Oscillation time is determined within television or videomonitor stimulators, and may be varied only in stimulators using mirror projections. Short oscillation times are then preferable. Attention must be given to illumination density and pattern contrast because they may be changed considerably over time by dust deposits on the stimulation field, by soot deposits on the projection lamp, by variable illumination, and by inadequate darkening of the room. These parameters therefore have to be controlled and recalibrated periodically. All stimulus parameters not only influence the amplitude significantly, but also the latency of the evoked potentials, and they are therefore decisive for the normative values.

During the examination of the patient, the build-up of the average potential and the unrefined signal is observed continuously in order immediately to eliminate sources of artifacts. Usually the component P100 is recognizable in crude lines after a few sweeps, and the examination may then be finished within a few min-

utes. If this is not the case, it must be ensured that the patient is really looking into the stimulation field. If this is not possible, for example because of markedly reduced visual acuity or because of disturbances of ocular movements (nystagmus), the stimulation field must be enlarged (by bringing the patient closer to the monitor) or the number of average sweeps must be increased. A not uncommon source of error in MS patients is α-waves which may occur during recording when patients are tired or unable to concentrate. Alpha waves have to be recognized immediately and the examination must be interrupted by frequent arousal and encouragement to attention. When interpreting the findings, it is important to define a positive maximum P100 following the first negative change (N75), even when a second positive maximum (P135) follows which may be even larger. Such W-configurations are a frequent cause of false-positive findings when the first positive peak is relatively small and therefore is not taken as P100. If such a situation is suspected, the examination has to be repeated with different conditions of stimulus and recording.

Visual evoked potentials are particularly

valuable in the diagnosis of MS because latencies remain pathological after subjectively healed optic neuritis. In this respect, they are even superior to subjective tests of color sense and contrast sensitivity, which may be more sensitive in the acute stage of optic neuritis. Visual evoked potentials therefore often allow verification of a subjective indication of possible optic neuritis. Even without subjective visual disturbances in the case history, pathological findings indicating a clinically silent lesion are often found. In MS patients this is the case in 60% to 90% of the eyes examined, and in 30% to 40% of patients without indications of visual symptoms in their case histories (Halliday 1994). In large series of definite MS patients, pathological VEPs on at least one side may be expected in 80% to 95% of cases (Trojaborg and Petersen 1979; Chiappa 1980; Halliday 1994).

The typical finding after optic neuritis is a markedly delayed response with only slightly reduced amplitude (see Fig. 8.4b). Latency may be delayed by 30 to 50 ms, and in extreme cases by up to 70 ms. If a delayed latency of P100 is found, opaque media, severe glaucoma, and uncorrected refraction anomaly on this eye must be excluded. Such ocular affections reduce the value of the moderately delayed latency as an indicator of a central lesion. Even though these affections primarily reduce the amplitude of VEP, they may often lead to a slight delay of latency which is more marked the smaller the stimulus pattern (see above). This holds true for other ocular affections (for example ischemic optic neuropathy) as well as for compressive optic nerve lesions: they all reduce amplitude primarily and may lead in addition to moderate delay of latency. Often no response at all may be recorded during the acute stage of severe optic neuritis, a finding which may also occur in acute occlusion of the central artery which may produce a similar clinical picture.

In addition to the above-mentioned tests of contrast sensitivity and color vision, the other psychophysical examinations of the visual system may be carried out using modern methods for the determination of visual fields and also by measuring flicker fusion.

Somatosensory evoked potentials

Somatosensory evoked potentials evoked by electric stimulation of nerve trunks at the extremities are well established in MS diagnosis. They produce reliable results without the need

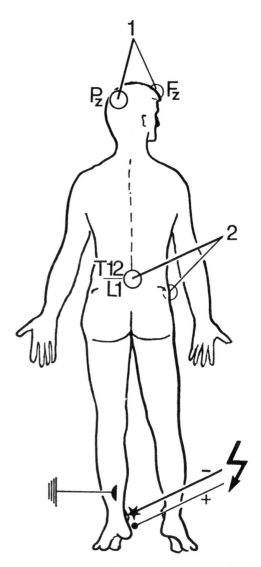

Fig. 8.5. Arrangement for stimulation and recording of SEPs from the tibialis nerve (tibialis SEPs). Stimulation behind the medial malleolus, lumbar recording (2) – best done using needle electrodes between spinous processes T12 and L1 (reference electrode over pelvis and abdomen) – and cortical recording (1) from midparietal with frontal reference.

for additional stimulus apparatus and within an acceptable period of time. Stimulus frequency of 2 to 3 Hz is sufficient, necessitating a duration of examination of 30 to 45 minutes for one nerve pair. By stimulating a mixed nerve slightly above motor stimulation threshold, stimulus frequency is adapted to the individual patient and is usually well tolerated (Figs. 8.5 and 8.8). By averaging 256 to 1024 sweeps, cortical re-

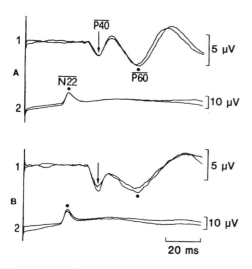

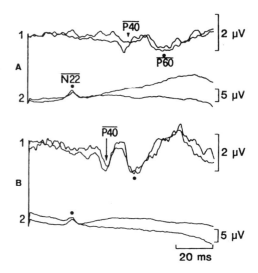

Fig. 8.6. Example of normal tibialis SEPs with cortical (1) and lumbar (2) responses following stimulation of the right (A) and left (B) foot. The components N22 (lumbar) and P40 and P60 are most suitable for determination of latencies. The latency difference P40 minus N22 is a measure of the afferent central conduction time (N22–P40), and is independent of the relatively variable length of the leg in contrast to the peripheral conduction time, N22. Two successive curves are superimposed in order to demonstrate reproducibility. (The same holds true for the following examples.)

Fig. 8.7. Example of pathological tibialis SEP of a patient with definite MS and sensory disturbances on the right side of the body. (Arrangement identical to that in Fig. 8.6.) When stimulating on the right side (A), the cortical response P40 (1) at 52 ms, and the central conduction time N22–P40 at 27.5 ms are markedly pathological, whereas the latencies are normal when stimulating left (P40 = 42 ms; conduction time N22–P40 = 18.7 ms). Note in comparison to Fig. 8.6 the larger amplification and therefore smaller amplitudes, in particular of the cortical response on the right side.

sponses are reproduced reliably even under pathological conditions, and in most cases even a peripheral response from brachial plexus and lumbosacral root entry zones may be obtained (Figs. 8.6 and 8.10). This is important in order to gain insight into peripheral conduction time, which is variable from person to person due to the different lengths of their extremities. Possible pathological situations which may influence central response indirectly are thereby recognized (Fig. 8.7). When stimulating a mixed nerve of the leg it is often possible to record a peripheral lumbosacral response (N22) by placing needle electrodes between spinous processes Th12 and L1 (see Fig. 8.5), in addition to the primary cortical response (P40) recorded by a scalp electrode. The difference in time between these responses corresponds to an afferent central conduction time over a relatively long distance. This distance may be divided further by additional cervical recording (N30) in order to calculate spinal conduction time. This is desirable for better localization in cases of delayed latency. In addition to clinical symptoms specific for a brainstem affection, pathological SEP findings may only be accepted as an indica-

tion of a silent second lesion if the delay of latency can be localized to the spinal region. However, it is not always possible to record this cervical component N30 by stimulating nerves of the leg, and in these cases, better localization of delay may be obtained by recording median nerve SEP in addition.

In median nerve SEP (Figs. 8.8 and 8.9), a cervical response can be recorded reliably in healthy people. This response is generated mainly on the cervical level and is recorded as component N13 over the spinous processes C5/C7. If spinal recording is performed with a frontal reference electrode, a caudorostral dipole component N14 generated within the medulla oblongata is added, and this can be avoided by using a ventral reference point at the neck (Desmedt and Cheron 1981). The complete lack of a spinal response, therefore, is a definite pathological sign and is due to a cervical lesion. Interestingly enough, in MS patients a cortical response, although reduced in amplitude and possibly delayed, may be recorded despite lack of a spinal response, indicating a relative integrity of thalamocortical projections. There are

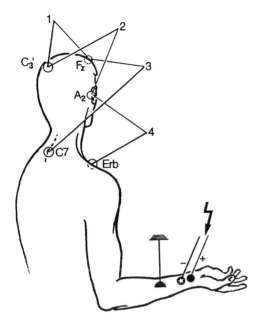

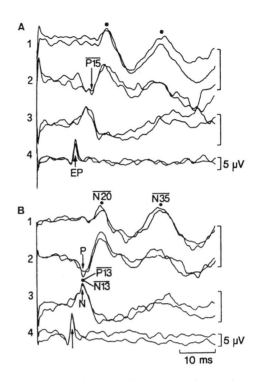

Fig. 8.8. Arrangement for stimulation and recording of SEPs from the median nerve (median SEP). Stimulation is at the wrist, recording supraclavicularly from Erb's point (4), from the neck over the spinous process C7 (3), and contralaterally from the scalp (2 and 1). The reference electrode lies frontal (1 and 3) or at the ear (2 and 4). Additional information may be gained by double cortical recording with different reference (1 and 2), because components of the potential which are visible only with an ear reference are of subcortical origin (so-called far-field components, see text).

Fig. 8.9. Example of normal median SEPs by stimulating the right (A) and the left (B) hands. Curves 1 to 4 correspond to the arrangement of recordings as depicted in Fig. 8.8. The most important components of potentials are indicated: the plexus potential or Erb's potential (EP) in 4, the cervical response N13 (3) and P13 (B2) and P15 (A2), respectively, which are recorded with an ear reference, the so-called far-field potentials, and finally the cortical primary complex N20 (1).

several reasons for this phenomenon. (1) In evoked brain potentials, stimulus responses occurring in temporal succession to a peripheral stimulus are not causally related because different afferents operating in parallel may produce potential components on different central levels of integration. (2) The relatively autonomous thalamus may react to a quantitatively weak afferent with a relatively strong thalamocortical projection, a property often described as amplification effect of the thalamus. In SEP it is probable that the spinal response requires a larger number of afferent impulses than the thalamocortical system.

In MS, the typical finding in SEP is again a marked delay of latency, often in combination with a more or less marked diminution of amplitude (Figs. 8.7 and 8.10). Compared to compressive lesions, for example due to a tumor, delay is relatively specific for MS because mechanical injury tends to reduce the amplitude,

and only minimal delay of latency or no potential at all may be obtained. In an individual case, this differentiation is often not reliable enough, and an anatomical depiction (MRI, myelogram) is required.

Somatosensory evoked potentials are particularly valuable in patients with sensory disturbances without objective signs, where the question arises of whether or not an organic lesion is present. In such cases, SEP may produce "hard" pathological evidence and indicate the direction for further investigations. Such situations are not rare, particularly in early stages of MS. On the other hand, normal SEPs are not proof of psychogenic disturbance!

Brainstem auditory evoked potentials

Brainstem auditory evoked potentials are usually evoked by clicks, i.e., short rectangular im-

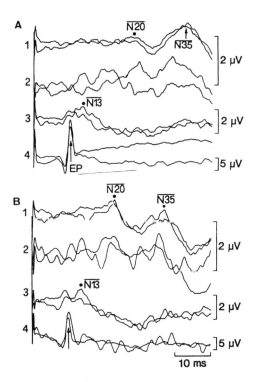

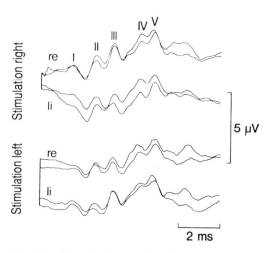

Fig. 8.11. Example of normal BAEPs by stimulation of the right (upper curve pair) and left (lower curve pair) ears and recording with the "different" electrode over the vertex (Cz). The peripheral cochlear component (I) is found only on the ipsilateral side with initially negative deflection (upward). Concerning the later central medullary (III) and pontomesencephalic (IV and V) components, the side of the recordings is not important in these far-field potentials.

Fig. 8.10. Typical pathological median SEPs of a 30-year-old patient with definite MS with variably marked paresthesias in the right arm for 6 years. Recording arrangement identical to that in Fig. 8.9. On the right side (A), markedly delayed cortical response N20 (latency = 43 ms) (1), diminished amplitude, and prolonged conduction time (N13–N20 = 29.6 ms). On the left-hand side (B), latencies and conduction time are normal (N20 = 22.2 ms; N13–N20 = 8.6 ms). Note the cervical responses which are deformed on both sides (3), a typical finding which, however, does not allow for any definite conclusions to be drawn.

pulses presented over headphones. Intensity of sound is best set at 70 to 80 dB above the threshold of this stimulus. Polarity of click stimulus is often chosen as alternating pressure and decompression stimulus in order to minimize stimulus artifacts. In addition, it should be possible to apply decompression impulses exclusively as such stimuli are often better at producing a discernible first cochlear response. Monoaural stimulation by masking of the contralateral ear is most commonly used. At least 1536 sweeps have to be summated because of the very small amplitudes. A relatively high stimulus frequency of about 10 Hz may be used.

Of the various components, the first five waves are of particular importance, usually numbered by Roman numerals (Fig. 8.11). The first component is generated by the auditory nerve and is therefore a peripheral cochlear stimulus response. The third component originates in the region of the medulla oblongata, the fourth and fifth components on the pontomesencephalic level. A reliable assessment of central responses requires the presence of the first component because latencies, and to some extent amplitudes, are related to this first component. If the first component is lacking, a delayed fifth component may not be taken as proof of a central lesion. In such cases, a peripheral cause has to be sought and the ear has to be inspected (for example for cerumen obturatum).

Of all the evoked potentials, the BAEPs are least suited to the detection of the second lesion so important for a diagnosis of MS. Apart from the visual disturbances and neuropsychological deficits, most central neurological syndromes may also be explained by a brainstem lesion. If pathological BAEPs are found in a patient with monoparesis, paraspasticity or internuclear ophthalmoplegia, they may indicate a second silent lesion which is, however, not necessarily distinct from the lesion producing the symptoms. Furthermore, pathological BAEPs are of-

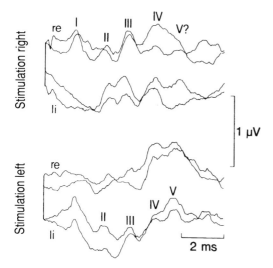

Fig. 8.12. Typical pathological BAEPs of a patient with longstanding MS. Identical recording arrangement to that in Fig. 8.11. Normal first cochlear response (I) on both sides and increased latency of all central responses, whereby component V on the right-hand side is not clearly delineated. Note the increased amplification in comparison to Fig. 8.11 (and therefore smaller amplitudes).

ten difficult to interpret because of their numerous components. There may be rather typical BAEP changes in cerebellopontine angle tumors. Despite claims to the contrary, specific pathological changes may not be defined in either MS lesions or in space occupying lesions, although typical delay of latency may be expected and observed (Fig. 8.12). Furthermore, BAEPs are relatively resistant and therefore rather less sensitive. An unequivocally pathological BAEP finding is therefore very important. For complaints which are difficult to define objectively, such as dizziness, BAEPs may produce the hard evidence justifying further investigations.

Examinations of reflexes

Lesions may be detected neurophysiologically by measuring reflexes. Reflexes with short central pathways and few synapses rarely yield positive findings, whereas more complicated reflexes with longer central pathways have the disadvantage of relatively high variability. Specific results for MS cannot be expected. Certain reflex examinations require special arrangements of equipment. These factors hamper their use in MS diagnosis, and therefore many

reflex examinations recommended for this purpose are not described in detail here; only the examinations which have proved to be most effective will be considered briefly.

Various brainstem reflexes are standardized electrophysiologically and may be measured: blink reflex triggered by supraorbital electrical stimulation of the trigeminal nerve is widely used because it can be performed with the equipment available in most laboratories. Comparing the first ipsilateral oligosynaptic response to the ipsilateral and contralateral polysynaptic late response, quite precise conclusions may be drawn as to localization. This reflex may also be triggered by physiological (acoustic or optic) means. Thus the considerable variability of these reflexes is further increased, and, in examinations of reflexes in general, a mean value of several (for example, eight) sweeps is determined. Electronic averaging, on the other hand, is less reliable. In MS, a relatively high incidence of pathological findings may be obtained (Khoshbin and Hallet 1981). Mechanically induced brainstem reflexes, for example masseter reflex, are less useful because of the large variability (Yates and Brown 1981). Acoustically induced stapedius reflex is well standardized. Its measurement, however, requires the special installation of impedance audiometry in order to detect mechanical response. It may detect subclinical brainstem lesions (Hess 1979).

Late reflex responses of extremity muscles (long latency reflexes) are of increasing interest in clinical diagnosis. They are induced either mechanically by a phasic stimulus or electrically by stimulating the corresponding mixed nerve at the motor threshold. Late reflex responses may be obtained by distal electrical stimulation of the skin (cutaneomuscular reflexes). The stimulus response consists of a modulation of the discrete voluntary tonic preinnervation and is measured via surface electrodes over the corresponding muscle after electronic averaging of several sweeps. Muscle activity recorded is rectified electronically in order to summate positive and negative deflexions. The rationale for using these late reflex responses in central neurological disorders is based on the assumption that late responses following the first segmental reflex response are due to a long reflex loop including transcortical pathways. This hypothesis is probably correct for certain types of investigations. However, it may not be accepted as a general assumption for late reflex responses, and awaits conclusive proof in individual cases. Nevertheless, in central lesions, and particularly in spastic pareses, typical changes have been observed in which the first segmental response is increased and the late reflex responses are diminished or lacking (Lee and Tatton 1975; Beradelli et al. 1984). This method may be widely used because electrically induced reflexes do not require the installation of equipment other than simple electronic rectifiers which are usually built into modern instruments. Electrically induced long latency reflexes after stimulation of the median nerve are established as a simple and practically useful screening method. The latency of the late (transcortical) reflex response is related to the simultaneously induced spinal H-reflex (Deuschl et al. 1988). Thus methodological problems of different arm lengths and additional peripheral neuropathies are elegantly avoided. Pathological findings can be determined by this method in 80% of definite and in 60% of probable MS cases (Deuschl et al. 1988).

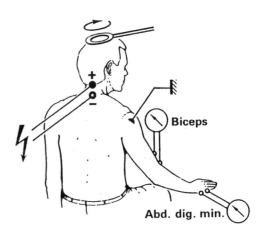

Fig. 8.13. Arrangement for stimulation and recording of central MEPs by transcranial cortical stimulation. Stimulation is in the form of single short magnetic pulses over the scalp and by short electric high-voltage stimulation over the neck. Recording by a surface electrode from abductor digiti minimi muscle and biceps brachii. By discrete voluntary preinnervation of both target muscles (spreading of the fingers, slight elevation of the forearm), a marked amplification of the motor compound potential is achieved.

Motor evoked potentials induced by transcranial stimulation of the cortex

Until a few years ago, neurophysiological diagnosis lacked the ability to examine central motor pathways directly. In MS, symptoms of disturbed motor control often occur at disease onset, and later may dominate the clinical picture. Merton and Morton (1980) were the first to succeed in stimulating motor cortex in awake individuals across the intact skull by electric high voltage stimulation. The latencies of the compound muscle potentials suggested activation of the rapid pyramidal system. Delays of latency of central motor impulse transmission were detected in MS patients by this method (Cowan et al. 1984; Mills and Murray 1985). Unfortunately, such high voltage stimuli applied to the skull are relatively painful, which limits the use of this method in routine examinations. Only by developing a strong generator of magnetic field pulses was it possible to stimulate motor cortex in awake individuals in the absence of pain (Barker et al. 1985). No serious side-effects have been reported so far. In patients at risk of epileptic seizures, a slight proconvulsive tendency should be considered. It is recommended that the hearing of children and adolescents should be protected since certain stimulation coils may produce an acoustic trauma. Patients with cardiac pacemakers and those with metallic devices inside their skulls have to be excluded from examinations. The examination is very simple and may be performed quickly because compound potentials of single stimuli are measured, and thus averaging is not necessary. In principle, motor evoked potentials (MEPs) have many applications.

Measuring central motor conduction by stimulating motor cortex with magnetic pulses is a relatively recent investigative technique, the actual value of which for clinical neurology has not yet been established. Most experience has been gained in MS, for which the diagnostic value of the method was first demonstrated (Hess et al. 1986a). It is therefore appropriate to describe briefly central MEPs.

By a surge of current within the stimulation coil applied to the skull, a short magnetic pulse is generated which by itself induces small currents in the brain (Hess et al. 1987c). Thereby current densities are produced which are not as high as in electrical high voltage stimulation. Muscle potentials evoked at the muscles of the extremities are recorded with surface elec-

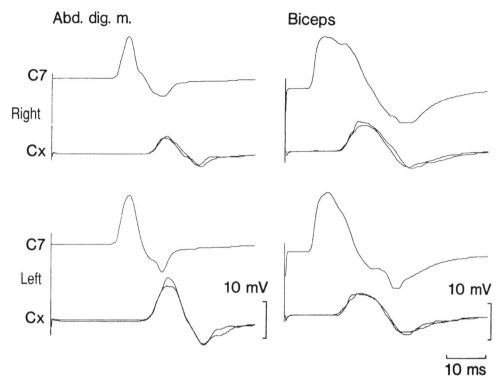

Fig. 8.14. Normal central MEPs from abductor digiti minimi and biceps brachii after stimulation over the cortex (Cx). Two single compound potentials are superimposed. By additional stimulation of the motor cervical roots (C7), a peripheral motor potential is evoked and a central motor conduction time can be calculated by subtraction of the latencies of both these potentials. A single cortical and cervical stimulating impulse is sufficient to produce a compound potential simultaneously in both muscles.

trodes, and are of the same order of magnitude as those evoked from peripheral nerves if the target muscle is slightly preinnervated voluntarily. In order to obtain a measure of central motor conduction time (CMCT), peripheral conduction time has to be subtracted from total corticomuscular latency. Peripheral conduction time can be calculated either by transcutaneous stimulation of motor roots at the neck and in the lumbosacral region (Figs. 8.13 and 8.14) or by determining F-wave latency. For stimulation of motor roots, a strong electric or magnetic stimulator is required. A stimulation electrode is applied over spinous processes C5–C7 and L5–S1, and the effective site of stimulation lies slightly outside the intervertebral foramina (Schmid et al. 1991). Depending on the stimulator and on the configuration of the body, it is not always possible to obtain supramaximal stimulus responses, particularly in the lumbosacral region.

Depending on the method used and the target muscle, CMCT in healthy individuals is 6 to 8 ms to the cervical region (Hess et al. 1986a), and 16 to 18 ms to the lumbosacral spinal cord.

Prolonged CMCT is found frequently in MS (Hess et al. 1986a; 1987d; Ingram et al. 1988; Jones et al. 1991; Fig. 8.15), and the degree of delay has been found to be unexpectedly large in certain patients (Hess et al. 1987a). In comparison to clinical findings on the extremity measured, a clearcut correlation was found with symptoms of spasticity or signs of pyramidal tract affection, much less so with pareses of the corresponding muscle. Pathological delays, however, were often found despite lack of motor pareses or spastic increase of tone, and even without exaggerated jerks. Even in extremities without any conspicuous clinical finding, prolonged motor transduction times were found (Hess et al. 1987d). Similar to the afferent

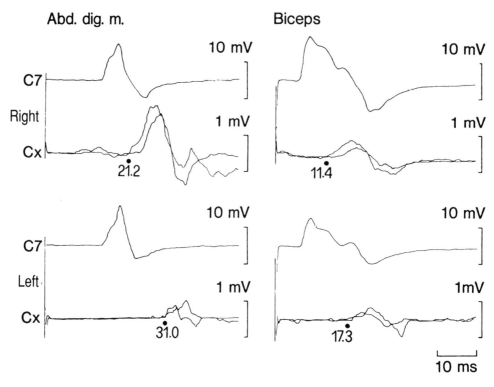

Fig. 8.15. Pathological central MEPs from the same MS patient as in Fig. 8.10. Arrangement of examination identical to that in Fig. 8.14. Whereas the motor compound potentials evoked by stimulation of the cervical roots are normal (C7), the potentials evoked by cortical stimulation show markedly pathologically increased latencies in both muscles on the left-hand side (Cx). Note the smaller amplitudes in comparison to Fig. 8.14, and the increased variability of the central motor responses (increased amplitude).

evoked potentials, clinically silent lesions may be detected in the efferent system. The MEPs prove to be equally as sensitive as SEPs in MS patients. It is rare, however, that MEPs are able to increase diagnostic certainty compared to SEPs or VEPs because they are less often capable of detecting clinically silent second lesions. Furthermore, MEPs do not provide findings which are pathognomonic for MS and they are even less specific than afferent evoked potentials in this respect. Marked prolongations of CMCT have been found in amyotrophic lateral sclerosis, in hereditary ataxias (for example Friedrich's ataxia), and in cervical myelopathy due to spondylosis (Hess et al. 1987b; 1987d; Claus et al. 1988; Schriefer et al. 1989; Eisen et al. 1990; Maertens de Noordhout et al. 1991). In these conditions, however, the extent of the delay is usually not as large as in many MS patients. The value of the method lies particularly in detecting clinically silent or doubtful disturbances in the pyramidal central motor system, rather than in the differential diagnosis of CNS diseases with motor symptoms. Motor evoked potentials provide a useful screening method as they require relatively modest equipment and are practical to use. In young patients with unspecific complaints which may suggest MS, clinical examination often reveals no hard evidence, probably only exaggerated muscle jerks. In such situations, pathological MEPs may indicate the right direction for further investigations.

Assessment of oculomotor disturbances by oculography

It is common clinical experience that oculomotor disturbances are particularly frequent in MS patients. It is therefore desirable in MS diagnosis that their exact analysis is made possible by the use of appropriate measuring equipment. Recording techniques have become more refined in order to find oculomotor disturbances which are typical for MS and to detect those which are not visible to the naked eye. The large corneoretinal potential is used which, as an axial dipole within the eyes, is easily measured by electrophysiological methods. In nystagmography, alternating current amplifiers are used which filter out low frequencies and therefore do not record slow movements. Thus, this method is not suitable for recording the position of the eyes, pursuit movements, and large saccades. Improved amplification techniques make it possible to record conjugated eye movements by direct current electrooculography. Analysis of saccades in MS provides pathological findings with the same frequency as VEPs (Mastaglia et al. 1982). However, examinations with DC electrooculography are relatively expensive and time consuming, particularly due to drift of electrodes and instability of the corneoretinal potentials in relation to illumination. Frequent calibration is thus often necessary. Furthermore, for reasons of symmetry, electrooculography does not allow independent separate recordings of both eyes (Hess et al. 1986b). This is a clear disadvantage for diagnosis since a separate recording would be desirable because dissociated (incongruous) saccades are a typical symptom of MS. Discrete internuclear ophthalmoplegia, so characteristic in MS (see Chapter 7), may be missed by clinical examination and may be detected only as a slightly slower velocity of saccades of the adducting eye.

Infrared reflection oculography, which has become methodologically more refined in recent years, is clearly superior to electrooculography for the separate examination of both eyes (Hess et al. 1986b). Reflection of the invisible infrared light is measured, and asymmetrical recording by electrodes is not necessary. Furthermore, examination with the infrared method takes markedly less time than with electrooculography.

It was possible to detect dissociated saccades in 58% of 80 cases of definite MS by infrared reflection oculography, a third of which were subclinical (Meienberg et al. 1986). Pathological findings were recorded in 80% of the cases if further oculographic parameters were considered. Again, these signs of brainstem lesions are less useful for the detection of clinically silent second lesions than VEPs. Nor are oculographic findings specific for MS. However, they may add valuable information when sub-jective disturbances have to be objectivated, or when a questionable finding has to be clarified and documented. The equipment required is expensive and will probably have to be confined to neurological centers.

Combined cystomanometric–electromyographic investigation of bladder and sphincter function

Bladder disturbances and resulting complications are common in MS and often give rise to the main problems of therapy and rehabilitation. They may result in reduced life expectancy, and quality of life is certainly compromised by urinary tract infection with the danger of chronic pyelonephritis and urosepsis. Bladder disturbances not only have to be detected in good time, but they also have to be identified precisely in order for them to be treated appropriately. This is not possible without auxillary diagnostic means. In MS, various forms of bladder disturbances caused by central lesions may occur depending on the different localizations of lesions in the CNS. The different forms may require different treatment modalities (see Chapter 7).

In combined cystomanometric–electromyographic investigation, pressure in the bladder and rectum is measured via a catheter, rectal pressure being a measure of intraperitoneal pressure. Muscle activity of the external sphincter of the bladder is measured electromyographically. According to our own experience, concentric or bipolar needle electrodes are most suitable because they allow muscle activity to be recorded constantly and free of artifacts, even during micturition. As a less invasive method for sphincter electromyogram, circular surface electrodes may be applied to the indwelling catheter which is placed as close as possible to the sphincter. However, the position of the electrode in relation to the sphincter is not always stable, and recording is less reliable. The internal bladder sphincter, being a smooth muscle, cannot be recorded electromyographically. Assessment of its contraction depends on morphological criteria of the bladder neck.

After clinical urological examination and determination of resting urine, the bladder is filled retrogradely with water containing contrast media. Pressure signals and tonic electromyographical activity are recorded continu-

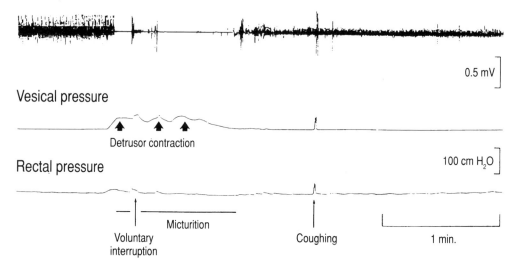

EMG Sphinct.vesicae ext.

0.5 mV

Vesical pressure

Detrusor contraction

Rectal pressure

100 cm H$_2$O

Voluntary
interruption
Micturition
Coughing
1 min.

Fig. 8.16. Recording of normal micturition during combined electromyographic-urodynamic examination. Sphincter EMG is recorded by needle electrodes; pressure in the bladder and rectum by indwelling catheters. The bladder was previously slowly filled with water containing a contrast agent until the patient felt the urge to urinate. After voluntary initiation of micturition, pressure within the bladder rises due to contraction of the detrusor, while tonic activity of the sphincter remains stable. The patient is capable of interrupting micturition by innervating the sphincter muscle. Coughing leads to prompt phasic increase of pressure in the bladder and rectum and to a short increase of activity of the sphincter (Venetz et al. 1989).

ously, and filling of the bladder is observed on the X-ray monitor. Reflexic phasic increase of sphincter activity and functioning of pressure measurement in the bladder and rectum are controlled by coughing and abdominal pressure. During the filling phase, uninhibited detrusor contractions, which may not be controlled voluntarily and which are typical of detrusor hyperreflexia in "neurogenic bladder," should be noted. They may be indicated by a sudden increase of pressure in the bladder while pressure in the rectum remains unchanged. With voluntary increased abdominal pressure, however, bladder and rectal pressure increases.

The patient should notify the first sensation of desire to urinate, but should only urinate when the desire is too strong to ignore and when the examiner asks him or her to do so. During micturition, it should be observed whether the external sphincter is relaxing normally, and, radiologically, whether the internal sphincter (bladder neck) is opening (Fig. 8.16). If this is the case, the patient is asked to interrupt micturition in order to assess whether prompt increase of phasic activity in the exter-

nal sphincter is present, indicating normal voluntary control of the striated sphincter muscle.

Urinary urgency, so typical in MS but also present in numerous other neurological conditions, is caused by uninhibited detrusor contractions occurring even with small bladder volumes during the filling phase. This so-called detrusor hyperreflexia may be due to lesions in various locations of the CNS: lesions lying in the suprasacral spinal cord, in the brainstem, or in the basal ganglia. Infravesical obstructions of outflow (hyperplasia of the prostate) may lead to detrusor hyperreflexia and have therefore to be excluded (see Chapter 7).

The syndrome of detrusor hyperreflexia has to be examined further for therapeutic reasons. Combined cystomanometric–electromyographic investigation allows further classification according to the behavior of the sphincter. In one type, the inner and outer sphincters relax during micturition. Patients may not be able to prevent a certain loss of urine by voluntary activation of the external sphincter; they are capable, however, of initiating normal micturition. This is called urge incontinence. These patients may profit from anticholinergic medication which

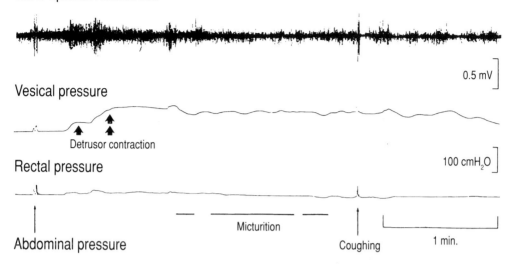

EMG Sphinct.vesicae ext.

0.5 mV

Vesical pressure

Detrusor contraction

Rectal pressure

100 cmH₂O

Micturition

Abdominal pressure   Coughing   1 min.

Fig. 8.17. Example of a typical detrusor–sphincter externus dyssynergia of an MS patient. Arrangement of examination identical to that in Fig. 8.16. During detrusor contraction, sphincter activity increases paradoxically and impedes micturition which initiates too late, occurs spasmodically and incompletely. The fact that rectum pressure does not show any relevant elevation proves that it is due to a true detrusor contraction and not to voluntary abdominal pressure, in which an increase of sphincter activity would be normal (Venetz et al. 1989).

supports the external sphincter and often prevents incontinence. In the second type, occurring in more advanced stages of the disease, either the internal or the external sphincter acts paradoxically during micturition by increasing phasic activity instead of relaxing, and thereby preventing loss of urine (Fig. 8.17). This detrusor sphincter externus dyssynergia leads to incomplete voiding and to backflow into the ureters when relatively high pressure is developed within the bladder. There is resting volume, and patients often suffer from urge incontinence. This diagnosis is of practical importance because of infectious complications and because ill-considered anticholinergic medication for incontinence may aggravate the situation. A pure internus dyssynergia may often be controlled by α-blockers. The treatment of externus dyssynergia is more difficult. Often self-catheterization leads to good results if the patient is capable of doing this. In male patients, surgical sphincterotomy may be performed as, although incontinence may be worsened postoperatively, urine can be collected in condom urinals (see Chapter 13).

It is important to consider the discomfort for the patient during the examination. Gross errors of assessment may result if a relaxed atmosphere is not created, and this requires skill on the part of the examiner. In the artificial situation in the laboratory, there is often a tendency to activate the external sphincter more markedly because of an unconscious reluctance to urinate when an examiner is present. This may lead to a false impression of detrusor sphincter dyssynergia. If asked to urinate, patients often use abdominal pressure, even though under normal conditions they would not do so. Thus the external sphincter is activated producing an erroneous result. Any impression of hurrying the patient should therefore be avoided, and the best position for the patient should be sought in order to make "normal micturition" possible. Only then can conclusive assessment of sphincter function be obtained.

MAGNETIC RESONANCE IMAGING
by J. Kesselring

Introduction

Magnetic resonance imaging is very sensitive for detecting lesions in the brains of MS patients. In the first study reported on the application of this technique in MS diagnosis (Young et al. 1981), 10 patients were examined, in 8 of whom diagnosis was clinically definite, and probable in 2. In these patients, 19 lesions could be detected on computer tomography (with and without contrast medium), all of which were also detected on MRI, as were 112 additional lesions. Since then, this method of investigation has become established in the diagnosis of diseases of the CNS, and in particular of the white matter, and of malformation in adults as well as in children. For detecting lesions in MS it is superior to all other auxillary investigations (Sheldon et al. 1985; Ormerod et al. 1986; 1987; Jacobs et al. 1986; Kesselring et al. 1989a; Miller et al., 1996). Computer tomography may still play a role in differential diagnosis where MRI is not readily available.

The basic principle of MRI is to bring the part of the body to be examined into a strong magnetic field. Nuclei with an odd number of protons build up a small magnetic moment due to their electric charge. The vectors of these small magnetic fields are distributed randomly at rest and produce a spin in a strong external magnetic field. The vectors of these spins line up in parallel to the external magnetic field and may be deflected from this arrangement by an additional electromagnetic impulse, thereby producing a precession motion which can be detected as an electromagnetic signal in the region of radio frequency. Similarly, a top spinning around its own axis which is deflected from this "resting motion" begins to rotate (precession). The relaxation of the nuclei which had been deflected out of the parallel arrangement by the electromagnetic impulse is exponential, and is characterized by two time constants, T_1 and T_2.

For imaging, hydrogen nuclei are normally examined because they are present in every tissue in abundance and because they produce a high MR signal.

Longitudinal relaxation time (T_1) is a measure of energy which is exchanged between the spin and its environment as it returns to the resting state (spin lattice relaxation time). T_1 may also be defined as the time after which 62% of the energy is exchanged. Body fluids and water in particular have long T_1 values because the chance of exchanging energy with the surroundings is smaller in such a homogeneous medium. In tissues with more compact and complex structures, it is much more probable that hydrogen nuclei exchange energy with their surroundings; therefore the T_1 relaxation time in such tissues is shorter. T_1 values, therefore, are quite tissue specific and give an indication of the water content. The fact that the exchange of energy between hydrogen nuclei and their surroundings occurs exponentially is made use of by examining tissue at certain time points after the application of the electromagnetic impulse. Shortly after the impulse, during the steep slope of the exponentially ascending curve, tissues with short T_1 values give a high signal (bright), whereas regions magnetizing slowly appear dark (T_1-weighted images).

Because molecules in a tissue contain small magnetic fields themselves, they determine the strength by which the magnetic field applied from outside may influence the rotating hydrogen nuclei. Precession frequencies therefore vary accordingly. Spins turn increasingly out of phase after the radio-frequency impulse due to this interaction (transverse or spin–spin relaxation time), thereby decreasing the signal emitted. This decrease of signal is again exponential, and is characterized by the time constant T_2. T_2 is always shorter than T_1 because the exchange of energy between hydrogen nuclei and their surroundings (T_1) contributes to the decrease of the signal emitted. In compound substances, T_2 is much shorter than T_1; they are of similar duration in homogeneous fluids.

The magnetic resonance signal emitted is quantified in MRI as gradations of gray. It depends on proton density and on the time constants T_1 and T_2 in the tissue examined. In normal brain, T_1 and T_2 values are shorter in the white matter than in the gray matter; both values are longer in CSF than in either gray or white matter.

This short introduction (for further information see, for example, Brant-Zawadzki and Norman 1987; Kesselring et al. 1989a; Miller et al., 1996) may suffice for understanding that magnetic resonance images may look very different according to the pulse frequency chosen and to the time after the impulse at which the emitted signal is read. Impulse frequencies are chosen in order to produce the strongest contrast possible in the regions of interest. Spin echo (SE) and inversion recovery (IR) are best established in the diagnosis of MS because they are able to depict plaques best. Differences in T_1 values, and therefore of anatomical detail according to different water content of the tissues, are best shown by inversion recovery. A spin-echo sequence, on the other hand, better depicts different T_2 values: in the case of MS, plaques, with their higher T_2 values, are shown as brighter areas surrounded by the normal-appearing white matter which looks darker in these images.

Magnetic resonance imaging appears to be without any danger of serious side-effects for the patient. Routine examination lasts about 20 minutes. Some patients find it claustrophobic to have to lie still in the narrow tunnel during examination, and some find the loud noise produced within the machine distressing. It is rare that an examination has to be terminated prematurely if patients are well prepared. The cost of these investigations is still very high.

Sensitivity

Lesions in the brains of MS patients are best depicted using moderately T_2-weighted pulse sequences, i.e., with a repetition time (TR) of 2000 ms, and an echo time (TE) of 60 to 80 ms. The new technique of MRI – fast spin echo – appears to be equally sensitive in lesion detection. It is to be expected that fast spin echo will supplant spin echo as the preferred sequence in MS. For patients undergoing repeated imaging, especially in treatment trials, it will save time and thus costs considerably (Miller et al., 1996). Over the last 10 years, hundreds of patients with clinically definite MS (according to the Poser criteria, see p. 88) have been examined by the NMR research group at the National Hospital, Queen Square, London, first with a magnetic resonance imager with a field strength of 0.5 Tesla (Ormerod et al. 1987; Miller et al. 1988; Kesselring et al. 1989b), and during the last 3 years with a field strength of 1.5 Tesla (Miller et al. 1996). Lesions in the white matter have been detected with a sensitivity of more than 90%. A normal magnetic resonance examination therefore does not exclude the clinical diagnosis of definite MS. In 98% of patients, lesions were located immediately adjacent to the ventricles; in 92.5%, lesions were also found away from the ventricles.

The anatomical distribution of the lesions is given in Table 8.2.

Lesions are less well depicted within the cortex because the cortex gives a higher signal than the adjacent white matter at the frequencies used.

Table 8.2 *Distribution of MRI lesions in the white matter of 200 patients with clinically definite MS (%).*

Periventricular	98
Cella media	97
Trigonum	86
Posterior horn	75
Inferior horn	66
Anterior horn	59
Isolated lesions in white matter	93
Cortico–medullary junction	65
Internal capsule	42
Cortex	13
Basal ganglia	8
Brainstem	66
Pons	52
Mesencephalon	36
Medulla oblongata	36
Fourth ventricle	53
Cerebellum	57

Kesselring et al. (1989a).

The characteristic magnetic resonance image in MS patients consists of multifocal irregular lesions within the white matter, particularly at the border of the lateral ventricles and in the region of the cella media (Fig. 8.18).

Most of the lesions visible on the magnetic resonance image are clinically silent, as apparent from clinicopathological comparative examinations. It is often possible, however, to detect isolated lesions on MRI, the localizations of which precisely account for clinical symptoms. Thus correlations between clinical picture and pathological changes may be detected to a degree that is not achieved by any other method (Kesselring et al. 1989b; Miller et al., 1996, Fig. 8.19).

By comparing magnetic resonance images with postmortem preparations, it may be proven that lesions of increased signal intensity on MRI correspond exactly to histologically defined MS plaques. It is not absolutely certain whether the increased water content in the lesions or the glia reaction is responsible for this.

Ringlike appearances in plaques are interpreted as due to the presence of paramagnetic free radicals in the macrophage layer forming the margin of acute plaques (Powell et al. 1992).

Specificity

Multifocal periventricular lesions in the white matter which cannot be distinguished from those seen in MS may be detected in cerebro-

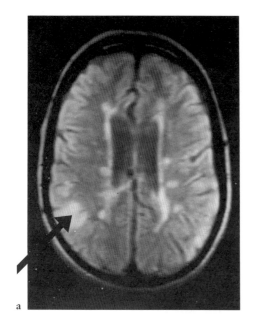

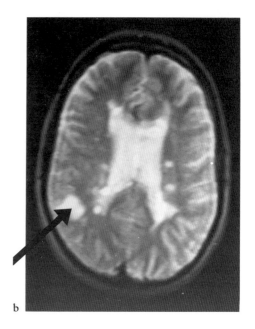

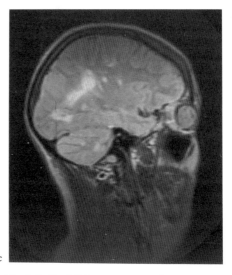

Fig. 8.18. Brain MRI of a patient with clinically definite MS (spin-echo sequence (SE): repetition time (TR) 2000 ms; echo time (TE) 60 ms). There are multiple lesions in the white matter, particularly along the lateral ventricles, as well as some discrete isolated lesions. The arrows point to a crescent-shaped subcortical lesion which is rarely seen outside the context of MS. (a) Axial "T_1 weighted" (TR 2000; TE 60). (b) Axial "T_2 weighted" (TR 2000; TE 120). (c) Sagittal (TR 2000; TE 60).

vascular disease (which, however, only rarely poses differential diagnostic problems), as well as in acute disseminated encephalomyelitis, in neurosarcoidosis, cerebral lupus, Behçet syndrome, and in tropical spastic paraparesis caused by HTLV-I. In all these conditions, which have to be differentiated from MS, lesions are rather less marked and their margins are quite smooth. In some cases, however, definite differentiation is not possible. In cerebral lupus, focal ischemic lesions may be seen on MRI; in neurosarcoidosis, there may be hydro-

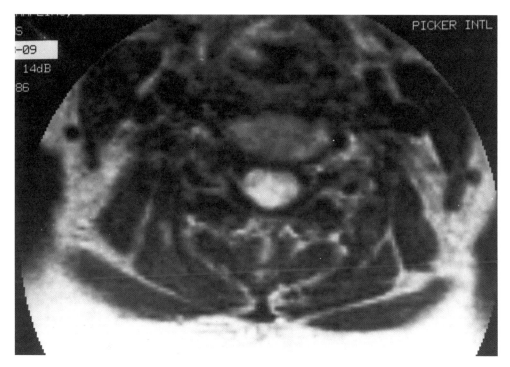

Fig. 8.19. Plaques in the posterior column of an MS patient with a syndrome of the "deafferented hand of Oppenheim" and unilaterally pathologically prolonged latencies in SEP.

cephalus or space occupying granulomata; and in Behçet syndrome, lesions in the brainstem region predominate. The evaluation of changes is complicated by the fact that similar lesions may be found in healthy people with increasing age. In controls who consider themselves to be healthy, unequivocal lesions in the white matter of the brain are found below the age of 50 years in 2%, below the age of 60 years in 24%, in the decade up to 70 years in 50%, and in all cases examined above the age of 70 years (Kesselring et al. 1989b). However, as long as the age and gender of the person examined are known, the danger of misinterpretation of periventricular hyperintensities on MRI is small (Yetkin et al. 1991).

Specificity may be significantly improved by accepting only a combination of at least three areas of increased signal and two of the following features, known as Fazekas' criteria: abutting body of lateral ventricles, infratentorial lesion location, and size greater than 5 mm (Offenbacher et al. 1993).

We have only seen crescent-shaped subcortical lesions (see Fig. 8.18) and multiple lesions in the cervical spinal cord in patients with definite MS (Fig. 8.20). Lesions in the corpus callosum, which are best depicted in sagittal sections with long repetition time and short echo time, appear to be particularly characteristic for MS, occurring in 93% of MS cases but only in 2.3% of control patients with other neurological diseases (Gean Marton et al. 1991).

For the diagnosis of MS, it is important to determine the age of the lesions visible on MRI. This is not possible with the naked eye, nor by measuring T_1 and T_2 relaxation times (Ormerod et al. 1987). Paramagnetic substances such as gadolinium DTPA play an important role in this respect. They change relaxation times within the tissue examined considerably, thereby improving contrast. The appearance of such an intravenously applied substance on the cerebral MRI indicates permeability of the blood–brain barrier (Fig. 8.21). Such contrast enhancement is found in most recent plaques in MS, whereas 4 to 6 weeks later it can no longer be detected (Miller et al. 1988a). Individual cases of MS have been reported in which enhancement was demonstrated in regions where no change could be observed on the unenhanced scan. Only 2 weeks later at the same site, a much

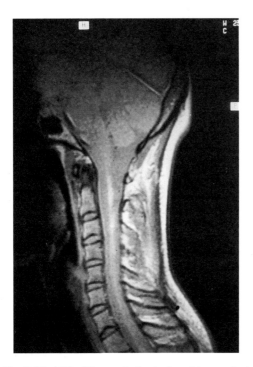

Fig. 8.20. MRI of the cervical spinal cord in a patient with clinically definite MS (TR 1500; TE 80; surface coil).

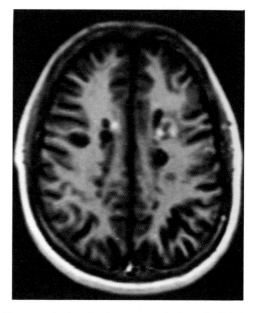

Fig. 8.21. Brain MRI of a patient with clinically definite MS. "Inversion recovery" after gadolinium-DPTA intravenously: single lesions enhance (bright), others do not (dark).

larger lesion was seen in an unenhanced T_2-weighted image (Kermode et al. 1990). This observation is important for the understanding of pathogenesis (see Chapter 5). It proves that opening of the blood–brain barrier is a prerequisite for the development of new plaques. Factors from the blood may penetrate into the CNS during this period of time. Disease activity as manifested by number, dimension, and age of the lesions may be followed by this method of serial examination with paramagnetic contrast agents (McFarland et al. 1992; Smith et al. 1993). A significant association can be demonstrated between periods of clinical worsening and MRI parameters including increases in total number, number of new lesions, and the total area of enhancement. Serial MRI with contrast enhancement contributes to a better understanding of pathogenesis (McDonald et al. 1992), and is a useful and reliable tool for evaluating therapeutic regimens (Gonzalez-Scarano et al. 1987; Willoughby et al. 1989; Miller et al. 1991; Barkhof et al. 1992). New lesions as detected by serial magnetic resonance examinations at 2-weekly intervals enlarge over 4 weeks

to their maximum dimension, and then shrink to a small signal change which cannot be distinguished from those seen in chronic lesions. The observation that new clinically asymptomatic lesions are detected so frequently on MRI points to the fact that the disease process, even with discrete clinical symptoms and signs, is much more active than was previously supposed. Therefore, serial MRI is extremely important for determining disease activity, and particularly for assessing therapeutic efficacy (Miller et al. 1991). Benign forms of MS are defined as cases with a score of less than three on the expanded disability status scale (EDSS, Kurtzke 1983a) 10 years after disease onset. They may be distinguished from chronic progressive forms on MRI by a smaller total area of the lesions and a more discrete tendency for confluence, and particularly by the fact that more clinically silent lesions are visible in benign forms. Chronic forms of MS differ considerably on serial MRI depending on whether they are primary or secondary progressive (secondary progressive cases are those in which relapses and remissions were present earlier in the disease course). In patients with secondary progressive MS, a mean of 18.2 new lesions per year have been found, 87% of which showed contrast enhancement. In the same number of patients with primary progressive MS observed over the same period of time, only 3.3 new lesions were detected, none of which was enhancing (A. J. Thompson et al. 1991). This study suggests that primary and secondary progressive forms of MS may be pathogenetically heterogeneous.

The future will show whether other techniques of magnetic resonance, such as magnetic resonance spectroscopy to detect different spectra within lesions of different ages (Arnold et al. 1990; Grossmann et al. 1992), or so-called lipid images for detecting myelin breakdown products (Hawkins et al. 1991), will allow for the more precise determination of the age of lesions and thus the activity of the disease.

A most important improvement in MR technology, as used in MS, is the examination of the spinal cord using multiarray coils and fast spin echo (Thorpe et al. 1993; Kidd et al. 1993). High resolution T_2-weighted sagittal images of the whole spinal cord may be obtained in about 5 minutes by this technique. Magnetic resonance imaging signal abnormalities within the spinal cord appear to be more specific for MS than cerebral white matter lesions, especially in subjects over 50 years old.

Without any doubt, MRI has facilitated the diagnosis of MS considerably, and has provided new insight into the pathogenesis of the disease (McDonald 1992; McDonald et al. 1992).

Magnetic resonance imaging in optic neuropathies and clinically isolated brainstem and spinal cord syndromes

The high magnetic resonance signal produced normally by fat tissue may be suppressed by using special sequences and specially adapted surface coils which focus the outer magnetic field onto the region of interest. For depicting the orbit and its contents, STIR sequence (inversion recovery with short inversion time) with surface coils has been developed. Isolated lesions within the optic nerve may be detected by this technique in over 80% of patients with acute or chronic optic neuritis (Miller et al. 1986; 1988b). Visual evoked potentials are more sensitive in this respect (see p. 93), but on MRI other pathological processes may be demonstrated which may lead to visual loss and delayed latency VEPs. Concerning recovery of visual acuity, prognosis of optic neuritis depends on the

length and localization of the lesion as visible on MRI: prognosis is worse for longer and intracanalicular lesions. Prognosis as to dissemination of the disease process cannot be determined by this anatomical detail (Youl et al. 1991).

In terms of diagnosis, and in particular prognosis, it is of interest to note that 60% to 70% of cases show lesions on MRI of the brain within the first few weeks after clinically isolated optic neuritis (Ormerod et al. 1987; Miller et al. 1988b). This method is far superior to all others for detecting separated lesions. The detection of these lesions in this way indicates a worse prognosis as far as further dissemination of the disease process is concerned. In serial examinations after 1 year, new lesions are found in over 50% of patients whose brain MRIs were abnormal at the time of the acute optic neuritis. Of course, not all of these lesions manifest themselves clinically. At follow-up after 5 years, progression to clinically definite MS occurs in over 60% of cases with an abnormal MRI at presentation, and only in about 3% of patients for whom initial brain MRI was normal (Morrissey et al. 1993).

Similar problems concerning diagnosis, differential diagnosis, and prognosis occur in isolated brainstem and spinal cord syndromes which also may be a first manifestation of MS. Multiple sclerosis lesions may be detected on MRI in the region of the brainstem and cervical spinal cord using special sequences, particularly T_2-weighted images with corresponding adapted surface coils (Thorpe et al. 1993; Kidd et al. 1993). It is of particular importance to detect lesions which are amenable to surgical therapy and which may produce a clinical picture similar to that of MS.

Changes described on MRI of the brain may be demonstrated at the time of first examination in one third of acute isolated spinal cord syndromes, in two thirds of chronic spinal cord syndromes, and in three quarters of cases with isolated brainstem syndromes.

CEREBROSPINAL FLUID

Production of immunoglobulins within inflammatory plaques in the CNS is part of the clinical picture of MS (see Chapters 2 and 3). Because these plaques are in contact with spaces filled with CSF, the examination of CSF provides information as to the amount and the qualitative composition of newly formed proteins. Instead of evaluating single findings of CSF examination, each requiring its own differential diagnosis, it is more useful to determine a CSF profile from the examinations of a large number of clinically definite MS cases or cases verified at post mortem. When the CSF profile as derived from definite cases is inconclusive in a single case, it has to be checked in long-term studies. Only in such cases are paraclinical investigations important for confirming the diagnosis or for indicating the prognosis.

The following parameters in CSF are best established by laboratory investigations supporting the clinical diagnosis of MS: oligoclonal bands of IgG, daily synthesis rate of IgG inside the blood–brain barrier, and dimensionless quotients which compare levels of albumin and IgG in serum and CSF. A slight pleocytosis, a change in the permeability of the blood–brain barrier, and the detection of myelin breakdown products such as MBP, do not differentiate clearly enough between MS cases and non-MS cases.

The combination of these elements of the CSF profile increases the predictability for MS to over 95% (Tourtellotte and Walsh 1984; Ebers 1984).

Cerebrospinal fluid profile in multiple sclerosis (Tourtellotte and Walsh 1984)

1. Appearance: clear and colorless.
2. Pressure: normal (<20 cmH$_2$O).
3. Number of cells: normal in two thirds of cases (<50 cells/mm^3).
4. Albumin: normal (<55 g/l) in 77%; (<65 g/l in 99%).
5. CSF IgG index {[IgG$_L$/albumin$_S$]}: >0.7 in 90% (normal <0.66). (L = CSF; S = serum).
6. Oligoclonal IgG (IEF, immune fixation, silver staining): present in $>90\%$.
7. IgG de novo synthesis per day (normal 3 mg/day): increased in 90%.
8. MBP in CSF: increased (depending on time of relapses) in 50% to 70%.

Comment

1. CSF in transverse myelitis may rarely be yellowish and opaque (Froin syndrome).
2. CSF pressure is almost always normal in MS except in transverse myelitis. It may be slightly increased during acute exacerbations.

3. More than 50 cells/mm^3 should raise doubts as to the diagnosis of MS. The cell number does not change significantly over the course of the disease.

4. An albumin concentration greater than 65 g/l in the CSF should raise doubts as to the diagnosis. Albumin within CSF is produced by capillaries in the choroid plexus and may be used as an indication of integrity of the blood–brain barrier. This is often slightly disturbed in the neighborhood of recent plaques.

5. A simple formula of the rate of intrathecally synthesized IgG and the integrity of the blood–brain barrier (Ganrot and Laurell 1974) is taken into consideration in the IgG index by comparing concentrations of IgG and albumin in CSF and serum respectively. Instead of giving a normal value (usually 0.66–0.7), which is exceeded in more than 90% of patients with clinically definite MS, this index may also be used for indicating diagnostic probability: the population with numerous diagnoses other than MS (n = 373) had significantly lower index values than the population with clinically definite MS (n = 93). Because of the overlap of both groups, it appears to be more sensible to determine for each value the probability for and against MS instead of fixing a limit between normal and pathological. At a value of 0.66, the probabilities for and against MS are equal. Increasing the index by 0.36 increases the risk of MS by a factor of 10 (Kesselring J and Ketz E, unpublished data, Fig. 8.22).

6. Oligoclonal bands not present in the serum may be detected in over 90% of cases with clinically definite MS on IgG electrophoresis of CSF (Fig. 8.23). These bands correspond to antibodies produced intrathecally by only a few plasma cell clones. It has only recently become possible to determine specificity of these antibodies. In single plaques, various oligoclonal bands may be found which are produced by various plasma cell clones (Mattson et al. 1980; Mehta et al. 1982). This fact alone does not prove that they are "non-sense proteins" due to an erroneous regulation of the immune system. Even after experimental immunization with a single antigen, various antibodies may be formed which produce heterogeneous oligoclonal bands in serum and CSF. These bands remain relatively constant in a patient over the course of the disease, and they are only slightly modified or diminished by immunosuppression.

RQ

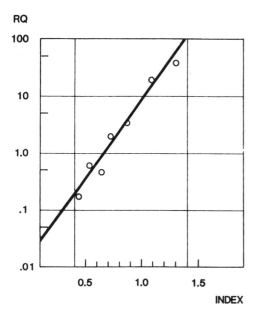

Fig. 8.22. Risk quotient (RQ) in relation to immuno-globulin index. An RQ of 1 means that the risks for and against MS are equal. With an RQ of 10, it is ten times more probable that MS is present than another condition (see text).

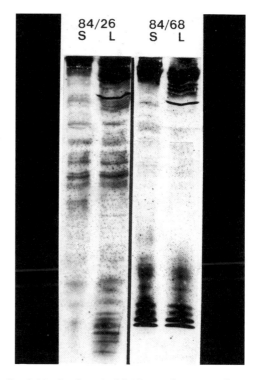

Fig. 8.23. Cerebrospinal fluid (l) and serum (S) electro-phoresis in a patient with MS (left, 84/26) and in a pa-tient with a disturbance of the blood–brain barrier (right, 84/68). Oligoclonal bands are visible only in the CSF of the patient with MS, whereas identical bands are visible in CSF as well as in the serum from the other patient. (With kind permission of the late Professor Claus Meier, Bern.)

Initially, determination of oligoclonal bands in CSF of patients with clinically definite MS (see p. 88) was mainly important for establish-ing the method of isoelectric focusing. Now it is more important to determine its value in early and possible MS cases and to know the differ-ential diagnosis of positive findings. In patients with monosymptomatic demyelinating lesions, dissemination of the disease process in those with oligoclonal bands in CSF more often oc-curs over a longer period of observation than in patients with similar lesions without this find-ing in CSF (Moulin et al. 1983). This is also true for isolated optic neuritis (see Chapter 7).

Oligoclonal bands are present in 80% of the rare cases (less than 10%) in which MS begins after the age of 50 years and may not be diag-nosed with established criteria (Poser et al. 1983; 1984) as it becomes manifest as chronic progressive myelopathy. Their presence sup-ports the laboratory diagnosis of probable MS (Noseworthy et al. 1983; see p. 88).

False-positive findings of oligoclonal bands in CSF occur in less than 10% of neurological diseases other than MS. The clinical differential diagnosis presents no difficulty in more than half of these cases. Differentiation from MS

may be difficult in cases which are also accom-panied by intrathecal immune reaction, such as viral meningitis and encephalitis, myelitis, para-neoplastic syndromes, sarcoidosis, lupus erythe-matosus, etc. (Ebers 1984; see also Chapter 11).

Apart from agar gel and polyacrylamide elec-trophoresis available in most laboratories in which CSF is examined, isoelectric focusing is more sensitive for detecting oligoclonal bands. Protein fractions of limited heterogeneity are particularly efficiently analyzed. This is there-fore the technique of choice for searching for oligoclonal bands in CSF of MS patients (Walsh and Tourtellotte 1983; Ebers 1984; Tourtellotte and Walsh 1984).

Two-dimensional electrophoresis of CSF (Wiederkehr et al. 1986) is a promising new de-velopment of the method which is still very ex-pensive but which allows more detailed analy-sis of CSF proteins occurring in MS.

7. Determination of IgG de novo synthesis within the blood–brain barrier (intrathecal) each day brings no significant diagnostic advantage compared to isoelectric focusing or the much easier determination of IgG index.

8. Myelin basic protein in CSF indicates the degree of demyelination within the CNS. It is found in over 80% of MS patients in close temporal relationship to a clinical exacerbation, and its concentration is said to parallel the severity of clinical symptoms (Thompson et al. 1985). Patients in whom MBP remains detectable during remission after an exacerbation (a quarter of cases) are at much greater risk of developing a new exacerbation than those in whom MBP was no longer detectable during remission.

Antibodies against antigens of neurogenic viruses such as measles, rubella, and herpes zoster are found in the CSF of 80% of MS patients (Felgenhauer et al. 1985). Their detection may be useful in differential diagnosis as they are not present in some other inflammatory CNS diseases.

Free light chains of immunoglobulins produced by separate cell clones may be found in CSF of MS patients. They do not appear in other neurological diseases, and their pathogenetic significance is not clear (Rudick et al. 1986).

The observation that terminal components of complement (C9) are significantly more often found to be low in the CSF of MS patients compared to patients with other neurological diseases (Morgan et al. 1984) is of particular interest. The quotient formed from analogy of this protein with the IgG index allows a clearer differentiation between patients with MS and those with other neurological diseases. The interest of this observation stems not only from its diagnostic usefulness, but also from its possible implications for a better understanding of pathogenesis. A reduction in the main component of complement in CSF of MS patients could indicate that it had been consumed during the formation of immune complexes against myelin sheaths within the CNS.

Examination of haptoglobin polymers in CSF which are mainly produced in the liver and not in the CNS is of importance for detecting disturbances of the blood–brain barrier (Takeoka et al. 1983). It may be shown thereby that the blood–brain barrier is often disturbed in MS patients (in approximately 50% of cases with recent plaques), as had been assumed by comparing serum and CSF concentrations of other proteins (see also Chapter 5).

Antibodies against a soluble cerebellar lectin (CSL) are reported to be found regularly (in 93.5% of cases) in MS and in less than 10% of controls below the age of 60 years (Zanetta et al. 1990). This finding would seem to be a characteristic of the disease which could be used diagnostically. However, it should first be confirmed in other laboratories. The CSL molecules form bridges between glycoprotein glycanes on the surface of myelin-forming cells in the peripheral and central nervous systems, and play an important role during normal myelination. Antibodies directed against CSL could be involved in demyelination.

Tumor necrosis factor alpha, so-called kachectin, appears to be a parameter of CSF which allows for the reliable differentiation between chronic progressive and stable MS (Sharief and Hentges 1991). This factor was found in other investigations to be an indicator for triggering exacerbations (Chofflon et al. 1992).

DISCUSSING THE DIAGNOSIS

There is no single opinion among physicians as to whether, when, and how patients should be told the diagnosis of MS. Those physicians who do not reveal the diagnosis – "Certainly it is not a brain tumor," "a sort of inflammation in the spinal cord," "Probably only a virus" – fail to do so in an attempt to avoid the anxiety and depression which follow the disclosure of the diagnosis of a chronic disease with an unpredictable course. Certainly, in such cases the fear of being unable to influence the course of the disease with an effective therapy may play a role. Also, many of these physicians know that the first reaction of a patient who is told the diagnosis may be to reproach the physician. Patients are often unable clearly to formulate their questions concerning the disease, particularly during its early phases. This may be interpreted by physicians as the patients' wish not to be informed more precisely. However, it is understandable that questions are imprecise, or are not asked at all, in the psychologically difficult situation which is produced when patients, following not particularly pleasant examinations, are confronted with a medical expert who gives them the diagnosis of an incurable disease, or when they are exposed on a medical ward to other patients or to a crowd of more or less involved physicians and students. However, it would be completely wrong to deduce from these experiences that patients do not want to know their diagnosis.

Convincing studies concerning this subject have been published (Gorman et al. 1984; Elian and Dean 1985). Patients with MS were asked about the time and the way in which they were told of their diagnosis. Less than 4% thought that they would not want to know the diagnosis, "because it does not matter anyway"; 13% gave no opinion. The overwhelming majority (83% of 167 people questioned) declared that the only acceptable way was for the physician concerned – "at best a competent neurologist" – to explain the diagnosis clearly as soon as it had been established: "The earlier the diagnosis is known, the better one can cope with the disease." Several declared in retrospect that they would have planned some things in their lives differently if they had known the diagnosis earlier. Others had not dared to ask for social support: "because a 'transient inflammation of the nerves' would not be a sufficient justification for that." For many patients, it is also important to know the correct name of their disease in order to explain themselves to relatives and other people who suspect "idleness, drunkenness or mental disease." Most patients who thought that the diagnosis should be openly told were of the opinion that everybody has the right to know "what is going on with them."

If physicians have asked themselves "Can the patient afford to know the diagnosis?", they have to ask themselves in the light of the patients' opinions, "Can the patient afford *not* to know the diagnosis?" (Elian and Dean 1985).

It is not good enough for patients if the diagnosis is concealed or if they discover it by chance. If the diagnosis is established according to the criteria and auxillary examinations described in this chapter, patients should be told of it by their physician in charge, preferably in the presence of a close relative or partner. The presence of other medical personnel at this moment is not desired by most patients (Gorman et al. 1984). It is not a satisfactory solution to tell the diagnosis to relatives and to conceal it from the person affected. It is an injustice to the latter, and too heavy a burden for the former. Enough time has to be set aside to answer the questions of patients and their relatives. It is often appropriate to organize a short hospital stay for this reason, to talk about the diagnosis and its consequences as much as necessary.

Undoubtedly, the process of adaptation to a disease such as MS will require much more time than is available even during a hospital stay. It is a long endeavor which, as with all adaptation processes after a loss, passes through different stages. In the case of MS, the loss of certain capabilities and future possibilities requires adaptation. The patient will go through stages of denial, anger, and resistance, possibly to final acceptance. It is important during this long process that the affected person can trust a physician who is prepared to support him or her. The physician's most important task only begins after the diagnosis has been revealed. In the time following this, and repeated discussion about its consequences on the life of the affected person, the basis of the future relationship between the physician and the patient is established.

If early symptoms are present which may be indications of MS but which do not allow for a definite diagnosis, for example optic neuritis or isolated spinal cord syndrome, the patient should be informed about the findings, but the differential diagnostic considerations should only be mentioned if asked about specifically. If, however, the diagnosis is established, there is no reason not to reveal it. However, it is particularly important that in the first discussions about the disease, not only is the diagnosis considered as a label, but a realistic picture of the disease be drawn which includes discussions of prognostically benign forms. These tend to be less extensively described in the medical literature and the lay press, which are likely to be consulted immediately by the affected person.

Not knowing the whole truth about this disease, and therefore being unable to tell it to the patient, our attitudes and actions should be guided by veracity.

9

Disease course

Studies of the natural disease course of MS are decisively dependent on the reliability of the diagnosis. Until 1983 (Poser et al. 1983; 1984), diagnosis was almost exclusively based on clinical criteria (Schumacher et al. 1965; McDonald and Halliday 1977; see also Chapter 8). In most earlier investigations into the course of the disease, diagnostic criteria were used which probably contained several sources of error when compared to pathological data. The quality of the conclusions drawn from earlier studies is limited by the inability to detect the early stages of the disease and to plan a true prospective investigation. Furthermore, it is unavoidable that individual cases cannot be followed and documented over a sufficiently long period of time by an individual observer. Even in particularly careful studies, errors of documentation may occur in 10% to 30%. Single studies describe heterogeneous groups of patients, with selection bias being introduced deliberately or due to external factors. Therefore conclusions drawn from studies of patients with relapsing remitting disease may not be compared directly with those from cases verified at post mortem or with information gained exclusively from military personnel or sampled in only one center. Despite these reservations, some facts concerning MS may be described, at least on a statistical basis.

It has been known since the first descriptions of the disease that MS may occur primarily with relapses and remissions, and may later run a (secondary) chronic progressive course, or, particularly when disease onset is in the higher age group, it may run a primarily progressive course without single separate exacerbations. It is therefore necessary to define terms such as relapse, exacerbation, remission, and progression, and to suggest how these may be quantified. The terms bout, attack, and episode are often used synonymously: the definitions of these terms are particularly important when they are applied in study protocols comparing various therapies.

AGE AT DISEASE ONSET

From the clinical standpoint, it is justifiable to define the onset of the disease as the point at which it manifests itself in such a way that the affected person contacts a physician who makes a "highly probable" diagnosis.

The first symptoms and signs of the disease most commonly occur in adults between the 20th and 40th years of age, and this was confirmed in a study in which 70% of patients developed the disease during this period of their lives (Confavreux et al. 1980; Fig. 9.1).

Comparable studies from areas with high prevalence show the frequency of disease onset rising steeply during adolescence, culminating around the 30th year of age (mean 29 to 33 years; Matthews 1991), and decreasing rapidly in the 4th and 5th decades. In women, the maximum frequency of disease onset is reached a little earlier than in men.

On average in our patients, disease onset was 32.4 (+/− 11.0) years. In women, onset was, at 31.6 (+/− 11.1) years, significantly (p < 0.005) earlier than in men, at 33.7 (+/− 10.7) years. In 10.9% of cases, disease onset occurred before the age of 20, and in 6.8% after the age of 50.

Age at onset in primary relapsing remitting forms was 28.8 (+/−3.3) years; in remitting progressive (secondary progressive) forms, 37.7 (+/− 10.4) years; and in primary progressive forms, 40.4 (+/− 11/3) years. Therefore, mean age at onset in relapsing remitting forms is highly significantly below that of secondary progressive forms, which itself is highly significantly below that of the primary progressive form. In 40% of the cases with disease onset

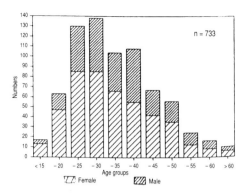

Fig. 9.1. Age at onset of disease.

after the 40th year of age, MS runs a chronic progressive course, whereas this form of the disease occurs in less than 10% of patients with disease onset below the age of 40.

In earlier studies, disease onset before the 10th year of age was assumed to occur in up to 10% of cases (Wechsler 1922). However, since the work of Muller (1951), the proportion has remained quite constant in all studies at 0.3%. There is the possibility that in retrospective studies like these, early symptoms may not be taken seriously by patients or may not be recognized by a physician who is considering a broad differential diagnosis. In the literature, convincing descriptions of individual cases can be found in which manifestations of the disease occurred in childhood and adolescence, and for which observation over a course of many years showed fulfilment of all the criteria of definite MS (Brandt et al. 1981; Hauser et al. 1982; Bye et al. 1985; Bauer and Hanefeld 1993). Female preponderance in childhood MS is even more marked than in adult cases (Izquierdo et al. 1985). Symptoms may differ in cases with earlier onset in that neurological deficits originating in the brainstem, and particularly dizziness as an initial symptom, occur more frequently. The diagnosis may be made even in this age group on the basis of clinical criteria with auxillary paraclinical findings, as in adult forms (Boutin et al. 1988).

As it is known from pathological studies made at post mortem that MS may be present in older people without any disease of the CNS having been apparent during their lifetime (Georgi 1961a; Phadke and Best 1983; Gilbert and Sadler 1983), it is important when counselling patients that they are made aware of the

benign forms of MS. These studies prove that the process leading to the typical pathological anatomical changes of the disease does not necessarily become manifest clinically. These factors indicate that MS may certainly be present in older people (Noseworthy et al. 1983; Lyon-Caën et al. 1985; Hooge and Redekop 1992). The precise frequency of such late cases cannot be assessed for the reasons mentioned. When considering reports that more than 10% of first manifestations occurring above the age of 40 years, or that the disease may start in individual patients at the age of 70 or more, it should not be forgotten that history taking in older patients is often not very reliable, and for most of them a broad differential diagnosis has to be applied as diagnosis is not always possible on clinical grounds alone. Even with the most reliable auxillary method of MS diagnosis (MRI), the differentiation between age-related "normal" changes and "typical" MS plaques is not reliable (Ormerod et al. 1987; Miller et al., in press; see also Chapter 8). Nevertheless, there is no doubt that cases of definite MS may become manifest for the first time in higher age groups (Noseworthy et al. 1983; Lyon-Caën et al. 1985; Hooge and Redekop 1992; Bauer and Hanefeld 1993), and differential diagnosis of CNS diseases deserves consideration in older people, particularly when there are progressive spastic gait disturbances (see Chapter 11).

RELAPSING REMITTING COURSE

McAlpine's definition of relapse (McAlpine 1972), reported in the new editions of his book edited by Matthews (1991), is as follows: the occurrence of a new symptom, or the recurrence of a symptom previously present. Symptoms should be considered to be an expression of a relapse if they can be explained as due to a new lesion within the CNS or to reactivation of lesions previously present (Poser 1980). Transient worsening of established deficits lasting only minutes or hours, such as occur with changes in temperature, fatigue, or psychological stress, should be differentiated. This differentiation is important for clinical assessment, and a limit of 24 to 48 hours' duration may be justified (Schumacher et al. 1965; Poser et al. 1984). Situations are well known in which visual disturbances of only a few hours' duration were followed by persistent delays of latencies of VEPs. Despite the only transient symptoms, these have to be viewed as an expression of a newly formed plaque if the activity of the disease process cannot be objectivated and measured. Arbitrarily defined assessment criteria, based on clinical experience, are still appropriate. Clinical manifestations are only accepted as being due to a new relapse if at least 4 weeks (Poser et al. 1983) or, more prudently, 6 months (Ormerod et al. 1987; Kesselring et al. 1990) have passed since the last relapse (see also Chapter 8).

Relapse rate

Very variable frequencies of relapses, as defined above, are reported within a given time period, for example 1 year. These differences, from 0.2 to 1.15 relapses per year, are not only due to the various disease forms, but also depend on the investigations applied. In general, systematic investigations confirm the clinical impression that relapse rate is highest in the first 5 years, and particularly in the first year, after onset of the disease, and decreases spontaneously thereafter (Muller 1951; Confavreux et al. 1980; Matthews 1991). As an example, Lhermitte et al. (1973) found 0.5 relapses per year in the first 5 years, and only half of that number (0.26 per year) in the following 5-year periods.

Overall, a relapse is a rare event over the whole course of the disease, and occurs on average between once per year and once every 4 years (Matthews 1991). Therefore, relapse rate alone is not an appropriate measure for determining disease activity or for assessing therapeutic effects.

Factors triggering or related to relapses

Considering the significance of a relapse in the life of the person affected, it is important to examine the factors triggering relapses. Retrospectively, factors may be recognized which have a close temporal relationship to a relapse. These are often considered to be causally related, although they are often events of only limited importance in normal daily life. Further studies are needed to clarify the role of trauma as a possible triggering factor.

Reliable indications may only be derived from prospective studies (Sibley et al. 1984). Relapses occur more frequently in spring and summer months, compared to fall and winter months. Although this seasonal difference may be accepted as a factor (Bamford et al. 1983), it cannot be explained in terms of a known infectious disease, nor by changes of disease intensity due to temperature according to the definition of a relapse given above.

Common infections such as influenza or unspecific diarrhea appear to be rarer in MS patients compared to controls. If they do occur, however, they often do so in close temporal relationship to a relapse (Sibley et al. 1984): nearly half of the relapses were registered within a period of risk (2 weeks before and 5 weeks after infection), and nearly half of the infections were followed by relapses. Extrapolated yearly relapse rate in such risk periods is three times as high as in periods in which no infectious diseases occur. Therefore, it may be inferred that even common infections may play a role in triggering MS relapses. Their place in the pathogenetic chain, however, has not yet been clarified.

Cases in which new relapses of MS occur after vaccinations often lead to considerable uncertainty. Although relapses may occur in close temporal, and probably causal, relationship to various vaccinations, this appears to be such a rare event that MS patients should not be advised against well-indicated vaccinations.

Since fertility is not compromised by MS, female MS patients carry as many pregnancies as healthy women (on average 2.04). The course of MS is influenced by pregnancies in a consistent way (Birk and Rudick 1986): an overview of studies concludes that during the period of pregnancy, significantly fewer relapses occur, and the last trimester, particularly, is a relatively protected period. This fact supports the assumption of immunopathogenesis of MS since several immunosuppressing mechanisms are active during pregnancy (Birk and Rudick 1986). However, during puerperium and the following months, manifestations of new relapses occur in 20% to 40% of patients. These do not influence the degree of disability in disease of long duration in comparison to patients who have not been pregnant, nor does the number of pregnancies influence the degree of disability in the long term (D. S. Thompson et al. 1986). There is no higher rate of malformation of children of mothers with MS.

The role of trauma in the development of MS and as a trigger for relapses was accepted in all retrospective investigations since, in McAlpine's series of 250 patients (McAlpine 1961), trauma was recorded in the case histories of 14%, and in only 5% of a control group of equal size. It may be assumed, however, that trauma occurring in close temporal relationship to the appearance of neurological symptoms will be remembered more easily than, for example, that occurring before appendicitis (Matthews 1991). More recent controlled and prospective studies (Bamford et al. 1981; Sibley et al. 1984) show that traumatic events are not found more often in the lives of MS patients than in those of comparable healthy people. Individual cases in which trauma has occurred in close temporal relationship to the onset of a relapse will be found repeatedly, leading to the temptation to accept a causal relationship. However, this is not upheld statistically. The same holds true for operations and lumbar punctures.

Often, psychological stress is mentioned as a triggering factor in MS relapses, but it is questionable whether such a common phenomenon may be responsible for causing a disease which, overall, is relatively rare. Differing reports are found in systematic investigations. In earlier studies, groups of patients with MS were compared to patients with other organic neurological diseases (Pratt 1951) or with healthy people, and no differences were found with regard to indications of specific psychological stress. However, more recent investigations (Warren et al. 1982; Grant 1986) have found a more frequent occurrence of factors in the life histories of MS patients which may lead to particular psychological stress (see Chapter 7).

Remission

It is more difficult to determine the end of a relapse and the transition to remission than to define its onset. Individual symptoms may increase in intensity during a phase of the disease, while others wane or remain the same. It is therefore impossible to define precisely the duration of a relapse, and figures ranging from 24 hours to 12 months may be found. As a rule, in an individual patient, subsequent relapses last longer than the initial one. A complete remission is reached when all manifestations of the disease which were observed during the relapse have completely disappeared. Remissions are often partial.

As a rule of thumb resulting from longer prospective studies (Kurtzke et al. 1968), a complete remission of manifestations of a relapse is found in half of patients, partial remission in a quarter, and no remission at all in a further quarter of cases. If clinical symptoms develop within 24 hours, complete remission can be expected to occur within 1 month in at least 70%.

Symptoms present for 2 months remit in 85% of patients, those present for 3 months in 30%, and those present for 6 months in only 10%. If symptoms persist for 2 years, remission cannot be expected (Kurtzke et al. 1968; 1977; Matthews 1991).

Sequelae of a relapse depend on the speed of development of clinical manifestations as well as on the duration and the severity of symptoms. Severe short-lasting deficits recover completely (95%) more often than milder ones (40%) of the same duration. Severe deficits recover better (29%) than milder ones (12%) when manifestations are long lasting (Kurtzke et al. 1968). For the patients, however, an incomplete recovery of severe deficits may be more disabling than the persistence of milder ones. Symptoms due to smaller plaques, such as optic neuritis, vertigo, double vision, and deficits of cranial nerve function in general, show a better tendency for remission. They become rarer with longer disease duration than do manifestations due to deficits of long tracts, and particularly of cerebellar function which, according to general experience (Matthews 1991), remit less completely. Sensory deficits may last for a long time; as a rule, they are less disabling because patients may become habituated. This, however, is not equal to recovery.

PRIMARY AND SECONDARY PROGRESSIVE COURSES

A primary progressive course of MS in which no individual relapses may be differentiated is found more often when disease onset is in the higher age group (Table 9.1, Confavreux et al. 1980; A. J. Thompson et al. 1991). Progressive spastic paraparesis (spinal MS) increases steadily over months and years, and may lead to increasing disability and handicap. In such cases, particular attention has to be paid to diagnostic differentiation from potentially curable causes of compression of the spinal cord (see Chapter 11). As with other forms of the disease, lesions may occur anywhere in the CNS and may lead to corresponding deficits. In more than half of the cases of isolated spinal cord syndromes

Table 9.1 *Clinical characteristics of exacerbating remitting and chronic progressive courses of MS*

	Primary exacerbating remitting	Chronic progressive
Frequency (%)	59*	18*
Gender (f : m)	1.9 : 1	1.3 : 1
Age at onset (years)	28	40
Main initial symptoms	Visual disturbances Sensory disturbances	Gait disturbances Pareses
Progression index (Kurtzke scale/ disease duration, see Chapter 10)	0.4	1.2

*23 percent remitting progressive (secondary progressive), i.e. exacerbating remitting course during at least ten years and then transition into chronic progression (gender relationship 1.3 : 1).

leading to progressive parapareses in which spinal cord compression has been excluded, multiple foci are found on brain MRI at the initial investigation (Ormerod et al. 1987). It may therefore be assumed that the majority of isolated chronic progressive spinal cord syndromes without compression are due to MS. It is much more probable that in isolated spinal cord syndromes the diagnosis of MS will be confirmed subsequently if oligoclonal bands are found in CSF at initial presentation (Moulin et al. 1983).

Secondary progressive or remitting progressive MS involves cases in which chronic progression of symptoms is observed at least 10 years after a pattern of relapses and remissions. These forms of the disease are found more frequently with longer duration of observation.

It is probable that the principal disease process of MS is chronic progressive, and that in relapses a threshold is crossed which makes clinical manifestations possible. The regularity of the basal progressive course may be described by mathematic models as linear, parabolic, or exponential. Clinical observations of an individual case may correspond to such models if continued over a sufficiently long period of time. Based on the dynamics of the disease during the first years in at least three quarters of cases, the further course may be extrapolated reliably.

FREQUENCY OF VARIOUS COURSES

In our epidemiological investigation of 1016 MS patients in the Canton Bern, Switzerland (Beer and Kesselring 1988; 1994), we found characteristics of primary and secondary progressive courses as described in Table 9.1. Based on extensive and detailed comparison with the literature, we consider this study to be representative.

10

Prognosis

LIFE EXPECTANCY

In the older literature on MS, disease duration from diagnosis to death is regularly reported as between 13 and 20 years (for overview, see Matthews 1991). The life expectancy of MS patients used to be considered to be reduced by 14 to 18 years compared to that of the average population. According to more recent studies (Confavreux et al. 1980; Phadke 1987), an average disease duration of at least 25 to 39 years may be expected; in a third of cases it is longer than 30 years. At the turn of the century, only 10 of 200 MS patients lived longer than 20 years, and only 2 of those longer than 30 years (Bramwell 1917). Nowadays, the average probable lifespan of MS patients 10 years after onset of the disease may be reduced by approximately 10 years in comparison to the normal population. Only in patients with disease onset after the 50th year of life is mean life expectancy 10 years after disease onset reduced, by 44% for men, and by 22% for women compared to members of the average population (Phadke 1987).

A good indicator of survival time after disease onset is the length of the interval between the first and the next relapse: of patients dying within 10 years after disease onset, all had had their second relapse within 2 years after disease onset, whereas in almost half of the patients alive 40 years after disease onset, the interval between the first and second relapse was more than 10 years (Phadke 1987).

Prognosis concerning the probability of survival after a certain period of time is determined most decisively by the actual degree of disability (Malmgren et al. 1981; Phadke 1987). The percentages of patients alive after 10 years are: 94% of those without disability; 80% of those with discrete disability; 69% of those with moderate disability; and only 28% of those with severe disability.

Brain MRI at presentation in clinically isolated syndromes suggestive of MS is a powerful predictor of the clinical course over the next 5 years (Morrissey et al. 1993). In clinically isolated syndromes of optic nerves, brainstem, or spinal cord, progression to MS had occurred in over 60% of cases with an abnormal initial brain MRI, and in only 3% of those with a normal MRI.

CAUSES OF DEATH

Only very rarely is MS the immediate cause of death, when a plaque in the respiratory center causes paralysis of respiration. In more than half the cases, the cause of death is due indirectly to the disease and more directly to bronchopneumonia, pyelonephritis, uremia, or sepsis (Leibowitz et al. 1969; Allen et al. 1978; Malmgren et al. 1981; 1983).

PROGNOSIS OF PROGRESSION

For affected people it is important to obtain reliable information about the risk of progression of the disease. For assessing disability we use (Beer and Kesselring 1988) the EDSS (Kurtzke 1983a; see also Appendix). The scale ranges from 0.0 to 10.0: a score of 0.0 means no disability; 10.0 exitus letalis due to the disease. For the calculation of progression of the disease, a progression index (PI) may be formed relating the Kurtzke scale to disease duration: PI = Kurtzke score/disease duration (years).

The following limitations have to be considered.

- No calculation of PI can be made during the first year of disease in order to avoid very high indices resulting from very short disease duration.
- No calculation can be made based on disability during a relapse because this would indi-

Table 10.1 *Initial symptoms and progression of MS*

Symptoms	Progression index
Gait disturbances	0.87
Pareses	0.83
Vertigo	0.82
Sensory disturbances	0.77
Sphincter disturbances	0.66
Visual disturbances	0.50

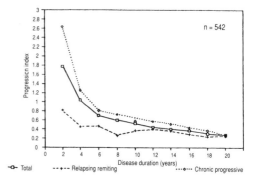

Fig. 10.1. Progression of MS in relation to disease duration.

cate a degree of disability which was temporarily unrealistically high.

In our large group of MS patients, a mean progression index of 0.67 was found, i.e., an average increase by 0.6 points on the Kurtzke scale per year. By extrapolation, this means that MS in our patients leads to wheelchair dependency on average after 10 years.

In a large group of MS patients in another hospital (Confavreux et al. 1980), 50% were ambulatory 6 years after disease onset, 25% after 15 years; 10% were severely disabled after 5 years, 25% after 10 years, and 15% after 15 years. In interpreting such figures it has to be considered that progression in patients from an epidemiological area is markedly slower and, on average, 0.2 points below patients examined in a hospital.

Progression indices differ significantly according to age at onset of the disease: with disease onset before the 30th year of age, PI is markedly lower (0.59) than with disease onset after the 40th year of age (0.92). The most rapid progression is found with disease onset after the 60th year (1.83). These differences are due to the fact that, in patients with a higher age at disease onset, the disease more often follows a chronic progressive course which itself is progressing more rapidly (see above).

The initial symptoms only partially facilitate an estimate of the further course and prognosis (Table 10.1). A more benign course is to be expected when the clinical picture is dominated initially by isolated brainstem symptoms (Phadke 1987), or optic neuropathy (Hutchinson 1976; Phadke 1987), and when initial symptoms appear rapidly and remit within 1 month (Kraft et al. 1981). Cerebellar and pyramidal deficits at disease onset are prognostically less favorable (Kraft et al. 1981; Visscher et al. 1984; S. Poser et al. 1986; Phadke 1987). As to the value of senso-

ry deficits as prognostic indicators, reports are contradictory in that more favorable (Visscher et al. 1984) and less favorable (Phadke 1987) prognoses are reported. In the latter, however, prognosis is probably determined more by pyramidal deficits present together with sensory dysfunctions.

The progression index depends significantly on the various disease forms: in our patient group it was 0.35 in relapsing remitting cases, 0.84 in secondary progressive, and 1.16 in primary progressive cases. In practical terms, these figures mean that for patients with primary relapsing remitting MS, wheelchair dependency is expected after an average of 20 years of disease duration, whereas patients with a primary progressive course may be disabled to the same degree after 6 to 7 years.

Figure 10.1 shows progression indices in relation to disease duration for relapsing remitting and chronic progressive forms. Differences concerning progression are highly significant during the first 10 years, chronic progressive forms progressing much more rapidly than relapsing remitting forms. There is no longer any significant difference after 10 years of disease duration. Factors influencing the prognosis of MS in a way which can be assessed by progression indices may be summarized as shown in Table 10.2.

With regard to prognosis concerning the degree of future disability, the "5-year rule of Kurtzke" (Kurtzke et al. 1977) is confirmed repeatedly: the degree of disability 5 years after disease onset corresponds on average to three quarters of the degree of disability after 10 and 15 years. A benign course within the first 5 years (0 to 2 points on the Kurtzke scale 5 years

Table 10.2 *Factors which influence progression of MS*

	PI<0.6	PI>0.6	Significance
Age at onset	<30 years	>30 years	p<0.0001
Initial symptoms	Visual disturbances	Gait disturbances Pareses Visual disturbances	p<0.01
Disease course	Exacerbating remitting	Chronic progressive	p<0.001

(Beer and Kesselring 1988.) PI, progression index.

after disease onset) indicates that the same will be found 15 years after disease onset in two thirds of cases, and in only 1 in 10 will there be very marked disability (more than 6 points). If, however, severe disability is present after 5 years, only in exceptional cases can improvement be expected after a further 10 years.

A similarly reliable indicator of the future prognosis is the presence or absence of cerebellar and pyramidal deficits 5 years after disease onset. If such deficits are lacking at this time, minimal disability (score of 0 to 2) will be present in 80% of patients after 10 years, in 55% after 15 years, and in only 6% can severe disability be expected after 15 years. On the other hand, in patients with severe cerebellar and pyramidal deficits in the first 5 years after disease onset, severe disability will be present in 90% after 15 years, and no patients will have a score below 3.

The fact that other members of a patient's family are affected by MS does not influence the progression index.

If the prognosis of MS is assessed according to working capacity after years, there are concordant reports that even after disease duration of 15 to 20 years, approximately 30% of patients are still (at least partially) able to work (S. Poser et al. 1986). Reduction of working capacity is due to spastic paresis in two thirds of cases, to incoordination in 40%, and to bladder disturbances in one quarter (Bauer and Firnhaber 1963).

A third of MS patients are able to work full time, and more than two thirds part time 5 years after disease onset. A quarter of affected people are working full time 10 years after disease onset, and at least 10% after this. After

such long periods of observation, the prognostic differences between patients examined in an epidemiological area on an outpatient basis and those examined at hospital disappear.

BENIGN COURSES

The extremes of the benign courses of MS comprise the cases in which the diagnosis is confirmed at postmortem examination without any signs of disease of the CNS having been present during their lifetime (Georgi 1961a; Mackay and Hirano 1967; Herndon and Rudick 1983; Gilbert and Sadler 1983; Phadke and Best 1983).

It is not possible to determine exactly how many cases never become clinically manifest during life and are diagnosed as MS only at post mortem. In careful neuropathological investigations, one case of definite MS without any clinical signs during life is found in 1000 randomly selected autopsies (Gilbert and Sadler 1983). Since this frequency corresponds exactly to the average prevalence rate of clinically diagnosed cases in regions with high disease risk (see Chapter 4), it is assumed that MS may remain completely silent in half of the cases. Furthermore, it may be inferred on the basis of cases verified at post mortem that 20% of clinically definite MS cases run a benign course which does not reduce life expectancy nor lead to significant disability after decades (Mackay and Hirano 1967). The increased detection of such benign cases by the newer methods of investigation (for example, MRI) may be a reason for the increased prevalence rates found in more recent epidemiological investigations.

From a clinical point of view, benign courses of MS are defined differently. Some authors consider only those cases with no disability after 10 years as benign. Thereby a considerable number of misdiagnoses may be included.

It appears to be more appropriate to define as benign, cases in which after 10 to 15 years a score below 2 to 3 on the Kurtzke disability scale is reached (Kurtzke et al. 1977; A. J. Thompson et al. 1986). These are the cases in which social and professional life is only marginally limited after disease onset (Bonduelle et al. 1979). McAlpine (1961), with his immense experience, estimated that a quarter of all MS cases will have a benign course after 10 years. Similar figures are reported by Kurtzke et al. (1977) and Bonduelle et al. (1979), whereas in other studies (Riser et al. 1971), 36% and, from Ireland (A. J. Thompson et al. 1986), even 42% of cases in a hospital population were reported to have a benign course. Indicators of significant importance for a benign course are early disease onset, long interval of remission after the first relapse, and, particularly, the lack of progression of symptoms. Prognostic indications may be gained from paraclinical tests only if values of MBP (see Chapter 8) are not elevated during remission. This indicates a benign course, whereas VEPs, IgG in CSF, or lymphocytes in peripheral blood are not reliable indicators (A. J. Thompson et al. 1986).

Even after many years and decades of a benign course, a rapid progression may occur (Bonduelle et al. 1979). From a clinical standpoint, therefore, it does not appear to be justified to separate benign forms as a single disease entity out of the whole spectrum of MS (Herndon and Rudick 1983).

MALIGNANT COURSES

The rare courses of MS leading to death or severe disability within the first 5 years after disease onset are called malignant. Cases leading to death during the first exacerbation due to a plaque in the region of the respiratory center are extremely rare (Matthews 1991). Death due to the disease is not to be expected in more than 5% of patients within the first 5 years after disease onset; however, severe disability may develop over this period of time in up to 10% of cases (Confavreux et al. 1980).

In such cases, the disease runs a more rapid course from onset, or leads, via relapses, to severe neurological deficits, and, more particularly, to dysfunction of the long tracts and cerebellum. An unfavorable prognosis is to be expected, particularly for those cases in whom deficits of higher mental functions dominate the clinical picture at the outset (Paty and Poser 1984). It is not known whether such cases result from the lack of certain protective elements or from an excessive disposition to causal factors. Particular care has to be taken with diagnostic differentiation in such cases (see Chapter 11).

PROGNOSTIC INDICATORS

Prognostic indicators for a more benign and more favorable course may be summarized as follows (after Kraft et al. 1981):

- walking capacity,
- minimal pyramidal and cerebellar deficits in the first 5 years of disease,
- rapid remission of initial symptoms,
- age at onset less than 35 years,
- monosymptomatic onset,
- rapid development of initial symptoms,
- short duration of previous relapse,
- lack of cerebellar deficits at disease onset.

A more recent investigation into prognostic factors with 25 years of follow-up (Runmarker and Andersen 1993) found a favorable long-term prognosis in patients with an acute onset, low onset age, high degree of remission at first exacerbation, symptoms of afferent nerve fibers, and onset symptoms from only one region of the CNS.

11

Differential diagnosis

INTRODUCTION

The multitude of symptoms and the variable course of MS often cause difficulties in its differential diagnosis, even for the most experienced clinicians. It is part of the confirmation of this serious diagnosis to exclude other diseases whose symptoms may be confused with those of MS.

The correct diagnosis is based on factors gleaned from various sources (see Chapter 8): clinical aspects – indications from the case history as to onset and course of the symptoms, findings of clinical examinations, therapeutic influences, etc.; electrophysiology – delay of latencies in various central tract systems; laboratory investigations – changes in CSF and serum; and imaging procedures. Each of these aspects has to be considered in the differential diagnosis before being accepted as part of the diagnosis.

In specialized MS centers (Murray and Murray 1984; Herndon and Brooks 1985), misdiagnosis of referrals occurs at a rate of 10% to 15%. It is a particular danger that during the initial period of observation, a diagnosis which is only under consideration becomes established and distracts the attention of the examiner from the differential diagnostic possibilities. When a diagnosis is established, almost all symptoms and signs should be explained by it, and further aspects of the differential diagnosis may be ignored. For this reason it is particularly important to reevaluate the established diagnosis at regular intervals and, in particular, the probable and possible ones. The most important diagnostic parameter in MS is the observation of the disease course. A misdiagnosis of MS has to be avoided at all costs, both because this diagnosis is always a heavy burden for patients, and because potentially curable diseases may be missed. This is particularly true for benign tumors of the CNS which are sometimes misinterpreted as MS (Bauer et al. 1975).

The following clinical parameters are warning signs of misdiagnosis. Although they may occur in the context of established cases of MS, they are so rare that they should act as a warning of a misdiagnosis and should lead to further reevaluation of the diagnosis and to further differential diagnostic considerations (Herndon and Brooks 1985; Rudick et al. 1986).

1. All symptoms and clinical signs may be explained by a single lesion in the posterior fossa. Tumors and malformations in the posterior fossa give rise to some of the most frequent and most portentious misdiagnoses of MS.
2. Progressive spinal syndromes, particularly if occurring in patients below the age of 35 years and without bladder or bowel dysfunction. The effects of steroid therapy may mimic remissions of symptoms, even in tumors.
3. No ophthalmological disturbances. MS plaques are so frequent in the visual system and in the coordination centers of ocular movements that doubt as to the diagnosis should arise if they are not present after a disease course of more than a year.
4. Normal CSF and marked elevation of cell number or protein. These are so rare in established cases that they should give rise to reconsideration of the diagnosis.

The following groups of diseases have to be considered in the clinical differential diagnosis of MS.

- Diseases leading to multiple lesions within the CNS.
- Diseases of the CNS with a relapsing remitting course.
- Systemic diseases of the CNS.

- Monotopic CNS lesions with a fluctuating or progressive course.
- Nonorganic syndromes.

The most important diseases which may become manifest in the ways described above and their differentiation from MS will be considered on the following pages.

VASCULITIC SYNDROMES

Systemic lupus erythematosus

Neurological complications were among the most significant causes of death in lupus before the introduction of steroid therapy. Since then, they have become the cause of death in only 20% to 50%. Neurological manifestations of cerebral lupus are manifold and variable (Kaell et al. 1986). Occurring in a third to three quarters of cases (Johnson and Richardson 1968; Hughes 1980; Lim et al. 1987; Futrell et al. 1992), they may be due to direct involvement of the CNS, or of other organs, or to drugs used to treat lupus. Psychopathological syndromes and migrainelike headaches are most common. Various deficits of cranial nerves, and in particular disturbances of visual acuity and ocular movements, cerebellar, spinal, and bulbar syndromes (Hutchinson and Bresnihan 1983), allow differentiation from MS. They usually accompany systemic manifestations of the disease, and may therefore be correctly classified. Even though, on rarer occasions, neurological syndromes may dominate the clinical picture throughout the course, other symptoms of the disease occur which facilitate the diagnosis.

Since no specific test for the diagnosis of lupus is available, it has to be based on a number of clinical and laboratory criteria which in combination make the diagnosis possible. The most useful criteria are: female gender, younger than 40 years at onset, livedo reticularis, loss of hair, allergies to drugs, high sedimentation rate, lymphopenia and thrombopenia, antinuclear and antimitochondrial antibodies in serum, elevated serum IgM, biologically false-positive lues reactions. Cold reactive lymphocyte antibodies occur in 80% of lupus patients; antineuronal antibodies occur in 75% of those with involvement of the nervous system (Hughes 1980).

In doubtful cases, a very high number of cells and an elevated protein content in CSF indicate vasculitis rather than MS.

On postmortem examination, perivascular infiltrations of lymphocytes are found in the white matter of the brain, in basal ganglia, and in the spinal cord, often with signs of ischemic necrosis. Lupus is not a primary demyelinating disease (Allen et al. 1979).

Primary Sjögren's syndrome

In Sjögren's syndrome, one of the most common collagen diseases, involvement of the CNS is said to occur in 20% of cases (Alexander et al. 1986). It may imitate MS in every respect, with relapsing multifocal deficits, delayed latencies in evoked potentials, and oligoclonal bands in CSF. The fact that peripheral neurological deficits may be detected in 40% of cases of Sjögren's syndrome with CNS involvement, and that oligoclonal bands in CSF disappear with steroid therapy, may be helpful for differentiation. Another basis for differentiation is the demonstration of the sicca complex (xerostomia, xerophthalmia, and relapsing enlargement of the salivary glands) followed by biopsy of a salivary gland, or a sural nerve for detection of accompanying vasculitis. It is not known whether the long-term prognosis is different from that for MS.

Primary Sjögren's syndrome occurs in 2 out of 64 patients, as proven bioptically (Miro et al. 1990), and this may indicate probability by chance, and is a sign of the problems surrounding definitions of disease of unknown etiology rather than of pathogenetic implications.

Behçet's syndrome

This syndrome is characterized by recurring oral and genital ulcers and hypopyon iritis. The CNS is affected in a third of cases (Morrissey et al. 1993). Cases occurring with signs of bulbar palsy, dysarthria, sphincter disturbances, and hyperreflexia may give rise to difficulties in differentiation from MS (Motomura et al. 1980). More often, the course is slowly progressive, and recurring forms with year-long remissions may occur. The greatest difficulties in differential diagnosis arise, as in lupus, with a combination of myelopathic syndromes and visual disturbances which may also be due to uveitis. A clearly elevated sedimentation rate, positive c-reactive protein, and pleocytosis in CSF may be arguments in favor of Behçet's syndrome. The differentiation from MS on the basis of elevated IgA and IgM values in CSF, as has been recommended, is not reliable.

Granulomatous angiitis of the nervous system

This rare form of vasculitis may lead to remittent, often painful, paraparesis, with confusion and cerebellar deficits (Rawlinson and Braun 1981). Apart from headache and meningeal irritation, typical lymphocytic pleocytosis and markedly elevated protein in CSF (more than 100 mg/dl) should be considered for differential diagnosis. The sedimentation rate is normal. No changes are found on angiogram since the disease process mainly involves small veins. Recurrent multifocal neurological deficits with pleocytosis, and elevated protein in CSF without systemic manifestations, should give rise to suspicion of this disease.

Panarteritis nodosa

Even though the CNS is involved, with multiple lesions, over the course of this disease in more than half the cases, there are fewer problems of differential diagnostic with regard to MS than there are with other forms of vasculitis. Neurological manifestations usually only occur late in the disease course, and then the correct diagnosis is usually made on the basis of involvement of other organs.

On MRI, vasculitic syndromes may produce pictures very similar to those seen in MS (Miller et al. 1987; 1996; Kesselring et al. 1989a). It may be helpful for differentiation that periventricular lesions in vasculitis tend to be rather less extensive than in MS, and that discrete lesions in the white matter without periventricular changes are almost unknown in MS (see Chapter 8). Infarcts in the vicinity of major vessels, and multiple cortical lesions, or focal cortical atrophies, favor a vascular basis.

INFLAMMATORY AND GRANULOMATOUS DISEASES

Sarcoidosis

Apart from isolated facial nerve palsies, involvement of the nervous system in sarcoidosis is rare, and occurs in less than 5% of cases (Stern et al. 1985). Intracranial granulomata present as brain tumors or with symptoms of a hydrocephalus, and rarely give rise to confusion with MS. Involvement of the basal men-inges may lead to progressive visual loss and optic atrophy. Usually, however, it is accompanied by symptoms which rarely occur in MS, such as diabetes insipidus or occlusion hydrocephalus. Diffuse involvement of the meninges in sarcoidosis may lead to mental disturbances, to epileptic seizures, and to lesions of the hemispheres and brainstem, and may therefore need to be differentiated from MS. This again is facilitated by additional symptoms such as olfactory disturbances, facial palsies, deafness, and progressive visual failure, which are more common in sarcoidosis than in MS. Remissions of earlier manifestations occur in both diseases, particularly with steroid treatment. However, spontaneous remissions of severe neurological deficits, which are typical for relapsing remitting forms of MS, are lacking in sarcoidosis.

Sarcoidosis may be the cause of optic neuropathy in various ways, and is therefore part of the differential diagnosis of MS. Papilledema may be due to uveitis or to raised intracranial pressure, as may optic atrophy. The latter may also be due to direct compression of the optic nerve by granulomatous involvement. Often, differentiation from optic neuritis in MS is possible when examining the eye: sarcoidosis leads to concentric limitations of the visual fields rather than to central scotomata, to rather less marked loss of vision, or to progressive loss of vision without remission. Almost always in such cases, signs of systemic disease are found, such as enlargement of hilar lymph nodes, erythema nodosum, parotitis, or iritis. When these aspects of the optic system and the general situation are considered, differential diagnosis should be possible in most cases.

It is more difficult in progressive myelopathic syndromes. In sarcoidosis, the spinal cord may be compressed by intradural or extradural granulomata, or may be interspersed by granulomatous tissue leading to progressive paraparesis, which often becomes manifest somewhat abruptly. Examination of CSF and myelography or spinal MRI may be useful for differentiation since neurosarcoidosis leads to elevated cell number and particularly to a persistently high protein content; compressing granulomata may also be visible on myelography or MRI.

Granulomata may be seen on computer tomography as hyperdense areas within the parenchyma or on the base of the skull. On MRI, extensive enhancement may be seen in the basal or spinal meninges in addition to granulomata or signs of hydrocephalus (Miller et al., 1996).

The following pathological laboratory findings favor a diagnosis of sarcoidosis: hypercalcemia, hyperglobulinemia, and particularly persistently high protein in CSF. The Kveim test is more often negative than positive in extrathoracal sarcoidosis, and a negative tuberculin test is not usually helpful for diagnosis. Overall, the manifestations of sarcoidosis outside the nervous system are particularly useful in its differentiation from MS.

Borrelia encephalitis

On rare occasions, a progressive encephalopathy with elevated antibody titers against borrelia in serum and CSF may give rise to confusion with MS, since the clinical picture may be almost identical with dysarthria, spastic tetraparesis, and ataxia (Reik et al. 1985; Masson 1987). In neuroborreliosis, there is always a markedly elevated protein and an elevated cell number in CSF. The etiology of CNS disease is not proven by a positive antibody titer against borrelia as it may occur in endemic regions in 10% to 20% of the normal population. A causal relationship should be assumed when various progressive neurological diseases and IgG as well as IgM antibodies are detected in serum and CSF. In these cases, therapy with high-dose penicillin is indicated. It is certainly not correct to infer from this that MS is due to spirochetes (Gay and Dick 1986), and the finding of reactive Lyme serology in an MS patient with no features suggestive of the infection is unlikely to indicate neurological Lyme disease (Coyle et al. 1993).

Acute disseminated encephalomyelitis

This clinical syndrome, developing acutely following infectious diseases or following vaccinations, is considered by some authors (Matthews 1991) to be equivalent to the early stages of MS since fever, headache, and confusion, with neurological deficits based on multiple lesions in the brain and spinal cord, are similar in both diseases. Although both are histologically identical (Lumsden 1970), their clinical courses are very different. Acute disseminated encephalomyelitis (ADEM) is monophasic, with a generally good prognosis when the acute stage is passed. Sequelae may persist, particularly when spinal cord and brainstem are signifi-

cantly involved during the acute stage. In the acute phase, mortality due to postinfectious encephalomyelitis may reach 20% following measles and rubella, and 5% following varicella (Johnson et al. 1985). In adult cases, problems of differentiation from MS may occur clinically and on MRI (Kesselring et al. 1990). Consideration of the initial symptoms and of previous infection or vaccination should indicate the right direction. Cell number in CSF is often more markedly elevated in ADEM than in MS. Oligoclonal bands may occur during the acute stage, and may, in contrast to MS, disappear.

Acquired immunodeficiency syndrome

Various neurological manifestations which occur in acquired immunodeficiency syndrome (AIDS) have to be considered in the differential diagnosis of MS. This is important because the nervous system may be affected at various sites at the same or at different times. Direct involvement of the brain by HIV leads to subacute encephalitis, manifesting as progressive dementia and focal neurological deficits. In the context of AIDS, PML, which used to be viewed exclusively as a paraneoplastic syndrome, has become more common, and may be seen in younger patients at ages of risk for the onset of MS. In particular, viral myelitis, due to HIV, cytomegalovirus, or herpes simplex type II virus, may give rise to confusion with progressive myelopathic syndromes. This is particularly so when disturbances of the eyes (periphlebitis and chorioretinitis) are present in addition (neuromyelitis optica). Antibodies against HIV in serum or CSF make differentiation possible. Because of the diversity and variability of neurological deficits occurring in the context of AIDS, and because of the rapid increase in its frequency, antibodies should be examined at least as frequently as serology against lues, which in most neurological clinics still forms part of routine examination. The person to be examined has first to be informed of the intention to examine them, and later of the results.

GENETIC AND METABOLIC DISEASES OF THE CENTRAL NERVOUS SYSTEM

Spinocerebellar degeneration

In most cases, differentiation between spinocerebellar ataxias and MS should be possible on clinical grounds alone. Onset of the former usually occurs in childhood or adolescence, the course is chronic progressive, the peripheral nervous system is also often involved, and a pattern of heredity may be discernible (Harding 1984). There are cases of progressive cerebellar ataxia with onset in adult life, and particularly of progressive spastic paraparesis (familial or sporadic) in which differentiation may be difficult. Differentiation is often not possible from electrophysiological findings (Pedersen and Trojaborg 1981) since the optic nerve may be involved in degenerative diseases as well. On MRI of the brain, differences from MS are often only discrete and unspecific (Ormerod et al. 1987; 1994). Examination of CSF is most reliable since it is regularly normal in degenerative diseases.

Leukodystrophies

X-chromosomal recessive adrenoleukodystrophy (Griffin et al. 1977), and in particular the variant of adrenomyeloneuropathy (Moser et al. 1984), may give rise to differential diagnostic difficulties with MS. There are cases known to begin only in adulthood, with progressive paraparesis and minor polyneuropathy (involving the autonomous system). Cerebellar syndromes, dementia, hemipareses, optic atrophy, and epileptic seizures have been described in late cases. Disease of the adrenal glands or manifestations in the nervous system may often be detected in the family history. Diagnosis is facilitated by the adrenocorticotrophic hormone (ACTH) stimulation test, which produces a decreased plasma cortisol level. Furthermore, very long-chain fatty acids are typically elevated in serum. Oligoclonal bands of IgG may occur in CSF. Magnetic resonance imaging may show diffuse involvement of the white matter. Metachromatic leukodystrophy may run an identical course. Over time, however, additional symptoms occur such as deafness, muscular atrophies, and peripheral neuropathies, which allow differentiation from MS even in those rare cases with onset in adulthood. Diagnosis is based on the detection of heterochromasia in the urine, leukocytes and fibroblasts, and diminution of arylsulfatase A in the urine.

Subacute combined degeneration

Subacute combined degeneration of the spinal cord due to a deficiency of vitamin B12 or folate is part of the differential diagnosis of chronic progressive myelopathic syndromes, which are not rare in MS, particularly with disease onset in the higher age group. Signs of an additional involvement of the peripheral nervous system are usually found. Indications of previous diseases or operations on the gastrointestinal tract, and determination of vitamin B12 and folate levels in serum point in the correct diagnostic direction. Since MS patients are often given vitamin B12 injections, it is more appropriate to perform a vitamin B12 resorption test (Schilling) than just to determine the vitamin B12 level. Whether vitamin B12 is of pathogenetic relevance in MS in general is still a matter of dispute (Reynolds 1993).

TUMORS AND MALFORMATIONS

Tumors and malformations in the region of the posterior fossa, and in particular in the region of the foramen magnum, may lead to difficulties in the differential diagnosis of MS. These regions may not always be depicted reliably enough on computertomography. Magnetic resonance imaging comprises a major advance, depicting the posterior fossa, cervical spinal cord, and pathological processes extremely well (Kesselring et al. 1989a; Miller et al., 1996).

Relapsing myelopathic syndromes may be due to spinal angiomata or to varicosis spinalis, which may be detected under certain circumstances only by myelography or selective angiography. If, in progressive spinal syndromes, VEPs show delayed latencies, and if oligoclonal bands are present in CSF, the probability of a spinal cord compression is so small that myelography may be avoided (Kempster et al. 1987).

CERVICAL SPONDYLOSIS

Cervical myelopathy due to spondylosis of the cervical spine leads to slowly progressive spastic paraparesis or tetraparesis which may not be differentiated from spinal forms of MS on clinical grounds alone. Patients with cervical myelopathy tend to be a little older, oligoclonal bands in CSF are lacking, and VEPs show normal latencies. Both diseases are said to occur simultaneously in some patients (Brain and Wilkinson 1957; Burgerman et al. 1992). Compressive laminectomy may relieve symptoms in cases of marked narrowing of the spinal canal, or may at least halt progression. Neurological symptomatology and its relationship to radiological changes of the cervical spine have to be taken into account if an operation is considered. Only if there appears to be a plausible causal relationship between the two is an operation indicated, and surgical intervention can then yield good results.

NONORGANIC DISTURBANCES

Pareses, sensory disturbances, vertigo, visual loss, unsteadiness of gait, etc., may occur as psychogenic disorders which require particularly careful differentiation from MS. They are often presented by patients with some knowledge of symptomatology, particularly frequently by medical and paramedical personnel. The complaints tend to be described imprecisely, and "deficits" such as gait disturbances and "pareses" are often different from those caused by organic lesions. For example, a patient cannot rise from a chair "because my legs are paralyzed," but may remain in a squatting posture for a long time which requires much more strength and force than walking. Alternatively, sensory disturbances alter several times during the course of a day, and may change sides and intensity; visual disturbances improve "by stroking the eyelid," falls to the

ground occur only when the patient is observed, etc. Obviously, psychogenic disturbances are not always easily diagnosed, and a careful diagnostic differentiation is indicated because they may accompany organic disease. A detailed case history and a thorough clinical examination are sufficiently useful diagnostic tools to make it possible in most cases to arrive at the correct diagnosis without more extensive examinations. It is a somewhat typical sign of psychogenic disturbances that different physicians are called upon again and again "because nobody understands me," and it is characteristic that the patients themselves often demand invasive diagnostic tests and interventions which not uncommonly result in self-mutilation. Electrophysiological and radiological investigations, CSF punctures, and MRI are performed to excess because too little trust is placed in the most basic forms of clinical diagnosis.

The field of psychogenic disturbances presents an immense task for physicians, who should not be dominated by patients but who should offer them adequate sympathy. Only then can treatment of these often very serious disturbances be made possible.

12

Assessment of performance, ability, and disability

The degree of disability resulting from a disease such as MS is recorded with varying degrees of accuracy. Therefore, conclusions based on such records are often inadequate and cannot be compared with each other. The International Federation of Multiple Sclerosis Societies (IFMSS) has therefore installed a working group with the task of producing a simple standardized protocol of examinations which would allow the disability of MS patients to be recorded in different clinical settings. This would lead to easier comparison of results of examinations and data from various sources. It is, for example, a prerequisite for epidemiological studies.

The entire protocol is constructed in such a way that it may be dealt with by electronic data processing. It contains quantified findings of neurological examinations in various systems which may be involved in MS (impairment). Furthermore, the degree of individual disability is recorded on a scale of ability or disability. Data for these two sections of the protocol are collected by physicians. Certain tasks important in daily life are also quantified, producing data on "incapacity." Finally, environmental status and social consequences of the disease are described. Careful evaluation of this protocol in various institutions has proved it to be easy to handle and to produce useful data, although it has been criticized (Willoughby and Paty 1988). Possibly a modified self-administered version of the minimal record of disability may represent a reliable instrument for obtaining a comprehensive profile of patients' abilities (Solari et al. 1993). In order to support distribution of this useful clinical instrument, a minimal record of disability is reproduced in the Appen-

dix (see p. 169). Various scales describing functional independence in daily life situations, or describing degree of disability, correlate well with the amount of time which has to be provided by a helper or with the affected persons' subjective indications of satisfaction with their own quality of life (Granger et al. 1990). The EDSS (Kurtzke 1983a) may be used as a predictor of impairment of functional activities of daily living. The criticism that it is heavily weighted in terms of mobility is reflected in the finding of a strong correlation between the EDSS and the total activities of daily living (ADL) disability level, where the ADL domain of "mobility" fully accounted for this relationship (Cohen et al. 1993). Novel approaches and improvements of assessment scales have been provided during the last few years, and these new instruments of recording have to be reconfirmed in centers other than those of the original authors (Confavreux et al. 1992; Mumford and Compston 1993).

For comparative studies on the spontaneous course of the disease, or on the effect of therapeutic endeavors, a point system may be used which has been elaborated on the basis of case histories of over 100 patients later confirmed at post mortem to have had MS (Poser et al. 1984): a point value corresponding to the percentage frequency (see Chapter 7) was accorded to clinically determined parameters.

Values are cumulative and are counted even when the corresponding clinical sign is no longer detectable. In addition, paraclinical data (see Chapter 8) are taken into consideration in this system.

Although various deficits may occur simultaneously at disease onset, only the highest val-

Table 12.1 *Point value system in the diagnosis of MS*

Clinical details	Point value
Age at onset (years)	
20–29	1
30–39	2
First symptoms	
muscle weakness	4
visual and oculomotor disturbances	3
paresthesias	
mental deficit	1
Remission	7
Symptoms/signs	
pyramidal tract	10
ocular disturbances	
delayed VEP	8
bladder disturbances	8
balance disturbances	8
vibration/posture	
delayed SSEP	7
nystagmus, delayed AEP	7
paresthesias	7
dysarthria	6
gait ataxia	6
mental/cognitive deficit	5
oligoclonal IgG bands in CSF	9
contrast medium enhancement on MRI or CT	5
Diagnostic scale	
MS definite	≥49
MS probable	36–48
MS possible	≤35

Poser et al. (1984). (SSEP, somatosensory evoked potential; AEP, auditory evoked potential.)

ue produced out of weakness, visual and oculomotor disturbances, paresthesias, and cerebellar deficits is taken into account. The initial symptom is considered again when evaluating the entire constellation of symptoms. As for the other parameters, descriptions given in Chapters 7 and 8 are valid.

Such a system of clinical aspects of disease may appear somewhat rigid and impractical to the clinician. However, it is valuable because it is validated on the basis of cases verified at post mortem and in various clinical series. A further advantage is the fact that only new symptoms and signs are included. They are more important for describing disease activity than the number of relapses. In the majority of cases (about 80%), no new symptoms are apparent during relapses but previously present manifestations are reactivated.

PART III

Management and therapy

A chronic disease such as MS, the etiology of which is unclear, precludes the possibility of causal therapy. On the other hand, it encompasses a wide range of symptoms, clinical signs, and associated complications, providing a great challenge for the treating neurologist or physician. An attempt is made in this section to describe some of the most important aspects of symptomatic treatments available for patients suffering from MS. In surveying treatment options, measures such as physiotherapy and occupational therapy, as well as drug treatment, are discussed. All of these measures can be unified under the heading of rehabilitation. In this context, the concept of rehabilitation should not be viewed too narrowly, attempting only to restore sensorimotor functions and the capacity to work. Comprehensive rehabilitation referred to here aims at the improvement, restoration, and maintenance of patients' overall quality of life, and maximum independence in all activities of daily living within their normal social environment.

To the average clinical practitioner, the mass of data on the postulated causes of MS and possible related therapies must appear confusing rather than informative. Thus, apart from discussing the aspects outlined above, it is necessary to give a critical overview of current attempts to find a causal therapy for the disease. A proper understanding of experimental treatments is absolutely necessary if the practitioner is to counsel patients. This is particularly important if additional damage to the patient, be it physical or psychological, is to be avoided. Such damage may result from situations in which, in the hope of finding a cure for their disease, patients turn uncritically to newly developed and not yet proven therapies.

A further aspect dealt with in this section is treatment through dietary measures.

13

Symptomatic treatment and nutrition

INTRODUCTION

A chronic disease such as MS, the etiology of which is unclear, precludes the possibility of causal therapy. On the other hand, this disease encompasses a wide range of symptoms, clinical signs, and associated complications, providing a great challenge for the treating neurologist or physician. The first chapter in this section attempts to describe some of the most important aspects of symptomatic treatments available for patients suffering from MS. In surveying treatment options, measures such as physiotherapy and occupational therapy, as well as drug treatment, will be discussed. All of these measures can be unified under the heading of rehabilitation. In this context, the concept of rehabilitation should not be viewed too narrowly, attempting only to restore sensorimotor functions and the capacity to work. Comprehensive rehabilitation referred to here aims at the improvement, restoration, and maintenance of patients' overall quality of life, and maximum independence in all activities of daily living within their normal social environment.

As experience with, and advances in palliative treatment of, MS have expanded, life expectancy and quality of life of patients have markedly improved. In the past, disturbances caused by the disease and its accompanying complications, for example respiratory weakness and pneumonia, urinary tract infections and renal failure, decubital ulcers and sepsis, often led to premature death. In recent times, however, the use of chemotherapy or antibiotics, as well as determined combating of disease-induced inactivity, have allowed for the control or prevention of such life-threatening complications. As a result, the life expectancy

of patients after the onset of the disease has risen considerably (Kurtzke et al. 1970; Confavreux et al. 1980; Hallpike 1983), bringing it to almost normal levels. In their study on the clinical course of the disease in, and disability of, over 1000 patients with MS, Weinshenker and colleagues (1989) found a median survival time of over 40 years. By using the Kurtzke scale to measure the increase in disability over the years (Kurtzke 1983a), they found a remarkably slow progression of the disease, with an average of 15.3 years before disability reached grade 6, and 46 years to achieve grade 8 (Fig. 13.1).

Previously, MS patients were often advised to avoid physical and, as far as possible, psychological stress. Relapses and rapid clinical progression of the disease were treated with weeks or months of bedrest, with physiotherapy limited to purely passive measures. Today we know that such treatment encourages the development of life-threatening complications; it has become clear that the inactivity caused by the disease must be combated. This can be achieved through intensive active physiotherapy, occupational and neuropsychological therapies, as well as through the greatest possible participation of patients in normal daily life. Such a treatment regimen helps to counteract the development of complications, such as inactivity-induced additional loss in neuromuscular functions, peripheral circulation disturbances and osteoporosis, and deterioration in mental health resulting from social isolation (Fig. 13.2). This modern management, as well as the use of drugs and methods to relieve symptoms such as spasticity or bladder disturbances, is the source of an impressive increase in life expectancy and a better quality of life for many MS patients.

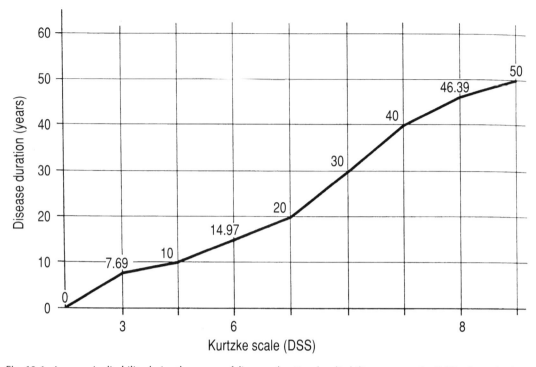

Fig. 13.1. Increase in disability during the course of disease in over 1000 Canadian MS patients, assessed using the Kurtzke disability status scale (DSS). (From Weinshenker et al. 1989.)

PHYSIOTHERAPY

Of the various options for treatment, physiotherapy is possibly the most important one for motor disturbances in the form of spasticity, paresis, and coordination deficits. The aims of such treatment are:

(a) to maintain the functional independence of the patient as far as possible,
(b) to promote the active patient by enhancing or restoring normal motor activity, or, in more advanced stages of the disease, to help with the development of compensatory functions and strategies,
(c) the prophylaxis or relief of secondary complications, such as contractures, decubital ulcers, posture changes, and osteoporosis.

Even today, the value of regular physiotherapy is often underrated, but an increasing number of doctors and patients are becoming convinced of its necessity. To quote an editorial remark by R.A.C. Hughes (1991): "Too little is made of physiotherapy. Uncontrolled observations suggest that experienced physiotherapists can reduce spasticity, improve gait patterns and increase functional independence. Little research has been devoted to the most effective types of physiotherapeutic supervision, benefits from physiotherapy, or into the efficacy of regular long-term physiotherapeutic supervision. Benefits from physiotherapy, occupational therapy and appropriate aids are self-evident. What is needed as much as research is an improvement in the provision of these services to patients."

Efficient physiotherapy for MS must promote the possibilities for functional repair offered by the plasticity of the CNS. This can be best achieved with the help of neurophysiologically based techniques. The most familiar methods are those which were developed for the treatment of hemiplegia, such as Kabat's proprioceptive neuromuscular facilitation (Knott and Voss 1981), and the spasticity-reducing and mobilizing methods of the Bobath concept (Bobath 1990; Mertin and Paeth 1994). Dependent on the patient's special needs, experienced physiotherapists tend to be pragmatic and often combine the two methods of treatment. Via facilitation of normal movement components and patterns, these treatment

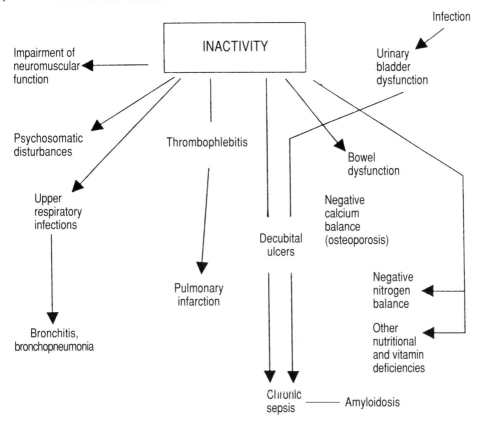

Fig. 13.2. Sequelae of neurological impairment in MS, and complications resulting from inactivity. (Bauer, referred to in Mertin and Paeth 1994.)

techniques serve to increase the active innervation and coordination of movement, and to strengthen unaffected muscle groups, thereby increasing muscular efficiency with respect to coordination, strength, and endurance. They include also integration of afferent pathways through the various stimulatory techniques which play an important role in the improvement of superficial and deep sensation, as well as of postural orientation. The inclusion of such afferent signals in the regulation of motor functions, controlled by cortical and subcortical centers and the cerebellum, is encouraged.

Through such specific demands on efferent and afferent pathways, improvement can be achieved of disturbed movement patterns caused by paresis, spasticity, and coordination disturbances.

It has been postulated that the learning capacity of the brain is also set into motion, allowing the development of new postural and movement pathways (Bobath 1990; Brooks 1986). In the case of many MS patients, this may be limited since they not only suffer from motor and sensory deficiencies, but also from cognitive disturbances which were underestimated until recently. Because of this, it is necessary for future concepts to be developed in which physiotherapy is combined with the use of neuropsychologically based learning strategies. This motor and sensory training should not be limited to mobilizing and stretching exercises and sensory stimulation techniques, but has to be determined by the tasks of daily living. It is only active participation that produces motor improvement or learning: "imposition of postures and movements can have no practical value" (Brooks 1986).

One of the main problems facing people with MS is the development of spasticity arising from an increase in phasic and tonic stretch reflexes. This usually presents as flexor (in the upper extremities) and as extensor and adductor spasticity (in the lower extremities) which, in the framework of associated reactions, can be accompanied by flexor spasms. The prevention of the inducing reflex activity is one of the main aims of physiotherapy. It can be achieved through correct positioning (the supine position increases spasticity, whereas lying on the stomach or on the side has the opposite effect), as well as through standing exercises, passive swinging and rotation, and facilitation of the movements of certain key points of postural control (Bobath 1990). Patients with only moderate spasticity can be taught by the physiotherapist to perform these exercises at home, either alone or with the help of a relative or friend. This helps to prevent an increase in spasticity and the development of additional complications (contractures).

Further possibilities for active physiotherapy arise when the treatment is carried out in water (temperature 28–32°C). The water's buoyancy and resistance facilitate the performance of movements of paretic muscles and in ataxia, for example through exercises aimed at the improvement of gait patterns.

Regular standing exercises, with the help of a standing board and other aids such as a standing frame, allow the patient who cannot stand unaided (perhaps supported by the application of leg splints) to combat circulation disturbances, contractures, and osteoporosis. They can also help to improve the mental state of bed- and wheelchair-bound patients. Such a positive psychological effect is also seen with hippotherapy, which, however, mainly serves to improve posture and balance, and reduce spasticity, as well as strengthening the back musculature. With this "physiotherapy with and on the horse," the transfer of rhythmic movements from the horse to the rider is exploited. Apart from having a positive effect on spasticity and ataxia, it also serves to improve breathing, circulation, and intestinal function.

In many patients – not just those with clinically advanced disease – a reduction in respiratory function (for example stress dyspnea, speech dyspnea) can be seen. As a result of their observations on lung function and cardio-respiratory tests, Olgiati and colleagues (1986) reported that the increase in energy used on walking led to a marked dyspnea and to tiredness of the legs, in which bad general condition, disturbed cardiovascular control, and

weakening of the respiratory muscles also played a role. In pilot studies, it was shown that respiratory weakness exhibited itself, for example, as a pathologically reduced respiratory pressure (maximal inspirational or expirational pressure). It was found that targeted respiratory muscle training could markedly improve this function (Olgiati et al., unpublished). Such training is carried out under physiotherapeutic control, and consists partly of relaxation and contraction of the respiratory and associated musculature, guided by the therapist, as well as breathing through a special mouthpiece which produces either expirational or inspirational resistance. Whether such training has a long-term effect on clinical parameters such as general condition and endurance, or even influences oxygen balance and thereby motor function and coordination, has still to be determined. There are patients who develop their own breathing exercises independently, and who are convinced of their positive effect. Indeed, one of the author's patients achieved a considerable therapeutic effect through regular playing of the mouth harmonica, an exercise whose therapeutic value was also reported by Vergith (1986).

A form of passive physiotherapy includes the application of ice packs or even ice baths to reduce spasticity and relieve pain. In the case of peripheral circulation and tropic disturbances, found particularly often in the case of paraparesis of the legs, treatment with ice can also be highly effective, as can water therapy or the techniques of lymphatic drainage.

In contrast to, for example, the patient with traumatic paraplegia, who can expect to achieve a lasting improvement in this condition, the success of treatment for MS patients is often questionable because of further disease-induced deterioration. Thus, functions regained and lost again through clinical relapse must always be learned anew. The frustration involved in this Sisyphean work makes it very difficult for the patient to muster or maintain the motivation needed for the active participation which determines the success of physiotherapy. In such a situation, it is the important task of the physiotherapist, as well as of the treating physician, nursing staff, and the patient's relatives and other carers, to encourage active participation and, when necessary, the regular performance of planned home-exercise programs.

The amount of physiotherapy, carried out either individually or as group therapy, must be tailored to the needs and capabilities of the patients, such that the initial level of exertion can be carefully increased in a stepwise manner which avoids overexertion. Treatment for spasticity should begin early in the disease, at a time when the spasticity is still limited, or in order to prevent the development of further spasticity-induced disability. In addition to outpatient physiotherapy, hospitalization in special rehabilitation centers is to be recommended for those with mild disturbances as well as for the seriously disabled. Such centers offer intensive physiotherapy and, if necessary, advice on physical aids (supports, splints, wheelchairs, etc.), as well as training in their use. To date, there is no indication that seriously disabled patients benefit from such intensive therapy with respect to measurable improvement in specific functions. However, if the treatment leads to stabilization which prevents further progression of disability, when this must also be seen as positive outcome. Thus, physiotherapy given regularly or at intervals plays an important role in the long-term care of patients in the advanced stages of the disease.

In a review of the application of the Bobath concept in MS treatment, Mertin and Paeth (1994) presented a hierarchy of the therapeutic strategies dependent on the clinical status of the patients. Accordingly, with a level of impairment/disability corresponding to points 0.5 to 5.5 on the Kurtzke EDSS scale, the therapy has to be targeted toward:

(a) normalization of postural control,
(b) inhibition or reduction of compensation strategies developed by patients themselves,
(c) facilitation of normal movement components and patterns,
(d) relearning of normal standing balance and gait,
(e) composition of a tailor-made home training program.

In more advanced stages of the disease, with impairment/disability corresponding to 6.0 to 7.0 EDSS points, therapy should be targeted toward:

(a) using the patient's compensation strategies and refining them to enable the patient to perform as efficiently as possible in the activities of daily living,
(b) selection of aids, and training in their use.

Compensatory motor strategies involve restricted and stereotypical use of muscle groups and of the joints. Therapeutic exploitation of such strategies necessitates the extension of the above treatment to the following:

(c) maintenance of the fullest possible range of movement,
(d) improvement of postural tone, especially in overused muscle groups such as the shoulder flexors,
(e) facilitation of normal movement components and patterns,
(f) maintenance of the best possible standing balance (for example by regular standing training),
(g) composition of a tailor-made home training program,
(h) training of carers.

In the case of even further advanced mobility loss (EDSS greater than 7.0), the treatment has to aim at:

(a) training of carers for positioning, transfers, stimulation techniques, and use of technical aids,
(b) prevention of the development of muscle/joint contractures and other complications such as decubitus or pneumonia,
(c) adaptation of the home training program to the more limited faculties of the patients.

Controlled efforts to counteract disease-inflicted inactivity are an important contribution to successful comprehensive rehabilitation therapy. Such therapy must become part of the daily 24-hour regimen developed in accordance with a conscious behavioral change, and initiated in the early stages of the disease (Mertin 1994).

Close cooperation between the treatment center, the treating physician, local physiotherapy department, and private physiotherapist should be a goal. Under physiotherapeutic guidance, a proportion of patients can learn to carry out home exercise programs, either alone or with the help of relatives. Such programs help to maintain the progress made during special therapy. The availability of diagrammatic instructions and of video films (Davies and Mertin 1989) offers support for such home exercise activities.

It is a regrettable weakness of physiotherapy, as a medical ancillary field, that no generally applicable scoring systems are used to determine functional status before and after therapy. Such schemes would help in the assessment of the short-term and long-term success of therapy. The lack of such a scoring system is certainly one of the reasons why the need for, and usefulness of, regular special physiotherapy is so frequently underestimated.

EXERCISE MACHINES

During the past few years, an increasing awareness of the importance of physical fitness has developed, which has led to exercising in such forms as jogging and aerobics. In addition, exercise machines have been developed with the purpose of increasing strength, endurance, and coordination. As a result, an ever-increasing number of patients with disabilities induced by disease of the musculature or nervous systems, and suited to treatment with physiotherapy, are turning to such exercise machines. There is thus a range of machines available, some of which, according to the manufacturers, are general purpose, whereas others are partially or specifically designed for the disabled. Such "fitness and therapy trainers" are often incorrectly viewed by MS patients as an alternative to physiotherapy. One of the aims of physiotherapy is to restore normal movement or, when this is no longer possible, to maintain the existing residual function. Normal movements include bending and stretching, abduction, adduction, and rotation. Exercise machines, however, are usually limited to bending and stretching, with the exclusion of abduction, adduction, and rotation. In addition, the bending and stretching movements are incomplete, for the apparatus is often used in a sitting position, thereby denying the opportunity for full extension, for example of the legs (including stretching of the hip joints). Such stretching is of great importance, particularly in cases of advanced spastic paresis or in order to prevent the development of contractures. For such patients, daily passive movements with full stretching, carried out with the help of relatives, the community (district) nurse or physiotherapist, are far more useful than an expensive exercise machine. In addition, the tactile stimuli afforded by physical contact between the patient and the helper carrying out the passive movements, cannot be replaced through the use of a machine.

However, exercise machines fulfil the promise made by their manufacturers: namely, improving the respiratory and circulatory functions which are important factors in the treatment of many MS patients. In doing so, such machines also perform a degree of thrombosis prophylaxis. If, however, the machine immobilizes the feet, thus preventing the necessary bending and stretching of the feet, then it will not serve to prevent deep vein thrombosis of the legs.

The conclusions to be drawn from the above are that exercise machines are too one sided in their usage, and therefore cannot replace physiotherapy. Their use as the sole form of therapy is inadequate, and can only lead to the introduction of incorrect and ultimately damaging changes in movement pattern. For patients in whom mobility is only moderately reduced, spasticity is not very pronounced, and regular special physiotherapy not required or available, such devices can be useful. However, for patients with more apparent disturbances, their use can only be seen as supplementary to the more important treatment through physiotherapy.

ERGOTHERAPY

The treatment options offered by ergotherapy have long surpassed those originally envisaged under the older term occupational therapy. Today, ergotherapy is a discipline of many aspects and tightly bound to the practice of physiotherapy and neuropsychology. It includes functional training of motor skills of the upper extremities (fine motor skills) and of the trunk (sitting control), schooling of superficial and deep sensation of the hands, neuropsychological practice in cases of, for example, concentration and perception deficits, and training in self-help for activities of daily living (eating, drinking, personal hygiene, writing, etc.). Within the framework of rehabilitation, and often in cooperation with welfare services, ergotherapists attempt to improve the patient's home situation. Thus, through analysis and reorganization of the household, the home situation is adjusted to the needs of the disabled, so that the patient may maintain the improvements achieved during a protracted stay in hospital. It is necessary to discuss these measures with the patient's relatives who, through a misguided wish to protect and to help, often question the changes introduced by the ergotherapist.

SPEECH THERAPY

The aims and logic of using speech therapy for patients with chronic progressive diseases of the nervous system are controversial. It follows that relatively little is known about the effectiveness of speech therapy as a treatment for MS patients. The motor speech disturbances encountered in MS patients include slurred dysarthric or scanning speech, or ataxic dysarthria. In advanced stages of the disease, these are often combined with speech dyspnea, as well as with chewing and swallowing disturbances, all of which can be treated using various methods of speech therapy. Such methods include therapy for motor disturbances of the tongue and mouth, through, for example, the use of myofunctional therapy (MFT), proprioceptive neuromuscular facilitation (PNF) methods, as well as phonation adjusted to breathing rhythm. The orofacial therapy described by Castillo Morales (1991) and Coombes (1992) is utilized by ergotherapists and speech therapists alike.

DRUG TREATMENT

In this section, the main areas for symptomatic treatment with drugs have been selected, i.e., spasticity, bladder disturbances and their complications, tremor, pain, epileptic seizures, and depression.

Spasticity

The mainstay of treatment of spasticity is active exercise under the guidance and control of specially trained physiotherapists and ergotherapists. Pharmacologic treatment with antispastic drugs may support physical therapy, but not replace it.

Before beginning medical treatment with such inhibitory substances, various aspects of the patient's condition should be considered. Thus, nociceptive stimuli from inner and outer surfaces, joints and tendons (increased urine retention and urinary tract infection, constipation, pain, incorrect posture, or a poor positioning in the wheelchair, etc.) can increase spasiticity or even make it apparent. Indeed, emotional changes can also have a negative effect on spasticity. The exclusion or reduction of these factors can make the treatment of spasticity with drugs unnecessary, or at least allow a reduction in the dosage given.

The pathophysiology of spasticity is not completely clear, with attempts at explanation often only tackling isolated aspects of the problem. Spinal and supraspinal lesions are thought to cause an imbalance between inhibitory and stimulatory pathways of the CNS (Eccles and Lundberg 1959). Sprouting of afferent pathways, leading to an increase in the influence of efferent impulses originating in muscle and skin on α-motoneurons (Benecke et al. 1990), may be another spasticity-inducing factor. The exact mechanisms of action of the various available antispastic drugs are unclear.

Diazepam and baclofen, as agonists of the transmitter substance γ-aminobutyric acid (GABA), could exert their spasticity-reducing effects via potentiation of the inhibitory action of GABA at the levels of presynaptic receptors located on afferent terminals, and of postsynaptic receptors located on interneurons and motoneurons. Tizanidin and pyridinolmesilat are used to inhibit the release of excitatory transmitter substances. In contrast to the above substances, which have their effects in the CNS, dantrolen has a direct influence on the contractile elements of striped muscles (Table 13.1).

The dosage of antispastic drugs and their administration over the day must be tailored to the individual – in close cooperation with the physiotherapist – beginning with a low dose followed by a stepwise increase in the amount given. However, it should be remembered that a certain degree of spasticity may be necessary in patients with paraparesis of the legs in order that they may stand and walk. Thus, with a complete loss of spasticity, or the development of muscular hypotonia (which may appear sporadically in patients not adjusted to their medication), it is necessary to reduce the dosage of drug given. In the case of spastic tetraparesis, it should be remembered that an increase in walking distance cannot be considered a treatment success if it is at the cost of movement and function in the arms and

Table 13.1 *Drugs in the treatment of spasticity*

Substance	Daily dose (mg)	Action
Diazepam	5–40	Inhibition of mono- and polysynaptic reflex conduction via enhancement of the inhibitory effect of GABA
Baclofen	10–100	
Tizanidine	6–24	Inhibition of mono- and polysynaptic reflex conduction via inhibition of the release of excitatory transmitter substances
Pridinolmesilat	8–32	
Dantrolen	50–400	Inhibition of muscle contraction

hands. The disturbing and often painful shooting spasms which frequently occur at night can be treated successfully with antispastic drugs, limited to a single dose given in the evening.

Side-effects of the antispastic treatment are initial tiredness, dizziness, vomiting or diarrhea, as well as an increase in ataxia or the occurrence of psychological disturbances (confusion, hallucinations). Micturition disturbances can also be increased in some cases. Some patients treated with baclofen have also developed epileptic seizures. Dantrolen treatment can lead to liver damage and photosensitivity, which then require the appropriate control measures (regular examination of liver function, avoidance of exposure to sunlight). The use of diazepam should be avoided whenever possible because of the many adverse side-effects of the drug, such as sleepiness and dependency, and it should only be used when other substances are ineffective or not tolerated. However, combining limited doses with, for example, baclofen or tizanidin, can sometimes increase its effectiveness.

The use of pumps for continuous intrathecal administration of baclofen should only be considered in cases of extreme spasticity, and has to be monitored at centers which are conversant with the neurophysiological methods necessary for diagnostic and therapeutic control. It may be the last resort for patients with extensive spasticity threatening severe complications and care problems for whom physi-

otherapy and medication have shown no signs of improvement. Some spasticity-related muscular contractures can be reversed through application by the physiotherapist of serial (plaster of Paris) casts.

Clinical trials in progress are examining the efficacy of tetrahydrocannabiol as a treatment for spasticity (Meinck et al. 1989).

Bladder disturbances

Almost two-thirds of MS patients develop temporary or permanent bladder disturbances during the course of the disease, which, apart from their various complications, often have a marked detrimental effect on the patient's social life. Bladder disturbances can arise from damage to cortical, subcortical, and spinal centers, and/or through interruption of the impulse conduction between these centers. The nervous coordination necessary for normal bladder function is based on a complicated circuit of regulation, which is understood only incompletely (see page 77). Thus, control involves sensory pathways which give awareness of bladder filling, together with parasympathetic, sympathetic, pyramidal, extrapyramidal, and spinally controlled motor stimuli which determine the activity of detrusor and sphincter muscles during filling and emptying of the bladder.

Control of the micturition spinal reflex arc can be reduced through the interruption of cortico–subcortical pathways and a resulting loss of supraspinal, partially voluntary, efferents. In addition, damage to afferent pathways, with subsequent sensory disturbances, can also play an important role. The resulting alterations in detrusor reflexes (hyperreflexia) cause bladder hypertonia, apparent as urgency, urge incontinence, and incontinence. Damage to the sacral spinal cord will, through abrogation of the spinal sympathetic–parasympathetic reflex arc, cause hypotonia of the bladder (inhibition of detrusor activity via beta-receptors) combined with failure in sphincter relaxation (alpha-receptors), giving rise to symptoms such as hesitancy, urinary retention, or overflow incontinence. Predominant parasympathetic stimulation, on the other hand, may result in hyperactivity of the vesical detrusor. Such a combination of miscarried innervation can lead to bladder disturbances like those in detrusor sphincter dyssynergia (concomitant stimulation of detrusor and sphincter musculature) through loss of extrapyramidal motor pathways.

A functional classification, as suggested by Duckett and Raezer (1976) and Parsons (1983), can provide guidelines for decisions on medical treatment of bladder disturbances. Briefly, bladder disturbances are classified as (a) weakness with incapacity for storage, (b) weakness with inability to empty, and (c) a combination of both disturbances.

Mild disturbances can often be treated successfully by the physician or neurologist on a trial-and-error basis. However, in the case of severe disturbances, the use of a combined therapy is often necessary, demanding prior careful urodynamic examination by an urologist.

In treating mild symptoms, it should be remembered that latent micturition disturbances often become relevant clinically only in the presence of additional complications. The most commonly encountered problems are urinary tract infection or spasticity of the pelvic floor musculature. The relevant treatment, with urinary antiseptics or antibiotics, or with antispastic drugs such as baclofen, can be sufficient to restore normal micturitional function.

When weakness or inability to store urine is present (Table 13.2), detrusor hyperreflexia can be influenced and symptoms reduced by the administration of anticholinergics such as propanthelinbromide, methanthelinbromide or emepromiumbromide, spasmolytics such as flavoxat, or GABA agonists such as diazepam. It is also possible to reduce detrusor tonus with levodopa or imipramin. Sympathomimetics such as phenylpropanolamin or imipramin (stimulators) or, conversely, phenoxybenzamine, reserpine or phentolamine (relaxants), can be used to influence sphincter function. Physiotherapy may also give improved emptying control, achieved through purely reflectory influence on the external sphincter by inward rotation of the legs. Simply balancing and controlling fluid intake can help to control incontinence and thereby reduce the resultant complications. The sleep disturbances caused by increased nightly frequency can be treated with drugs which reduce urine production, such as the vasopressin derivative desmopressin, which can be given in the form of a

Table 13.2 *Drugs used in the treatment of bladder disturbances*

Disturbance	Substance	Action
Inability/weakness to store	Propanthelinbromid, Methanthelinbromid, Emepromiumbromid	Anticholinergic, inhibition of detrusor activity
	Flavoxat, Nifedipin	Spasmolytic
	Levadopa, Imipramin	Decrease in detrusor tone
	Phenylpropanolamin, Imipramin, Noradrenalin	Stimulation of sphincter activity (alpha-adrenergic)
	Desmopressin	Reduction in urine production
Inability/weakness to empty	Carbachol, Carbamoylcholine chloride, Distigminbromide, Neostigmin, Bethanediol	Cholinergic, stimuation of detrusor activity
	Phenoxybenzamin, Guanethidinsulphat, Reserpin, Phentolamin activity	Alpha-sympathicolytic, inhibition of sphincter
	Baclofen, Tizanidin, Diazepam	Reduction of spasticity of sphincter muscle

nasal spray (Hilton et al. 1983; Kinn and Larsson 1990).

Chronic urinary tract infections may be prevented by acidification of the urine, or by protracted treatment with the urinary antiseptic methenamin, as hippurate or mandelate (Tourtellotte et al. 1983).

If medication should prove ineffective, or lead to unacceptable side-effects, and the above-cited methods also prove insufficient, then bladder emptying may be brought under control by intermittent (self-)catheterization, by the insertion of an indwelling catheter, or by surgical intervention (suprapubic catheter, incision or resection of the sphincter, ileal conduit). Bladder stones can be a particular problem in patients with an indwelling or suprapubic catheter. They may not only lead to blockage of, and eventually damage to, the catheter, but can also be a cause of hemorrhage. In order to prevent the development of stones, patients must be encouraged to drink plenty of fluids (a daily intake of 2 to 3 liters). Smaller stones may be excreted spontaneously or removed via the urethra, whereas larger ones must be removed surgically.

Pain

The prevalence rate of clinically significant pain in MS has been reported to be about 50% (see Chapter 7; Vermote et al. 1986; Stenager et al. 1991), although no distinction is made in this estimate between peripherally induced and central pain.

Nociceptive musculoskeletal pain, including back pain, results secondarily from disease-related clinical phenomena and/or their complications, such as spasticity, osteoporosis, urinary tract infection, etc. Central acute paroxysmal and chronic pain are caused by lesions in the posterior column, spinothalamic tract, posterior roots, and possibly also in the spinal ganglia.

Whereas paroxysmal pain, including trigeminal neuralgia, painful tonic seizures, and painful Lhermitte's sign, is a relatively rare event, chronic central pain in the form of dysaesthetic or pseudoradicular pain is reported more frequently.

Trigeminal neuralgia occurs in 4% to 5% of patients with MS (Österberg et al. 1993), and is caused, unlike peripherally induced idiopathic trigeminal neuralgia, by inflammatory lesions or demyelination in the brainstem area, with damage to the trigeminal root and short-circuiting of axons.

Central pain cannot be influenced by standard pain-relief treatment employing nonnarcotic analgesics and nonsteroidal antiinflammatory drugs which exert their main effects in the periphery. It can only be dealt with by agents which influence CNS functions, such as antiepileptic and psychotropic drugs.

In most MS patients suffering from trigeminal neuralgia, treatment with antiepileptic drugs will successfully suppress recurrent neuralgic pain, or at least diminish its severity. The first-line drug carbamazepine, given initially at a low dose of 100 mg tds and subsequently increased gradually to up to 1000 mg daily, can be the cause of aplastic anemia, agranulocytosis, thrombocytopenia, or liver damage. Thus, weekly, and later monthly, examination of blood counts and liver function is essential. A mild and constant leukopenia is acceptable. As with other antiepileptics, it is to be expected that a sudden cessation of treatment may result in epileptic seizures. Thus, it is preferable to reduce the dosage slowly and in a stepwise manner. For patients who fail to react to carbamazepine, treatment with phenytoin, clonazepam or biperiden may be attempted. Success has also been achieved with baclofen (alone or in combination with carbamazepine), its levo-form appearing to be superior to the commonly used mixture of levo- and dextro-baclofen (Fromm and Terrence 1987). Surgical interventions, such as glycerol injection or coagulation, are usually not helpful in drug-resistant cases of trigeminal neuralgia in MS.

Carbamazepine is also effective in the other forms of central paroxysmal pain. The painful Lhermitte's sign usually only occurs as a short episode in acute relapse, and therefore does not often require prolonged treatment. In contrast, the effect of carbamazepine or other antiepileptic drugs on chronic central pain is only marginal, and psychotropic substances, antidepressants, and/or neuroleptics, have to be prescribed. Combination of such drugs allows relatively low dosages to be used, thereby minimizing their well-known adverse effects, e.g., a combination of clomipramin (10–25 mg tds), haloperidol (0.5–1.0 mg tds), and carbamazepine (100–200 mg tds) has proven to be effective in a number of patients with a long history of dysaesthetic pain. Such combined treatment should also begin with the use of the drugs at the lower doses.

In the management of chronic pain, psychological interventions, such as psychotherapy or relaxation, and biofeedback methods may be useful, but as yet experience with such approaches in MS has been limited.

Nociceptive pain arising from MS symptoms and their related complications has to be managed primarily by treatment of its sources. Thus, for example, active physiotherapy, passive physical treatment (for example with ice), combined with the administration of muscle-relaxant drugs, are recommended in the case of spasticity-related pain. Physiotherapy is also the main approach to combat the pain arising from degenerative alterations of the vertebral column or joint abnormalities which result from fixed neurological deficits; additional treatment with nonnarcotic analgesics or nonsteroidal antiinflammatory drugs is often unavoidable. The latter should be used with care, since it has been reported that the use of indomethacin can result in activation of the disease (Niewodniczy and Posniak-Patewicz 1973; Rudge 1985), possibly via an interference with prostaglandin action in immunoregulatory circuits (Mertin and Stackpoole 1981).

Tremor

Ataxic and intention tremor can be so marked that an MS patient free of spasticity and paresis can still be made virtually helpless. Even when tremor is relatively mild, it can still play a significant role in disability. There is no known medication with predictable success in treating this problem, although propranolol, diazepam, chlorpromazin or tetrabamat can sometimes have an inhibitory effect. Therapeutic trials with the tuberculostatic substance isoniazid (INH), a drug which increases GABA levels in the CNS, have shown a positive effect in some patients, particularly in those with postural tremor. However, at a daily dosage of 600–1600 mg, the adverse side-effects of the drug are unacceptably high in comparison to its modest effects on tremor. Preliminary results of treatment with glutethimide were positive (Aisen et al. 1991), and should now be followed up in controlled therapeutic trials. In particularly difficult cases, neurosurgical stereotactic intervention may be necessary.

Epileptic seizures

It is to be expected that the tendency to develop epileptic seizures is increased in MS patients with lesions tangent to or in the cerebral cortex (see Chapter 7). The frequency of epilepsy in MS has been reported to lie between 0.5% and 10%. Epileptic seizures associated with cerebral lesions are usually of the grand mal type, but may also occur in the form of focal seizures. In most cases they can be well controlled by longterm antiepileptic treatment with carbamazepine or phenytoin. These drugs are also effective in the suppression of other types of seizures, which are believed to be tonic brainstem attacks. Such seizures can present as painful muscle cramps, paroxysmal tachycardia or dysarthria, or as unbearable dysaesthesia.

Depression

Depression comprises another important problem facing the MS patient (Joffe et al. 1987). It is often difficult to differentiate between an endogenous MS-unrelated depression and a reactive depression arising out of the confrontation with the illness and its associated psychological and social problems, and grieving over lost health. An endogenous depression would best be treated with antidepressants, whereas reactive depression requires psychotherapy and sociomedical intervention.

Schiffer (1987) has observed that all the psychotherapeutic strategies used were successful for patients in whom depression was associated with a clinical deterioration leading to feared dependency. In contrast, depressed patients in remission did not react to physiotherapy, and had to be referred to a psychiatrist. Although the clinical course of the latter group of patients was milder than that of those with active disease, they appeared to encounter more difficulties in coping with their disease and needed more help. In addition, there was a greater fear of disease-related social disadvantages than of loss of independence.

Nutrition

There are two different aspects concerning nutrition in MS. First, many MS patients suffer from chronic constipation resulting from a combination of spinal lesions, a poor fluid intake, and disease-induced inactivity. Change in dietary habits (combined with bowel training and increase in physical activity) is an important approach to the management of this problem. Second, nutritional factors have been examined in the context of MS etiology and pathogenesis, and there is some evidence supporting the assumption that dietary treatment or supplementation of the diet with certain dietary factors may have a beneficial effect on the course of the disease.

Prevention and therapeutic success in the treatment of chronic constipation (and obesity) can best be achieved through a fiber-enriched diet which does not exceed the daily caloric requirement and includes plenty of fresh vegetables (partly in their raw form), salad, and fruit. Lean meat and offal, fish, skimmed milk products, and eggs will provide the necessary protein intake, while brown bread (best as wholemeal) and potatoes are an ideal source of carbohydrate. The dietary fat content should be reduced in relation to carbohydrate and protein, and should originate primarily from plant sources (rich in polyunsaturated fatty acids: cold-pressed oils, seeds, nuts). Such a balanced diet which is rich in fibers, vitamins, and minerals is also recommended for the prevention of vascular disease and its complications. Therefore, family and friends can also benefit from it and this ensures that social isolation ensuing from chronic disease is not unnecessarily increased through exclusive dietary regimens.

Other measures against chronic constipation include physical activity and physiotherapy, and a regular intake of linseed (two to three teaspoons swollen in water and then mixed with yoghurt, soft cheese, or muesli), or oral laxatives such as glycerine or senna.

Several dietary factors have been implicated in the pathogenesis of MS. It has been suggested that the methanol and formaldehyde released in pectin metabolism intiate autoimmune reactions, and are the cause of the myelin damage seen as the disease progresses. As a consequence, a diet free of pectin-containing foods has been recommended. Those in favor of a gluten-free diet believe that hypersensitivity to this grain-based protein contributes to the etiology of MS. The interest in food allergy as a source of various diseases (including psychoses) has led to the reemergence of the discussion on the use of allergy-free diets in MS. Apart from the fact that there is no concrete evidence to support the recommendation of such diets, it should be remembered that they can easily result in the development of a variety of dietary deficiencies.

The theory that deficiency of a dietary constituent is responsible for the etiology and pathogenesis of MS is best supported in the case of essential fatty acids (EFAs). Linoleic acid and α-linoleic acid, the progenitors of the n-6 and n-3 families of polyunsaturated long-chain fatty acids (PUFAs), cannot be synthesized by mammals. Thus, they are an essential component of the diet, with the daily requirement for a healthy adult estimated to be 15–25 g. From these EFAs, the body is able to synthesize long-chain carbon compounds with a high level of conjugated double bonds. The PUFAs comprise an important structural and functional component of membrane phospho-lipids (arachidonic acid) and myelin (eicosa-pentanoic and docosahexanoic acids). The EFAs are also progenitors of important physioregulatory substances, namely prostaglandins, thromboxanes, and leukotrienes.

Several biochemical investigations have shown that MS patients have reduced levels of EFAs and related PUFAs, not only in the CNS, but also in serum, leukocytes, erythrocytes, and thrombocytes. Based on these findings, R.H.S. Thompson (1975) postulated that MS resulted from an "inborn error of lipid metabolism." This theory is supported by the epidemiological observation that the incidence of MS is raised in areas in which the inhabitants eat primarily animal (saturated) fats (meat, cows' milk) in comparison to areas in which the diet is rich in plant or fish oils (unsaturated fat: Mertin and Meade 1977). R.H.S. Thompson (1975) assumed that an inborn disturbance in fat metabolism would make itself apparent, or not, depending on the type of fat taken in the diet. Based on the above suppositions, Millar and coworkers (1973), and thereafter other groups, performed double-blind controlled studies to examine the therapeutic effects of an n-6 EFA-enriched diet (15–25 g in addition to the EFAs already present in the diet) on the progression of MS. They observed a slight, but significant, improvement in clinical course, particularly in those patients starting the treatment at an early stage of the disease when there was little or no permanent disability (Dworkin 1984). A double-blind study of 292 patients examined the effectiveness of n-3 EFAs and produced similar results (Bates et al. 1987). It was noted, however, that n-3 did not appear to be as effective as n-6 EFAs. Further trials in which dietary supplementation with EFAs is combined with immunosuppressive therapy are underway in the U.S. and Europe. Awank and Brewer Dugan (1990) analyzed the clinical course in 144 patients whom they had treated with a (saturated) fat-reduced diet for 34 years. They found that those patients restricting themselves to a diet low in animal fats and supplemented with plant and fish oils had a significantly slower disease progression and a lower mortality rate than patients less concerned with dietary intake. Best results were obtained when the diet was started early in the disease, at a time when there was minimal disability.

Millar and coworkers (1973) based their

studies upon the assumption that they were affecting the uptake of EFAs by the CNS and, thereby, encouraging a stabilization of myelin. However, later experimental studies demonstrated that EFAs exert their effects through their immunoregulatory function (Mertin 1980). Thus, it is not EFAs as such, but rather their prostaglandin derivatives which are responsible for the observed immunological effects (Mertin and Stackpoole 1981; Mertin et al. 1985; Mertin and Mertin 1988).

There is no specific MS diet. However, patients should be encouraged to adhere to the above-mentioned fiber-, mineral-, and vitamin-enriched dietary regimen. Such a diet is usually sufficient to ensure regular gut and bowel function. It can be enriched with cold-pressed oils which are rich in EFAs. When preparing foods, these oils (for example sunflower, corn, or thistle oil) must not be heated, and should be stored under cool and dark conditions. Their intake should not be a problem if they are added to salads, to vegetables after cooking, to soft cheese, or yoghurt. An EFA-enriched diet increases the requirement for antioxidants, so that vitamine E supplements are to be recommended

For additional medical treatment, the available EFA capsules usually contain no more than 0.5 g of EFA and are not therefore able to provide the necessary daily intake of, for example, 15–26 g of linoleic acid. Such capsules can provide, at best, a supplement to the EFAs taken in the diet.

Concluding this chapter, it has to be pointed out that rehabilitation therapy with activity-promoting and complication-preventing special physiotherapy, ergotherapy, home training, and suitable sports activities should not be reserved for patients with more or less advanced disease, but has to start with diagnosis, in the framework of the necessary behavioral changes. In the long-term care of very disabled people with MS, be it within the family or in a suitable institutional home, the whole range of physical and medical rehabilitation measures needs to be exploited to avoid complications, promote stabilization, and ensure thereby the patients' highest possible quality of life. Cognitive impairment is a prominent feature in MS symptomatology (Comi et al. 1993) and greatly contributes to disability and handicap. Here, too, rehabilitation is possible, for example with special techniques including cognitive retraining of basic deficits (Prosiegel and Michael 1993).

14

Therapy

INTRODUCTION

In recent years we have witnessed significant progress in the search for treatments targeted to influence the pathogenetic process in MS (Hughes 1994; Ebers 1994; Wolinsky 1995; van Oosten et al. 1995). This progress has been hastened by our increased knowledge of MS pathogenesis, by better means of monitoring the disease process, advances in the design of therapeutic trials, and by the introduction of new therapeutic agents. In line with the increasing evidence supporting a crucial role of the immune system in MS pathogenesis, nearly all the therapies discussed in this chapter are targeted at different parts of the immunoregulatory network.

ASSESSING DISEASE EVOLUTION AND THERAPEUTIC EFFECTS

Since the first description of MS, more than 100 different therapies have been applied, and all of them – although based on different etiological and pathophysiological assumptions – have claimed improvements, sometimes by as much as 100% (Schimrigk and Schmitt 1988; Sibley 1992). These contradictory and unsatisfactory results have led to an increasing awareness of the problems associated with the assessment of therapeutic effects in this disease. Committees chaired by Schumacher (1965) and by Brown (1979) defined the main problems as: inprecise diagnosis, a variable and unpredictable disease course with frequent spontaneous remissions, lack of a direct method to assess disease activity, the masking effect of already existing persistent damage on new activity, psychological disturbances, and sometimes hysterical tendencies in some patients. While in most cases the problem of diagnosis is solved by applying the diagnostic criteria defined by the committee of Schu-

macher et al. (1965), or their extension by Poser et al. (1983), unpredictability and frequent spontaneous remissions can only be overcome by the inclusion of large groups of patients and randomized assignment to parallel therapeutic groups. Due to the chronicity of the disease, the patients have to be followed for longer periods of time (more than 2 or 3 years) if an effect on the course of the disease is to be assessed. The vulnerable function of partially demyelinated fibers predisposes the performance of MS patients to be significantly influenced by positive or negative expectations and mood. Not only patients but also their neurologists are susceptible to bias when assessing neurological function (Noseworthy et al. 1994a). Only a double-blind design controls for this important variable. Large-scale multicenter trials, with good quality study design involving adequate patient numbers, are now accepted as standard, and the only way to achieve genuine therapeutic progress (Noseworthy et al. 1989). But even in this setting, the main problem remains the accurate and valid assessment of disease evolution. When applying clinicial measures in order to do so, we face both test-inherent and disease-inherent problems. Figure 14.1 shows that even the best clinical measures will not necessarily mirror the "real" pathogenetic process. Other methods of assessment, such as neuroimaging, electrophysiological and immunological tests, may help to complete the picture by depicting specific parts of the pathogenetic process. As MS can strike nearly every part of the central nervous system, there is an immense quantitative and qualitative variability of symptoms which is nearly impossible to assess with one rating scale. Some of the symptoms may be directly due to structural change in the CNS, some reflect nonpermanent or functional changes which may fluctuate from hour to hour. Some symptoms may be easily measur-

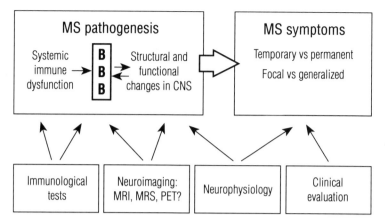

Fig. 14.1. Relation of MS pathogenesis, MS symptoms, and methods for their assessment. BBB, blood–brain barrier; MRI, magnetic resonance imaging; MRS, magnetic resonance spectroscopy; PET, positron emission tomography.

able, for example a paresis; others may be more difficult to assess, such as neuropsychological disturbances, or be ill-defined, such as disease-related fatigue. Comprehensive scales may lose sensitivity for change in single relevant independent dimensions of MS symptomatology. Because of the long duration of the disease, many patients will have only minor changes during periods of 2 or 3 years.

Stability or even improvement of symptoms may occur spontaneously or as an effect of treatment. Stability may be "real," i.e., reflect a stable phase of the inflammatory demyelinating process, or "delusive" because the demyelinating process is going on at "clinically silent" sites of the CNS. Serial MRI studies have clearly shown this discrepancy. Although in the long run what counts is the clinical symptomatology, disability, and impairment, additional "nonclinical" measures are indispensable in order to assess the whole range of MS-related pathology (see Fig. 14.1).

Clinical scales

Requirements for clinical outcome measures have recently been summarized as a result of a meeting (Table 14.1; Whitaker et al. 1995b). Several different clinical scales have been used in MS (some of them are listed in Table 14.2).

The longest established and most widely used scale is that of J.F. Kurtzke (Kurtzke 1965; 1983; see Appendix, p. 169). Its range is from 0 to 10 in 19 steps of 0.5 points. Based on a complete neurological examination, dysfunction is

measured in different neurological systems ("functional systems"): vision, brainstem, pyramidal, cerebellar, bladder and bowel, cerebral, and other. A total score (EDSS) is calculated on the basis of the functional system scores. In the upper part, from 5.0 upwards, the EDSS score is nearly exclusively dependent on ambulation. Several disadvantages of this scale have been depicted by its critics: it is not linear (e.g., a change from 1.0 to 2.0 is not equal to a change from 6.0 to 7.0); if applied to an unselected population of MS patients, it has a bimodal distribution, as illustrated in Table 14.3 (Weinshenker et al. 1991). Patients tend to remain longer in certain steps of the scale so the probability of change will be lower in patients on certain scores. Other shortcomings are low intrarater and even lower interrater reliability (Amato et al. 1988; Noseworthy et al. 1990; Goodkin 1991; Francis et al. 1991; Verdier-Taillefer et al. 1991), insensitivity to cognitive decline and fatigue, and poor assessment of upper limb function (Willoughby and Paty 1988).

Despite this critique, an international panel recently concluded that the EDSS system provides "the best compromise at present for use in multicenter trials" (Whitaker et al. 1995b). Attempts have been made to improve the reliability of the scale by standardization of the neurological examination (which should include walking with the patient) and by better definitions of the terms and algorithms used to determine the score (Lechner-Scott et al. 1995). Specific tests that cover those functions under-

Table 14.1 *Requirements for MS clinical outcomes measures*

Criterion	Explanation
Sensitivity	The measure should be sensitive to disease worsening over a relatively short time interval
Realiability	The score should be derived using objective criteria and should have a high intra- and interrater reproducibility
Validity	Test instrument measures impairment caused directly by the disease and disability that is clinically relevant
Measure contains components that reflect the independent dimensions of MS	Test instrument measures the principal independent dimensions of the disease, but contains minimally redundant components
Measure is applicable to the range of MS impairments	Available scores should allow classification of all patients and avoid ceiling effects
Ease of administration	The measurement instrument should be easy and quick to administer
Cost-effectivness and efficiency	The measurement instrument should be conservative of time and resources

R. Rudick, cited in Whitaker et al. (1995b).

Table 14.2 *Scales used in multicenter trials*

Name	Author
Expanded Disability Status Scale (EDSS)	Kurtzke (1955, 1983)
Scripps score	Sipe et al. (1984)
Neurostatus	Kappos et al. (1988a)
Ambulation index	Hauser et al. (1983)
QENF	Potvin and Tourtellotte (1976, 1985)
9-hole peg test	Mathiowetz et al. (1985)

Table 14.3 *Average time at each level of DSS*

EDSS step	n-progressing	Time at DSS step (y)		
		x	SEM	Med.
1	854	4.1	0.2	1
2	675	2.8	0.1	1.5
3	539	2.0	0.1	1
4	467	1.2	0.1	1
5	444	1.3	0.1	1
6	292	3.1	0.2	2
7	114	3.8	0.3	3
8	32	2.4	0.4	2
9	14	2.5	0.6	2

Weinshenker et al. (1991) (n = 1037).

represented in the EDSS system should be added and, together with the EDSS, should form a kind of "composite measure" (Goodkin et al. 1995). This composite measure would include a quantified test of upper limb function, e.g., 9-hole peg test (Mathiowetz et al. 1985), a scale assessing fatigue (Krupp et al. 1994) and quality of life (Ware and Sherbourne 1992; Gill and Feinstein 1994), and ideally a short neuropsychological assessment (Fernell and Smith 1990; Beaty et al. 1995; Rao 1995). For treatments aimed at halting the development of impairment/disability, the best criterion for assessment would be time to sustained change in one of these measures in a survival curve analysis. Usually a change of one full step in the EDSS (with the exception of 5.5 to 6.0, 6.0 to 6.5 and 6.5 to 7.0 which are regarded as equivalent to full steps: Multiple Sclerosis

Study Group 1990) is accepted as "relevant difference," but generally accepted criteria have not yet been established for other scales in such a composite measure. "Sustained" is usually defined as a change that is confirmed at a second examination 3–6 months later.

"Surrogate" markers

The term surrogate is used to indicate a nonclinical test that might replace clinical change in the evaluation of treatment effects. Such a marker should be reliable, sensitive, and objective. Ideally, in a disease like MS, a surrogate marker should also allow prediction of ulti-

Table 14.4 *Effects of different therapeutic agents on MRI parameters*

	Effects on	
Agent	Gd enhancement	T2 lesion load
Steroids (high dose)	+	+/−
rIFN-β-1b	(+)	+
rIFN-β-1a	+	(+)/?
rIFN-α	(+)	−
Azathioprine	?	(+)/?
Cyclophosphamide	?	?
Mitoxantrone	+	(+)/?
Cladribine	+	?
Linomide	(+)	?
Deoxyspergualin	−	−
Anti CD4	−	?
Cyclosporin A	?	−

+ established effect, (+) uncontrolled evidence and/or small controlled trial, − no effect, ? no data available.

mate clinical change in the long term, reflect established pathology of the MS lesion, and help to elucidate pathogenesis. Up to now, no nonclinical marker is thought to fulfil all these requirements.

MRI

Brain MRI now has a prominent place as an outcome measure in therapeutic trials. The use of high field scanners, standardized acquisition of images in thin slices, and a uniform imaging processing, as well as blinded assessment, preferably by the same raters, are necessary prerequisites (Miller et al. 1991). Frequently used outcome parameters are number and area of gadolinium-enhancing lesions in T_1-weighted scans, occurrence of new or enlarging lesions on T_2 scans, and assessment of lesion load (hyperintense areas) on T_2 scans, or (recently) hypointense areas in T_1 scans. For the calculation of areas, more-or-less operator-interactive computer methods are used (Paty et al. 1992; Wicks et al. 1992; Filippi et al. 1995a, 1995b).

Most researchers in the field agree that serial MRI, especially frequent (monthly) gadolinium scans, may be useful in early phase II trials as a primary outcome measure (D.H. Miller et al. 1991; Whitaker et al. 1995b). Serial MRI allows assessment of the potential impact of new treatments on parts of the inflammatory process during lesion evolution, and identification of agents which should then be tested in de-

finitive trials. It should, however, be kept in mind that some treatments could affect disease in a fashion not reflected by the available MRI parameters (McDonald et al. 1994). As already discussed in Chapter 8, correlation of established MRI parameters with clinical disability has been significant but disappointingly low (Kappos et al. 1987; McDonald et al. 1994; Filippi et al. 1995c). The *predictive value* of MRI is also a matter of debate. New techniques, such as spinal cord imaging (atrophy seems to be closely correlated with disability: Kidd et al. 1993), magnetization transfer imaging (MTI: Dousset et al. 1992; Gass et al. 1994; Hiele et al. 1995), or proton spectroscopic imaging (Wolinksy and Narayana 1991; David et al. 1995; Roser et al. 1995; Schiepers et al. 1995), may allow more detailed and clinically/prognostically meaningful analysis of the MS lesion. Table 14.4 provides an overview of available information on the effects of various treatments used in MS on two MRI parameters: gadolinium enhancement, and T_2 lesion load.

Evoked potential

Actually evoked potentials are not considered as important nonclinical measures of disease evolution to be used in clinical trials. They seem to be displaced by the enthusiasm for MRI (Whitaker et al. 1995b), although (as shown in Fig. 14.1) they may add important information relating to the functional consequences of the disease process (Capra et al. 1989; Nuwer 1990; Bednarik and Kandanka 1992) – information that is not made redundant by MRI or clinical examination.

Laboratory measures

If systemic immune dysregulation is an important constituent of MS pathogenesis, one would anticipate that immune parameters in the peripheral blood or other body fluids should provide important insights into both the pathogenetic process and the possible effect of treatment. Indeed, levels of cytokines or of mRNA for TNFα, IL-2, IL-6, IL-10, TNFβ, and TGFβ have been described to correlate with phases of disease activity or remission (Rieckmann et al. 1994; Rieckmann et al. 1995a). Different standards used in different laboratories and variability of results still preclude the use of such measures outside of controlled settings. The same is true for soluble receptors such as sTNFR, sIL2R, sICAM1, VCAM and selectins (Hartung et al. 1993; Rieckmann et al. 1995). Even more disappointing were data from CSF studies (Andersson et al. 1994). Recently, analysis of urine samples for neopterine has revealed a correlation with MRI and clinical disease activity (Giovannoni et al. in press). Raised urine MBP was associated with a change from relapsing remitting to secondary progressive disease and may gain importance as a predictive parameter (Whitaker et al. 1995a).

TREATMENTS DIRECTED AT THE MS DISEASE PROCESS

Depending on the clinical course and the phase of MS, different possible targets of treatment can be defined.

a) To shorten the duration and improve recovery from acute relapses of the disease.
b) To prevent relapses: if this is not possible, to delay their occurrence and reduce their severity.
c) To stop or retard progression of residual disability/impairment.
d) To improve function of damaged areas of the CNS (ameliorate conduction, enhance remyelination).

In patients with relapsing remitting disease without progression between relapses, (a) and (b) and perhaps (d) will be ideal treatment tar-

Table 14.5 *Effects of glucocorticoids (GC) possibly relevant to MS treatment*

- Form with intracellular receptor GC–receptor complex which enters the nucleus and acts as transcription factor, turns on or shuts down other genes.
- Most immunologically relevant effects are transmitted by interaction with NF-κB, a transcription factor which regulates many cytokine and cell adhesion molecule genes by:
  direct competitive inhibition of NF-κB,
  increased IκBα-production (IκBα holds NF-κB in inactive form).
- These complex molecular interactions result in:
  reduced expression of adhesion molecules on endothelia and reduced lymphocyte attachment to endothelial cells → less perivascular infiltration in CNS;
  inhibition of T cell proliferation and production of Th1 cytokines (IL-2, TNF-α, IFN-γ);
  inhibition of immunoglobulin synthesis;
  increased release of IL-4, activation of TGF-β genes (Th2 response).
- Induction of T-cell apoptosis (high dose GC).
- Inhibition of phospholipase A results in decreased availability of arachidonic acid → decreased synthesis and release of prostaglandins and leukotriens, proteolytic enzymes and proinflammatory cytokines by macrophages and other immune cells.
- Direct effect on CNS tissue function:
  improved conduction (ACTH),
  increased neuronal regeneration ? (ACTH),
  direct antispastic effect (GC)

References: Drews (1990); Marx (1995); Auphan et al. (1995); Scheinmann et al. (1995); Zettl et al. (1995).

gets. For patients with relapsing progressive or secondary progressive disease, (c) will be the most important treatment goal, while (a) and (b) and of course (d) may also contribute. For patients with primarily progressive disease, (c) and (d) would be the appropriate targets.

Treatment of relapses

Since their first use in the late forties, glucocorticoids remain the mainstay of relapse treatment in MS (Troiano et al. 1987; Beer and Kesselring 1991; Kupersmith et al. 1994). Both their antiinflammatory/antiedematous and their immunosuppressive activities seem to be important (Table 14.5 Troiano et al. 1987; Beer and Kesselring 1991). Direct effects on CNS tissue function, especially improved conduction and perhaps increased neuronal regeneration, have been ascribed to adrenocorticotrophic hormone (ACTH), but their relevance for MS remains unconfirmed (Arnason and Chelmicka-Szave 1974; Levin et al. 1974; McEwen et al. 1986; Funder and Sheppard 1987). Several controlled studies have shown that treatment with steroids, either with ACTH or with glucocorticoids, hastens recovery from MS relapse (Table 14.6; for review see Beer and Kesselring 1991; Myers 1992). Usually, the positive effects of treatment on the clinical status were no more detectable as compared to controls if patients were reexamined after 6 or 12 months (Tourtellotte and Haeven 1965; Rose et al. 1970; Frequin et al. 1994). Therefore most authorities conclude that steroids do not have an influence on long-term disease prognosis. Open studies with serial MRI have shown that high-dose i.v. steroid treatment of acute relapses is followed by accelerated reduction of gadolinium enhancement (Kappos et al. 1988c; Burnham et al. 1991; Barkhof et al. 1991, 1992; Miller et al. 1992). Gadolinium enhancement may recur in some of the lesions after cessation of steroids (Burnham et al. 1991; Miller et al. 1992; Barkhof et al. 1994). The rate of recurrence may depend on abrupt discontinuation versus taper, or on the dosage and duration of high-dose treatment. In our own study with 0.5 g for 5 days and oral taper, no recurrence was observed; Barkhof et al. (1994) mention 4% recurrence after a treatment with 1 g for 10 days without taper; Miller et al. (1992) 39% after 1 g for 3 days. Definite conclusions from such comparisons are not possible because all these MRI studies have been without a control group and with different timing of treatment and MRIs. No consistent effect on number and volume of *nonenhancing T₂ lesions* has been shown after steroid treatment of acute relapse (Kesselring et al. 1989; Barkhof et al. 1994). Whatever the effects of steroids on blood–brain barrier leakage may be, they do not seem to influence those parts of the pathogenetic process that lead to T_2 abnormalities. There is quite definite evidence that low-dose chronic treatment with either ACTH or oral steroids does produce significant adverse events, but that it neither retards progression nor reduces relapse rate (Millar et al. 1967; Myers 1992).

A short course of i.v. steroids may also improve neurological symptoms in some secondary progressive patients, but this effect is only minor and does not last for long (Milligan et al. 1987). The effect in secondary progressive patients may be related to a direct, possibly peripheral antispastic, action which has also

been observed with intrathecal steroid treatment. Intrathecal administration has been favored by some groups (Neu, 1982; Rohrbach et al. 1988a, 1988b; Heun et al. 1992). Three or four intrathecal injections of Triamcinalone acetonide crystaline suspension have been found to be superior to oral steroid treatment in one small double-blind trial (Rohrbach et al. 1988a, 1988b), but comparisons with high-dose steroids have not been performed. Intrathecal treatment has been abandoned because of potential hazards and inconvenience to the patients (Nelson et al. 1973; Bernat 1981).

Direct comparative trials of ACTH and high-dose i.v. steroids suggest that the latter lead to more reliable and rapid onset of improvement with fewer adverse events. This is due to the fact that adrenal secretion of glucocorticosteroids in response to stimulation with ACTH is highly variable, especially in MS patients, both intraindividually and interindividually (Maida and Summer 1979; Snyder et al. 1981). There is no evidence that other adrenal hormones which are also stimulated by ACTH – besides producing unpleasant side-effects – have a positive role in MS (Myers 1992). Thus we may conclude that the use of ACTH and its analogues should be abandoned as long as the relevance of their direct effects on nerve conduction or regeneration remains poorly substantiated.

A large North American trial in optic neuritis compared i.v. methylprednisolone 1 g for 3 days followed by oral prednisone 1 mg/kg body weight for 11 days, with oral prednisone 1 mg/kg body weight for 14 days and placebo, and included 457 patients with acute optic neuritis of recent onset (less than 8 days: Beck et al. 1992). The results (Fig. 14.2) have an important impact on the use of steroids for treatment of MS relapses in general. In this trial, oral prednisone was not superior to placebo. Intravenous methylprednisolone treatment was accompanied by a higher rate of function recovery, but at 3 and 6 months results for all three groups were very similar (see Fig. 14.2). Interestingly enough, over a period of 2 years, the number of patients with monosymptomatic optic neuritis who then fulfilled diagnostic criteria for MS was significantly lower in the i.v. methylprednisolone group: 10 out of 389 in the i.v. methylprednisolone group, 19 in the oral prednisone group, and 18 in the placebo group. This difference, favoring pulse methylprednisolone was most pronounced in pa-

Table 14.6 Controlled clinical trials with ACTH and glucocorticoids in MS relapse (adapted from Myers, 1992)

Protocol	Phase	Number treated				Comments	Reference
		Total	Better	Same	Worse		
60 U i.m. bid x 7 d, then 40 U i.m. bid x 7 d	Relapse	22	11	8	3	Double-blind, randomized. ACTH significantly better than saline placebo at 3 weeks.	Miller et al. (1961b)
Saline placebo	Relapse	18	4	7	7		
40 U im. bid x 7 d, then 20 U bid x 4 d, then 20 U qd x 3 d	Relapse	103	84	14	5	Double-blind, randomized. ACTH significantly better than placebo at 1, 2, & 3 weeks but not at 4 weeks, little justification for ACTH.	Rose et al. (1970)
Inert placebo	Relapse	94	65	18	11		
MP i.v. 20 mg/kg/d x 3d, then 10 mg/g/d 4 d, then 5 mg/kg/d x 3 d, then 1 mg/kg/d x 5 d	Relapse	30	21	9	0	Open, randomized. No significant differences at end of treatment or 18 months later. MP regarded as useful.	Abbruzzese et al. (1983)
ACTH synthetic 0.5 mg i.v. bid x 15 d	Relapse	30	22	8	0		
MP 1g i.v. qd x 7 d	Relapse	14	NS	NS	NS	Blind observer, randomized. MP group better than ACTH group at 3, 7, & 28 days but not at 3 months.	Barnes et al. (1985)
ACTH i.m. 60 U, 40 U, 20 U each x 7 d	Relapse	11	NS	NS	NS		
MP i.v. 15 mg/kg/d x 3 d, then 10 mg/kg/d x 3 d, then 5 mg/kg/d x 3 d, then 2.5 mg/kg/d x 3 d, then 1 mg/kg/d x 3 d	Relapse	11	10	1	0	Double blind, randomized. MP significantly better than placebo at end of treatment.	Durelli et al. (1986)
Placebo	Relapse	10	4	6	0		
MP 500 mg i.v. qd x 5 d	Relapse	12	11	1	0	Randomized, double blind. MP significantly better than placebo, no long-term benefit.	Milligan et al. (1987)
Placebo	Relapse	9	2	6	1		
MP 500 mg i.v. qd x 5 d	Progressive	13	6	7	2	Randomized, double blind. MP significantly better than placebo, no long-term benefit.	Milligan et al. (1987)
Placebo	Progressive	15	0	13	0		
MP 1 g i.v. qd x 5 d	Relapse	15	12	3	0	Open, randomized, 5 days effective, 1 day not effective.	Bindoff (1988)
MP 1 g i.v., qd x 1 d	Relapse	17	0	14	3		
MP 1 g i.v. qd x 3 d	Relapse	15	12	3	0	Double blind, randomized, no significant differences at 3, 7, 14, 18, or 84 days except fewer adverse effects with MP.	Thompson et al. (1989)
ACTH 40 U i.m. bid x 7 d, then 20 U bid x 4 d, then 20 U qd x 3 d	Relapse	17	0	14	3		
MP i.v. 1 g/d x 3 d, then prednisone 1 mg/kg/d x 11 d, 20/mg/d x 15 d, 10 mg/d x 16 and 18 d	acute ON	151	80	NS	NS	Randomized, partially blinded. MP group significantly higher rate of recovery at day 4, 15, month 1 and 6. Prednisone and placebo equal. Lower rate of conversion to MS with MP at 2 years.	Beck et al. (1992, 1993)
Prednisone 1 mg/kg/d x 14 d; 20 mg/d x 15 d, 10 mg/d x 16 and 18 d	acute ON	156	74	NS	NS		
Placebo d 1–18	acute ON	150	75	NS	NS		

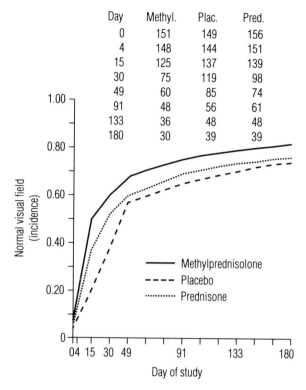

Day	Methyl.	Plac.	Pred.
0	151	149	156
4	148	144	151
15	125	137	139
30	75	119	98
49	60	85	74
91	48	56	61
133	36	48	48
180	30	39	39

Fig. 14.2. Optic neuritis study (Beck et al. 1992). Life-table analysis showing cumulative rates of recovery of normal visual function over the 6-month follow-up period, according to treatment group. The number of patients in each treatment group without recovery to normal before each visit is shown. Methly., methylprednisolone; Plac., placebo; Pred., prednisone.

Table 14.7 *Optic neuritis treatment trial: cumulative percentage of patients with clinically definite MS by treatment group (Beck 1995)*

Time period	i.v. MP (n = 134)	Placebo (n = 126)	Oral prednisone (n = 129)
6 months	3.1	7.4	7.2
1 year	6.4	13.4	10.5
2 years	8.1	17.7	15.6
3 years	17.3	21.3	24.7
4 years*	24.7	26.9	29.8

*Follow-up not complete.

tients with higher numbers of hyperintense lesions in T_2–MRI scans at presentation (Beck et al. 1993). Although this putative preventive effect on the occurrence of further episodes of demyelination was nearly lost in the third year of follow-up (Table 14.7; Beck 1995), this observation may encourage early and perhaps less stringent indication of i.v. methylprednisolone in MS relapses.

The potential benefits of treatment with i.v. steroids (modest but reproducible relief of acute symptoms, putative preventive effect) must be weighed against the side-effect profile of such treatment. Side-effects are usually mild and transient, most being related to the physiological effects of this hormone. It appears that use of short courses of high-dose steroids has even reduced the incidence of steroid-typical side-effects (Lyons et al. 1988; Myers 1992). Serious complications of high-dose i.v. steroids are fortunately very rare: epileptic seizures in patients at risk; aseptic bone necrosis (which seems to be much less frequent than in patients receiving pulse steroid treatment for other indications, where an incidence of up to 1% has been reported); and anaphylactic reactions. Cardiac arrests not related to allergic reactions have been reported, but only after rapid injection. Although the risk of ulceration of the gastrointestinal tract may have been overestimated (Spiro 1993), many neurologists prescribe a H2-receptor antagonist prophylactically when treating patients with high-dose steroids. The use of oral hydroxy vitamin D and calcium supplementation has been proposed as a prophylaxis of steroid-induced osteoporosis, but should only be considered in patients at risk or in the case of repeated or prolonged steroid courses. We usually prescribe low-dose benzodiazepine for a few days in order to treat steroid-related insomnia and restlessness. As long as the optimum dosing regimen of pulse treatment has not been established, we administer either 1 g per day for 3 days or 0.5 g methylprednisolone or equivalent for 5 days, preferably in the morning, followed by oral steroids (prednisone or equivalent) for 14 days (approximately 1 mg/kg b.wt). If at the end of high-dose treatment no satisfactory response is achieved, pulse treatment may be prolonged or repeated for another 3 to 5 days. From the endocrinologic point of view, a taper would not be necessary as the hypothalamic–pituitary–adrenal axis recovers within 120 hours after a 5-day course of high-dose steroids (Myers 1992; Wenning et al. 1994). Although there have been no comparative trials with and without oral taper of prednisone, observations with serial gadolinium-enhanced MRI and in EAE (Reder et al. 1994) suggest that an oral gradual taper during 2 to 4 weeks after high-dose i.v. steroids would be the preferred option (see p. 153).

It is not always easy to distinguish a relapse from fluctuations due to intercurrent illness (usually infection with or without fever, sometimes depression, or even increased dosage of antispastic agents which results in weakness). The decision may be especially difficult if the relapse is not characterized by new symptoms, but by worsening of already apparent complaints. In such cases, a MRI scan showing recent inflammatory activity with contrast-en-

hancing lesions may help; but MRI activity alone should not be the deciding factor for treatment.

There are still several questions regarding steroid treatment that should be answered by means of controlled trials:
What is the best dosage and treatment schedule?
Could i.v. treatment be replaced by equivalent oral doses? (Alam et al. 1993.)
What is the impact of repeated courses of i.v. steroids on relapse rate and disease progression? Preliminary evidence shows that such treatment may be well tolerated, but data on efficacy do not seem to be overwhelming.
Is the time to the next relapse in patients treated with i.v. steroids longer as compared to placebo? The optic neuritis study by Beck et al. provides evidence that this could be the case in the setting of isolated optic neuritis, but we do not know if it applies also to established disease.
What is the effect of repeated relapse treatment with i.v. steroids as compared to placebo treatments?

Other agents

Antiedematous treatment with mannitol may produce an improvement of neurological function in patients with MS (Stefoski et al. 1985). The effect is transient and such treatment has not been widely used. Recently, a trial with an inhibitor of platelet activating factor (gingkolide B) failed to demonstrate any advantage as compared to placebo in the treatment of acute relapses (Brochet et al. 1995). Blockade of cell adhesion molecules, administration of metalloprotease inhibitors (Leppert et al. 1995a, 1995b) or antagonists of proinflammatory cytokines (Debets and Savelkoul 1994) theroretically should have a therapeutic effect in relapses, but have not yet entered clinical practice.

Treatments aimed at reducing relapse rate and halting progression

Treatments aimed at reducing relapse rate and those that are intended to halt progression are discussed together because there is significant

Table 14.8 *Agents aimed at reducing relapse rate and halting progression*

I Nonselective immunosuppressants (cytostatic agents) 　　azathioprine 　　methotrexate 　　cyclophosphamide 　　mitoxantrone 　　cladribine
II Selective immunosuppressants/immunomodulators Chemically defined substances 　　cyclosporine 　　rapamycin 　　FK506 　　15 ± deoxyspergualin (DSG) 　　linomide Cytokines and cytokine antagonists 　　IFN-β-1b and IFNβ-1a 　　other IFN (α, ω) 　　TNF-α antagonists 　　TGF-β Monoclonal antibodies against T-cell subpopulations, activation markers Various: plasma exchange; high-dose Ig
III Activation of endogenous regulatory circuits 　　CoP-1, altered peptide ligands 　　oral myelin 　　T-cell vaccination

overlap, although both the results of recent therapeutic trials and knowledge about the pathogenesis of the disease indicate that efficacy regarding relapse rate does not imply efficacy regarding progression, and vice versa (McDonald et al. 1994). Table 14.8 gives an overview of the substances discussed in this chapter. It must be kept in mind that the use of immunosuppressive and immunomodulating agents is based on more or less detailed hypotheses on the role of autoimmune processes in MS pathogenesis. As long as these hypotheses are not beyond doubt, treatment is at least partly empirical. On the other hand, evidence of efficacy or inefficacy of certain treatments may help to elucidate the pathogenesis of the disease.

Nonselective immunosuppressants

Nonselective immunosuppressants act mainly through their antiproliferative cytostatic action and reduce the pool of possibly autodestructive immune cells, but also, at least to some extent, "normal" or counterregulating immune cells. Some selectivity is achieved by the higher vulnerability of rapidly proliferating cells and by still poorly understood differential effects on some immune cell subpopulations.

Azathioprine

The immunosuppressant drug most commonly used in MS has been azathioprine. Its main metabolite 6-mercaptopurine is a purine antagonist that acts as an S-phase-specific antimetabolite. The exact mode of its immunosuppressive activity is not yet completely clear (Oger et al. 1982; Spina 1984; Elion and Hitchings 1990). It has a wide range of effects, particularly on T-cell function. It is assumed that it acts mainly on rapidly proliferating immature cells of the immune system, whereas mature cells are less susceptible (Spina 1984; Kappos et al. 1989). Since its first use in MS patients (Aimard et al. 1966), several uncontrolled and a few controlled studies have been reported. For more comprehensive reviews, the reader is referred to Kappos (1990), Yudkin et al. (1991), and Hughes (1992). As shown in the metaanalysis of controlled trials by Yudkin et al., there is a significant but minor reduction of relapse rate after 2 to 3 years of treatment as compared to placebo, and also a slight reduction of progression as measured with the EDSS (about 0.2 units over 2 years). This small benefit, which is smaller than the variation which may occur in some patients during a day, seems not to be clinically relevant. On the other hand, such a difference, if it were sustained for several years, might gain importance in a chronic disease like MS. The proof for such long-term efficacy would be prospective controlled studies over 10 or even more years, which do not seem to be feasible. In a matched-pairs comparison of azathioprine and no immunosuppressive treatment over 10 years, we found evidence supporting an important long-term effect of azathioprine treatment, but the results are compromised by the retrospective design and possible bias in the selection of patients treated (Kappos et al. 1990b). No conclusive studies on changes in serial MR scans are available. Several questions concerning azathioprine in MS await answers from prospective controlled studies:

Could the modest effect be better with early treatment?

What is the relative efficacy as compared to IFN-β?

Would azathioprine be a suitable partner in combination, for example, with IFN-β?

Side-effects. About 10% to 20% of patients have gastrointestinal intolerance which precludes long-term treatment with this drug. Regular (weekly, then monthly) blood tests are necessary because of possible leukopenia (Ventre et al. 1985; Kissel et al. 1986). As with every effective immunosuppressant, increased susceptibility to infections may occur, but is only rarely a problem in patient management. With the exception of one report of Lhermitte et al. (1984), several long-term observations (sometimes more than 10 years) have not substantiated an increased risk of malignancy in MS patients treated with azathioprine (WHO 1981; Kappos et al. 1985; Kappos 1990). The only exception could be malignant lymphoma. Data from transplantation or treatment of rheumatoid arthritis are not directly applicable to MS because of disease-specific and treatment-specific confounding variables (Kinlen 1985; Penn 1986).

The dosage recommended is 2.5 mg/kg b.wt per day. After 3 to 6 months of treatment, either a slight leukopenia or an increase of mean cellular volume (MCV) of the erythrocytes (≥ 10% from baseline) should occur (Wickramasinghe et al. 1974; Haas and Patzold 1982; Witte et al. 1986). If this is not the case, a dosage increase should be considered. The macrocytosis is not related to vitamin B12 deficiency, but may be a slight sign of liver toxicity.

Methotrexate

The long-known cytostatic agent methotrexate is a potent inhibitor of dihydrofolate reductase, with consequent effects on folate-requiring reactions in the biosynthesis of thymidilate and purines. It has a relatively selective action on DNA synthesis and inhibits replication and function of both T and B cells. Stimulated by positive results with low-dose methotrexate (7.5 mg given once a week) in rheumatoid arthritis (Kremer et al. 1994; Markham and Faulds 1994), two small studies have recently been conducted. While the first pilot study failed to show any effect in chronic progressive disease and found only a tendency favoring treatment in relapsing remitting disease (Courrier et al. 1993), the second study by Goodkin

et al. (1995), which included 60 patients (18 primary progressive, 42 secondary progressive), used a sensitive composite measure of disability (EDSS, ambulation index, upper extremity function), and found a significantly lower rate of progression. Fifty-two percent of the 31 methotrexate-treated versus 83% of the 29 placebo-treated patients reached the predefined criteria for treatment failure in one of the parts of this composite measure for two examinations separated for more than 2 months (p = 0.01). If only the EDSS had been used – as in most other studies – only a trend favoring methotrexate-treated patients would have been detectable. Also here, the modest effect must be weighed against possible side-effects such as hepatic fibrosis or even cirrhosis, and, rarely, nonseptic pneumonitis. Preliminary evidence suggests that folate supplementation could decrease the side-effects without compromising the immunosuppressive activity of the drug (Shiroky et al. 1993; Morgan et al. 1994). Before the use of this drug is recommended in MS, further controlled studies are necessary.

Cyclophosphamide

Cyclophosphamide is a well-known alkylating agent, which is activated by the hepatic cytochrome P450 system. Its active metabolites crosslink DNA and preferentially kill rapidly dividing cells, including lymphocytes (Lando et al. 1979; Kovarsky 1983; Hengst and Kempf 1984; Miyawaki et al. 1984). Most studies in MS have been conducted with dosages of up to 8 g given i.v. over periods of 10 to 20 days with the intention of inducing moderate leukopenia (Hommes et al. 1975; Gonsette et al. 1977; Hauser et al. 1983). This treatment was in most cases combined with ACTH or glucocorticoids. While most open uncontrolled and several single-blinded randomized studies show a reduction of disease progression, after a few months the disease starts to progress again (Weiner et al. 1993). The Canadian Cooperative Multiple Sclerosis Study Group (1991) compared i.v. cyclophosphamide (1 g every other day until white blood cells fell below 2000 cbmm, on average 5 g), oral prednisone (40 mg for 16 days) with oral cyclophosphamide (1.5 to 2.0 mg/kg b.wt per day for 22 weeks), oral prednisone for 22 weeks, weekly plasma exchange for 20 weeks, and placebo including sham plasma exchanges. No significant differences were observed between the groups throughout the 2-year study period. There was a (nonsignificant) tendency towards better results in the active treatment groups in the first 6 to 12 months, but in the second year this was reversed. Overall, progression in the placebo group was rather low, although patients were selected for progression of at least 1 point in the EDSS in the year before randomization. Side-effects of cyclophosphamide treatment are significant, including transient alopecia, hemorrhagic cystitis, amenorrhea, oligospermia, as well as nausea and vomiting. Longterm risks are carcinoma, especially of the bladder (Pederson-Bjergaard et al. 1985; Samra et al. 1985; Baltus et al. 1990). In order to improve the tolerability of the treatment, Mauch et al. (1989) have used lower dosages (8 mg/kg body weight every 4 days until lymphocyte count was reduced by 50% of the initial value). The reported positive effects with this and similar regimens (Goodman et al. 1990) in nonrandomized trials await further confirmation.

In conclusion, there is little evidence that the potential benefit could outweigh the hazards of cyclophosphamide treatment.

Mitoxantrone

Mitoxantrone is an anthracycline derivative with much less cardiac toxicity than doxorubicin (Henderson et al. 1989; Faulds et al. 1991). It stimulates the formation of strand breaks in DNA, mediated by topoisomerase II. It also intercalates with DNA. It inhibits B-cell proliferation both directly and by effects on macrophages. In T-cell compound, CD4 cells seem to be inhibited, while suppressor activity is not affected or even augmented (Fidler et al. 1986a; 1986b). Several preliminary open studies have shown stabilization of secondary progressive MS using dosages of 10 to 15 mg/m^2 body surface every 3 to 4 weeks for 3 to 6 months (Gonsette and Demonty 1989; Kappos et al. 1990a; Mauch et al. 1992; Noseworthy et al. 1993). In most of these studies, a pronounced effect on contrast enhancement in serial MRIs was observed (Kappos et al. 1990a; Noseworthy et al. 1993; Krapf et al. 1995). An early phase II French randomized study including 42 patients with very active secondary progressive disease confirmed these findings, comparing monthly methylprednisolone with monthly methylprednisolone plus 20 mg mitox-

antrone for 6 months (Edan et al. 1995). A European multicenter controlled study including 191 patients compares placebo with two dosages of mitoxantrone given every 3 months for 2 years (12 mg/m^2 and 5 mg/m^2). While the acute toxicity compares favorably with cyclophosphamide (fewer gastrointestinal side-effects, nearly no alopecia), cumulative dosages of 130 to 160 mg/m^2 are associated with an increased risk of cardiotoxicity (Janmohammed and Milligan 1989). Patients having mitoxantrone treatment should be closely monitored for cardiotoxicity (Villani et al. 1989). Prolonged amenorrhea has also been reported (Shenkenberg and Von Hoff 1986; Noseworthy et al. 1993). At present, treatment with mitoxantrone could be considered in ambulatory patients with active secondary progressive disease, but should be reserved to centers experienced in immunosuppressive treatments of MS.

Cladribine

Cladribine is a purine analogue which is resistant to intercellular metabolism (Beutler 1992). It has a relative specificity for lymphocytes, inducing apoptosis, and seems to be equally effective against dividing and resting cells (Plunkett and Saunder 1991). Sipe et al. (1994) conducted a double-blind matched crossover study involving 51 patients with progressive MS and comparing four monthly treatments with cladribine (0.7 ml/kg b.wt i.v. through an indwelling central catheter) with placebo. They described a significant difference, favoring active treatment both for quantified neurological function and gadolinium-enhancing lesions in MRI. A double-blind placebo controlled trial has now started in the U.S. and Canada, using a more feasible subcutaneous application of the drug (Lilemark et al. 1992; Sipe et al. 1995). Until the results of this study are available, treatment with cladribine should not be given outside of clinical studies. Profound and longlasting bone marrow suppression is the main adverse effect (Beutler et al. 1994).

Total lymphoid irradiation

While a study by Cook et al. (1987) found reduced progression as compared to placebo with total lymphoid irradiation according to a protocol which is used in the treatment of Hodgkin's disease, a recent study by Wiles

(1994) using the same treatment regimen failed to show any significant clinical benefit in the treated group.

Selective immunosuppressants/ immunomodulators

Chemically defined substances

The chemicals to be discussed in this section have less of a generalized cytostatic activity and act by functional inhibition of certain categories of immune cells rather than by decreasing their numbers. The first drug in this category, *cyclosporin A*, was investigated extensively in three multicenter controlled studies, two comparing cyclosporin A with placebo (Rudge et al. 1989; The Multiple Sclerosis Study Group 1990), one with azathioprine (Kappos et al. 1988a, 1988b). As compared to azathioprine, no advantage was found regarding clinical efficacy, but there was a twofold increase in side-effects. As compared to placebo, a very modest effect was found, but also significant toxicity. At least as a single agent, cyclosporin does not have a place in the treatment of MS. *FK506 (tacrolimus)* has a similar mode of action. It suppresses the expression of proinflammatory cytokines such as IL2 and IFN-γ (Macleod and Thompson 1991; Sigal and Dumont 1992). No conclusive evidence about its usefulness in MS is available (Bolton 1992). *Rapamycine* interferes with growth factor and cytokine production during the phase between activation and proliferation of T-cells (Sigal and Dumont 1992). A potent synergistic effect with other immunosuppressants has been described, but its potential usefulness in MS has not yet been tested.

15 ± Deoxyspergualine (DSG) acts later in the immunological cascade. The substance inhibits maturation of antibody-secreting B- and cytotoxic effector T-cells (Nishimura and Tokunaga 1989; Morris 1991; Nadler et al. 1992); without having an effect on activation marker expression or proliferation, it functionally inhibits CD4-positive T cells (Jung et al. 1994). Its effect on macrophages is controversial. Two double-blind placebo controlled studies started in 1992 and were completed at the end of 1995 (Kappos et al. 1992, 1996). Although the final evaluation of these studies is not yet available, interim results concerning change of gadolinium-enhancing lesions in monthly MRIs and also T_2 lesion volume did not show significant differences, although the rate of clinical progression tended to be lower in the active treatment groups.

Linomide is a synthetic immunomodulator (quinoline-3-carboxamide) which enhances natural killer cell activity and activates some lymphocyte subpopulations in experimental animals and humans (Karussis et al. 1993a; 1993b). In addition, it interferes with antigen presentation. Two small studies with about 30 patients have been conducted, one with secondary progressive, the other with relapsing remitting disease (O. Anderson: personal communication; Karussis et al. 1995). A slight clinical improvement was observed, and also less active inflammation in the MRIs performed. Two controlled studies, including about 300 to 400 patients each, started in January 1996 to compare linomide with placebo in secondary progressive disease and in relapsing remitting disease.

Cytokines and cytokine antagonists

There is increasing evidence that cytokines play a crucial role in the evolution of the MS lesion (Kirk 1991; Olsson 1994; Cannella and Raine 1995; Weber and Rieckmann 1995). The cytokines most extensively investigated in MS are the interferons.

Interferon β

Mode of action of interferon β. The use of IFN-β in MS is another paradigm of how clinical therapeutic research may stimulate basic science, which then hopefully will help to accelerate therapeutic progress (Panitch 1992; Jacobs and Johnson 1994). Although two controlled therapeutic studies have demonstrated a partial benefit to patients with relapsing remitting MS by treatment with recombinant IFN-β, we are still lacking a widely accepted explanation for the observed effects. At the molecular level (Farrar and Schreiber 1993; Johnson et al. 1994; Weinstock-Guttman et al. 1995), it is now clear that IFN-β binds to a specific membrane receptor. This binding activates intracellular tyrosine kinases and janus kinases, which phosphorylate STAT molecules (signal transducers and activators of transcription), which then – together with another protein – induce messenger RNA transcription in the cell nucleus.

How this results in an effect in MS is still unknown, but clinical immunological investigations provided evidence that IFN-β antagonizes IFN-γ effects. It downregulates MHC class II gene products, suppresses IFN-γ synthesis by T-cells, reduces lipopolysaccharide receptor expression on monocytes and macrophages, and downregulates inflammatory mediator production by macrophages (Arnason and Reder 1994; Goodkin 1994; Weinstock-Guttman et al. 1995). In addition, IFN-β inhibits T-cell proliferation and restores suppressor T cell function, mainly by shifting the balance towards T-helper 2 (Th2) type responses. Blood–brain barrier permeability is also decreased. The available evidence argues against the relevance of virostatic activity, which was the initial rationale behind testing interferons in this disease (Arnason and Reder 1994).

Table 14.9 gives an overview of the available IFN-β preparations. Other interferons, especially recombinant IFN-α-2a and IFN-ω, may also have a place in the treatment of MS. Recombinant *IFN-α-2a* was studied in a small trial with 20 patients and seems to have effects similar to IFN-β-1b (Durelli et al. 1994). More pronounced neurological or neuropsychological side-effects may decrease its value. Interferon-ω, which seems to have a profile somewhere between IFN-β and IFN-α, has not yet entered phase II studies in MS (Adolf 1995).

Interferon β-1b

In summer 1993, 14 years after the first pilot study by Jacobs et al. (1982; 1994) with human fibroblast IFN-β given intrathecally to MS patients, recombinant *IFN-β-1b* was the first drug to be approved by the FDA for the treatment of relapsing–remitting MS. The decision was based on the results of a 2-year study including 372 patients, randomized to treatment with placebo or two different dosages of recombinant IFN-β-1b (Betaseron®, 1.6 million IU or 8 million IU s.c. every other day) (Paty et al. 1993; The IFN-β Multiple Sclerosis Study Group 1993). In the high-dose group, the annual relapse rate over 2 and 3 years was significantly lower than with placebo (0.84 versus 1.27). Also, severity of relapses, time to first and second relapse, or number and duration of hospitalizations favored the high-dose group. Comparison of annual MRIs showed that after 3 years, placebo-treated patients had an increase of 20% in the lesion area, whereas the lesion area remained unchanged in the 8 Mio IU group. Only a trend favoring the high-dose group but no significant difference from placebo was found regarding change in disability as measured by the EDSS. The 4- to 5-year follow-up of the patients essentially confirmed the results of the first 2 to 3 years (The IFN-β Multiple Sclerosis Study Group, The University of British Columbia MS/MRI Analysis Group 1995). After a median follow-up of 46 (placebo) and 48 (8 million IU) months, 46% of the placebo patients and 35% of the patients in the high-dose treatment arm had reached confirmed progression (persistent increase of 1 or more EDSS steps, confirmed on two consecutive evaluations separated by at least 3 months). Side-effects of the treatment were local reactions at the injection site, flue-like symptoms, mild lymphopenia, and liver enzyme increase. Fluelike symptoms after injection decreased from 52% initially to 8% after 1 year of treatment. Injection site reactions decreased less (from 80% initially to about 50% at years 4 and 5). Injection site necrosis occurred in about 1% to 3% of the patients at some time. A matter of concern was the development of neutralizing antibodies to IFN-β-1b in 38% of the patients (The IFNB Multiple Sclerosis Study Group, The University of British Columbia MS/MRI Analysis Group 1995). Once patients developed neutralizing antibodies, their exacerbation rate approached that found in the placebo group. Although this analysis is retrospective, it is very probable that neutralizing antibodies do have a clinical significance and may abrogate the favorable effects of IFN-β treatment.

Interferon β-1a

Results of a second multicenter trial, including 301 patients with relapsing remitting MS, have been presented (Jacobs et al. 1994; 1995). This study compared recombinant mammalian cell-line-derived glycosylated IFN-β-1a, 6 Mio IU given i.m. once a week for 2 years, and placebo. The main efficacy parameter was progression of EDSS by 1 point, persisting for at least 6 months. Twenty-two percent of the IFN-β-1a-treated and 35% of the placebo-treated patients reached this endpoint during the 2-year treatment period. The difference was statistically significant. The annual relapse rate over 2 years was also significantly lower in the treated group (0.62 versus 0.9). The num-

Table 14.9 Overview of IFN-β preparations

Preparation	Brand name	Cellular source	Chemical description	Glycosylation	Recommended dosage/route	Other dosages under investigation
rIFN-β-1b	Betaseron® (Berlex) Betaferon® (Schering)	E. coli	165 amino acids (ser-17 instead of cys-17, no N-terminal methionine)	−	8 MIU every other day s.c.	5 MIU/m² every other day s.c.
rIFN-β-1a	Avonex® (Biogen)	CHO (Chinese hamster ovary cells)	166 amino acids (sequence identical to human)	+	6 MIU every week i.m.	12 MIU every week i.m.
rIFN-β-1a	Rebif® (Serono)	CHO (Chinese hamster ovary cells)	166 amino acids (sequence identical to human)	+	–	6 MIU every week s.c. 6 MIU 3 times/week s.c. 12 MIU 3 times/week s.c.
nIFN-β	Frone (Ares-Serono)	Natural (human) fibroblast	166 amino acids (sequence identical to human)	+	–	9 MIU 3 times/week s.c.

ber and area of gadolinium-enhancing lesions on annual T_1-weighted MRIs were also significantly lower in the IFN-treated group, whereas lesion area in unenhanced scans did not show statistically significant differences to placebo. Reported side-effects were well tolerated by almost all patients; injection site reactions were minimal. The reported incidence of neutralizing antibodies was 22% at 2 years.

Three smaller studies that looked at gadolinium-enhancing MRIs as the primary endpoint have also been presented. One study with 12 relapsing remitting MS patients compared serial monthly gadolinium MRIs before and after treatment with 8 Mio IU IFN-β-1b (s.c. every other day) and found a significant reduction of the number of enhancing lesions (Stone et al. 1995).

The second study, with 68 relapsing remitting MS patients (Fieschi et al. 1995), compared a 6-month run-in period with monthly gadolinium MRIs to a 6-month treatment period with either 3 or 9 Mio IU recombinant IFN-β-1a (Rebif) (s.c.) on 3 days per week. The number of gadolinium-enhancing lesions was reduced by 49% and 73% respectively.

The third study by Fernandez et al. (1995) included 58 patients; 29 were treated for 12 months with 9 Mio IU natural IFN-β (Frone) 3 days per week s.c., while the other 29 patients had a 6-month waiting period and were then treated with the same dosage for 6 months. Also here, a reduction of gadolinium-enhancing lesions was demonstrated. In these two studies, the reported side-effect profile resembled that of the initial Betaseron study.

In summary, these studies demonstrate that recombinant IFN-β is definitely not a cure for MS. But both IFN-β-1b and IFN-β-1a have a gradual effect on relapse rate, and also a perceivable effect on accumulating disability/impairment in patients with relapsing remitting disease. If this effect is really sustained over longer periods, the advantage to the patients would be significant.

At present, it is not clear if the favorable effects observed in relapsing remitting patients may also be found in secondary progressive MS. This is the reason why rIFN-β treatment is only recommended for ambulatory patients with a relapsing remitting course of their disease and one or more exacerbations per year (The Quality Standards Subcommittee of the American Academy of Neurology 1994). Two

placebo controlled studies involving 700 and projected 800 patients are investigating the role of recombinant IFN-β-1b in secondary progressive MS (Polman et al. 1995). Another study, including more than 600 patients, is investigating the role of recombinant IFN-β-1a (Rebif), also in secondary progressive MS (Sandberg-Wollheim et al. 1995). Another is comparing IFN-β-1a, 6 Mio IU s.c. once a week, with placebo in patients with a first episode suggestive of MS (Comi et al. 1995).

The optimal dosage and root of administration have not yet been established. Experimental evidence suggests that even oral IFN treatment could be feasible (Brod and Burns 1994). Comparative trials will be necessary in order to confirm this, and also to find out if IFN-β-1b or IFN-β-1a should be preferred. The role of neutralizing antibodies and possible strategies to prevent their occurrence must be assessed in the near future. Existing evidence also fails to answer the question of how long treatment with IFN-β should be continued.

Other cytokines

Tumor necrosis factor-α (TNF-α) is regarded as a key player in inflammation and demyelination in the MS lesion (Selmaj et al. 1991; Vassalli 1992). Several agents that counteract its activity or inhibit its production, such as pentoxifylline, a xanthine derivative (Nataf et al. 1993; Myers et al. 1995), rolipram, a selective type IV phosphodiesterase inhibitor (Sommer et al. 1995), or soluble TNF receptor, are currently being investigated.

Transforming growth factor-β (TGF-β) and recombinant interleukin 10, both antiinflammatory downregulatory T-helper-2 cytokines, are also promising agents which are entering phase I and II studies (Moore et al. 1993; Rowe 1994; Calabresi et al. 1995; Skias and Reder 1995).

Monoclonal antibodies against T-cell subpopulations and activation markers

It is tempting to try selectively to eliminate specific players in the immune network with specific monoclonal antibodies (Weiner et al. 1986; Hafler et al. 1988; Waldmann 1992). Side-effects of such treatment, especially sensitization against xenogenic immunoglobulin, have been reduced by the introduction of humanized or chimeric antibodies, composed of human immunoglobulin constant region coupled to a murine variable region. Small uncontrolled studies (Lindsey et al. 1994; Moreau et al. 1994) have been published which describe a positive effect on serial gadolinium-enhanced scans. The only double-blind controlled study with chimeric anti-CD4 antibodies, including approximately 80 patients (Miller et al. 1995), did not show any significant benefit as compared to placebo regarding gadolinium enhancement and also clinical parameters, although a profound and lasting reduction of CD4 cells was achieved. Other more specific targets of monoclonal antibodies are certain activation markers, adhesion molecules, or cytokines such as TNF-α. Studies with such antibodies have been conducted in rheumatoid arthritis (Elliott et al. 1994a, 1994b) and are entering phase I studies in MS.

Various approaches

Plasma exchange. There is some evidence from controlled studies that plasma exchange may improve and hasten recovery in acute relapses of MS (Warren et al. 1982; Weiner et al. 1989). The results were not impressive and would usually not justify the risks and expense associated with this procedure (Rostami 1991).

Intravenous immunoglobulin. There are two possible ways that i.v. immunoglobulin could exert therapeutic effects in MS: through immunomodulation, which would result in reduced relapse rates and perhaps less disease progression, and by a direct effect that promotes remyelination. Both are supported more by data from animal experiments and mostly uncontrolled evidence in MS (Rothfelder et al. 1982; Achiron et al. 1992; Tenser et al. 1993). Controlled studies have already started or are in preparation (Noseworthy et al. 1994b, 1994c).

Activation of endogenous regulatory circuits

Copolymer 1 (CoP-1) is a synthetic polypeptide prepared from L-alanine, L-glutamic acid, L-lysine, and L-tyrosine. It was initially produced to mimic the antigenic properties of MBP, but was then found to downregulate experimental autoimmune encephalomyelitis and to inhibit MBP-specific murine and also human T-cell lines ("increase suppressor activity") (Bornstein et al. 1982; Bornstein and John-

son 1992). Recent data suggest that CoP-1 may bind directly to MHC class II receptor and inhibit binding or even displace MBP peptides in the trimolecular complex (Schroth et al. 1992; Teitelbaum et al. 1992). Three controlled studies have been performed with this substance. Bornstein et al. (1987) included 49 exacerbating remitting patients in a 2-year trial. The group treated with CoP-1 (20 mg s.c. every day) had statistically fewer exacerbations. In a second study (Bornstein et al. 1991), including 106 patients with chronic progressive disease, there was a trend favoring CoP-1 but no significant difference compared to placebo. In the third study, including 251 patients with relapsing remitting disease and an EDSS score of 1.0–5.0, a significant decrease of the annual relapse rate over 2 years was observed (0.84 placebo versus 0.59 CoP-1; see Fig. 14.3). There was also a statistically significant difference in the number of patients having worsened by one or more grades in the EDSS from baseline to month 24 (see Fig. 14.4). No conclusive data from serial MRIs are available. The treatment was well tolerated; some injection site reactions occurred, but they were less pronounced than with IFN-β-1b. About 15% of the CoP-1-treated patients had a transient selflimited "systemic reaction," which consisted of chest pain or tightness with or without anxiety, flushes, sweating, palpitation, or perceived difficulty with breathing. The favorable effect of the treatment was more pronounced in patients with low disability at entry (Wolinsky 1995).

Oral tolerance

Evidence from EAE has shown that oral administration of a putative autoantigen such as MBP elicits T-helper 2-type responses in gut-associated lymphoid tissue (Brod et al. 1991; Weiner et al. 1994). The generated regulatory cells seem to have a site specificity depending on the ingested autoantigen (e.g., with collagen being orally administered, regulatory cells migrate to the joints; with a CNS antigen like MBP, they migrate to the CNS, where they release suppressive cytokines such as TGF-β and interleukin 4; Miller et al. 1991a; 1991b; 1993). The suppression is not specific for the autoantigen that was given orally, but also for other proteins from the target tissue. For example, in EAE it was possible to suppress proteolipid protein-induced disease by feeding MBP. After an inconclusive pilot trial in MS (Weiner et al. 1993a), a multicenter con-

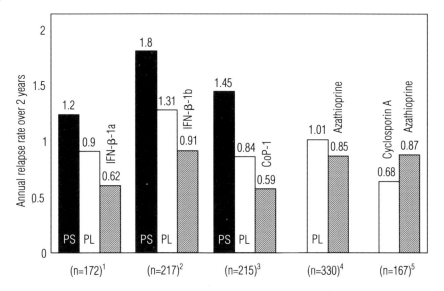

Fig. 14.3. Annual relapse rate of 2 years in recent controlled studies in relapsing-remitting MS patients. [1]Jacobs et al. (1995): only patients with a complete follow-up of 2 years included. [2]The IFN-β-1b Multiple Sclerosis Study Group (1993): only 8 million IU and placebo groups with complete 2-year data included. [3]Johnson et al. (1995). [4]British and Dutch: the study includes about 35% of patients with (mainly secondary) progressive course. [5]Kappos et al. (1988a). About 30% with (mainly secondary) progressive course. No information is available about prestudy relapse rate. PS, prestudy, both treatment groups; PL, placebo. (Adapted from Kappos (1995), with permission.)

trolled trial is now underway in the U.S. involving approximately 500 patients with relapsing remitting MS.

T-cell vaccination

Inoculation of specific T-cells that recognize a putative autoantigen can specifically prevent the induction of EAE (Lider et al. 1988; Offner et al. 1988). This protective effect is due to an anti-T-cell response against these potentially autodestructive cells. Once learned, this reaction should prevent attacks by these autoreactive cells. Three small studies have shown that this approach is feasible and tolerated by the patients. The available data do not allow any conclusion about clinical efficacy (Hafler et al. 1992; Zhang et al. 1993), although the most recent study with eight patients claimed some beneficial effect, as shown by MRI lesion size (Medaer et al. 1995). A more elegant approach would be to vaccinate MS patients not with attenuated T-cell lines but with T-cell receptor peptides (Howell et al. 1989; Bourdette et al. 1994) or with altered peptide ligands, which can interact with the MHC product and the T-cell receptor, but then induce not a TH1 but a TH2 response (Martin et al. 1995; Brocke et al. 1996). The main problem with these attempts at specific immunosuppression is that there is no good evidence that the antigen-specific T-cell repertoire is really restricted in MS. At least up to now, intensive studies of all three components of the trimolecular complex (T-cell receptor, MHC class II product, and antigen) failed to reveal real and consistent restriction (Pette et al. 1990a; 1990b; Martin et al. 1992a; 1992b; 1993; Valli et al. 1993; Meinl et al. 1993). This implies that specific immunosuppression would have to be tailored to each individual MS patient, or that it would only be a useful tool if the suppressive effect shows some kind of generalization, as discussed with oral exposure to antigens.

Combinations of treatments

We are in the favorable position of having more than one agent with partial efficacy in *relapsing remitting MS*, which is substantiated through controlled studies (Table 14.10; Figs. 14.3 and 14.6). These agents are: recombinant IFN-β-1b, recombinant IFN-β-1a, CoP-1, azathioprine, and, in the treatment of acute relapses, high-dose glucocorticosteroids. On the other hand, partial efficacy implies the need for improvement. As in other diseases such as

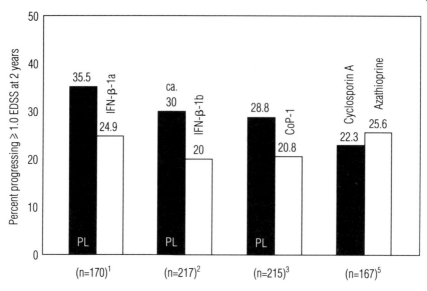

Fig. 14.4 Proportion (%) of patients progressing 1.0 or more units on the EDSS after 2 years in recent controlled studies with immunomodulating or immunosuppressive agents in relapsing remitting MS. [1]Jacobs et al. (1995): only patients with a complete follow-up of 2 years included. [2]The IFN-β-1b Multiple Sclerosis Study Group (1993): only 8 MU and placebo groups with complete 2-year data included. [3]Johnson et al. (1995). [5]British and Dutch: the study includes about 35% of patients with (mainly secondary) progressive course. No information is available about prestudy relapse rate. PL, placebo. (Adapted from Kappos (1995), with permission.)

Table 14.10 *Overview of the therapeutic armamentarium in MS: agents with partial or possible efficacy in relapsing–remitting and in secondary progressive disease*

Agents with partial efficacy
In relapsing remitting disease
  high-dose steroids
  rIFN-β-1b
  rIFN-β-1a
  CoP-1
  azathioprine

Agents with possible efficacy

In relapsing remitting disease	In secondary progressive disease
methotrexate	IFN-β-1b and IFN-β-1a
mitoxantrone	azathioprine
cladribine	methotrexate
CyA and analogues	mitoxantrone
linomide	cladribine
deoxyspergualin	CyA and analogues
TNF-α antagonists	linomide
TGF-β	deoxyspergualin
oral myelin	TNF-α antagonists
i.v. Ig	sTNF-αR
plasma exchange	i.v. Ig
monoclonal antibodies	monoclonal antibodies

*Follow-up not complete.

cancer, a combination would perhaps help to improve the modest favorable effects of single drugs. The combination of steroids with global immunosuppressants or with recombinant IFN-β has been used widely and seems to be safe. Theoretical and also in-vitro evidence suggests that CoP-1 and recombinant IFN-β could have additive or even synergistic effects. There could also be an additive effect of combining azathioprine or methotrexate with one of the immunomodulating agents. However, it should be kept in mind that combinations harbor several disadvantages: it is even more difficult to assess the differential effects of treatments; therapeutic regimens could be too complicated; more side-effects could occur; and also there could be an explosion of the treatment costs. So candidates for combination treatments should be selected according to theoretical or in-vitro evidence for additive or synergistic effects; a partial efficacy should be documented for each agent separately; no negative interactions should have occurred; and the side-effect profile should be compatible.

In *secondary progressive MS*, no single treatment has really convincing evidence supporting its effectiveness. Treatment aimed at the disease process in these patients is more or less experimental and should preferably be discussed and coordinated with some center active in MS research.

For patients with *primary progressive disease*, no convincing evidence exists at the moment that any treatment is able to hold or decelerate the disease process. Patients with primary progressive disease may profit from treatments aimed at improving conduction in demyelinated areas and perhaps even at stimulating remyelination.

IMPROVEMENT OF CONDUCTION, ENHANCING REMYELINATION

4-Aminopyridine, an agent interacting with the sodium channel, has been shown to reduce disability in about 30% of patients as compared to placebo (Stefoski et al. 1991; Van Diemen et al. 1992; Bever et al. 1994). The dosage used was up to 0.5 mg/kg b.wt. If serum levels of the substance are kept below 100 mg/ml, treatment is usually well tolerated (Polman et al. 1994; Bever et al. 1995).

Although results from tissue cultures have been encouraging about the possibilities of induction of myelin repair, possible candidates for clinical studies have not yet been identified in MS. Only recently, a prospective trial was started in order to assess the efficacy of i.v. immunoglobulin in promoting recovery of myelin (Noseworthy et al. 1994b, 1994c).

Appendix: Assessment Scales

NEUROLOGICAL ASSESSMENT KURTZKE FUNCTIONAL SYSTEMS (FS)

1. Pyramidal functions
0 Normal
1 Abnormal signs without disability
2 Minimal disability
3 Mild to moderate paraparesis or hemiparesis (detectable weakness but most function sustained for short periods, fatigue a problem); severe monoparesis (almost no function)
4 Marked paraparesis or hemiparesis (function is difficult); moderate quadriparesis (function is decreased but can be sustained for short periods); or monoplegia
5 Paraplegia, hemiplegia, or marked quadriparesis
6 Quadriplegia
9 Unknown

2. Cerebellar functions
0 Normal
1 Abnormal signs without disability
2 Mild ataxia (tremor or clumsy movements easily seen, minor interference with function)
3 Moderate truncal or limb ataxia (tremor or clumsy movements interfere with function in all spheres)
4 Severe ataxia in all limbs (most function is very difficult)
5 Unable to perform coordinated movements due to ataxia
9 Unknown

3. Brainstem functions
0 Normal
1 Signs only
2 Moderate nystagmus or other mild disability

3 Severe nystagmus, marked extraocular weakness, or moderate disability of other cranial nerves
4 Marked dysarthria or other marked disability
5 Inability to swallow or speak
9 Unknown

4. Sensory functions
0 Normal
1 Vibration or figure-writing decrease only in one or two limbs
2 Mild decrease in touch, or pain, or position sense, and/or moderate decrease in vibration in one or two limbs; or vibratory (c/s figure writing) decrease alone in three or four limbs
3 Moderate decrease in touch, or pain, or position sense, and/or essentially lost vibration in one or two limbs; or mild decrease in touch or pain, and/or moderate decrease in all proprioceptive tests in three or four limbs
4 Marked decrease in touch, or pain, or loss of proprioception, alone or combined, in one or two limbs; or moderate decrease in touch, or pain, and/or severe proprioceptive decrease in more than two limbs
5 Loss (essentially) of sensation in one or two limbs; or moderate decrease in touch or pain, and/or loss of proprioception for most of the body below the head
6 Sensation essentially lost below the head
9 Unknown

5. Bowel and bladder functions: rate on the basis of the worse function, either bowel or bladder.
0 Normal
1 Mild urinary hesitancy, urgency, or retention

169

2 Moderate hesitancy, urgency, retention of bowel or bladder, or rare urinary incontinence (intermittent self-catheterization, manual compression to evacuate bladder, or finger evacuation of stool)
3 Frequent urinary incontinence
4 In need of almost constant catheterization (and constant use of measures to evacuate stool)
5 Loss of bladder function
6 Loss of bowel and bladder function
9 Unknown

6. **Visual (or optic) functions**
0 Normal
1 Scotoma with visual acuity (corrected) better than 20/30
2 Worse eye with scotoma with maximal visual acuity (corrected) of 20/30 to 20/59
3 Worse eye with large scotoma, or moderate decrease in fields, but with maximal visual acuity (corrected) of 20/60 to 20/99
4 Worse eye with marked decrease of fields and maximal visual acuity (corrected) of 20/100 to 20/200; grade 3 plus maximal acuity of better eye of 20/60 or less
5 Worse eye with maximal visual acuity (corrected) less than 20/200; grade 4 plus maximal acuity of better eye of 20/60 or less
6 Grade 5 plus maximal visual acuity of better eye of 20/60 or less
0 Unknown
   Record #1 in small box for presence of temporal pallor

7. **Cerebral (or mental) functions**
0 Normal
1 Mood alteration only (does not affect DSS score)
2 Mild decrease in mentation
3 Moderate decrease in mentation
4 Marked decrease in mentation (chronic brain syndrome – moderate)
5 Dementia or chronic brain syndrome – severe or incompetent
9 Unknown

8. **Other functions:** any other neurological findings attributable to MS.
a) Spasticity
0 None
1 Mild (detectable only)
2 Moderate (minor interference with function)

3 Severe (major interference with function)
9 Unknown

b) Others
0 None
1 Any other neurological findings attributed to MS: Specify _____
9 Unknown

NEUROLOGICAL ASSESSMENT KURTZKE EXPANDED DISABILITY STATUS SCALE (EDSS)

0 Normal neurological exam (all grade 0 in FS*)
1.0 No disability, minimal signs in one FS* (i.e., grade 1)
1.5 No disability, minimal signs in more than one FS* (more than one FS grade 1)
2.0 Minimal disability in one FS (one FS grade 2, others 0 or 1)
2.5 Minimal disability in two FS (two FS grade 2, others 0 or 1)
3.0 Moderate disability in one FS (one FS grade 3, others 0 or 1), or mild disability in three or four FS (three or four FS grade 2, others 0 or 1) though fully ambulatory
3.5 Fully ambulatory but with moderate disability in one FS (one grade 3), and one or two FS grade 2; or two FS grade 3; or five FS grade 2 (others 0 or 1)
4.0 Fully ambulatory without aid, self-sufficient, up and about some 12 hours a day despite relatively severe disability consisting of one FS grade 4 (others 0 or 1), or combinations of lesser grades exceeding limits of previous steps; able to walk without aid or rest some 500 meters
4.5 Fully ambulatory without aid, up and about much of the day, able to work a full day, may otherwise have some limitation of full activity or require minimal assistance; characterized by relatively severe disability, usually consisting of one FS grade 4 (others 0 or 1) or combinations of lesser grades exceeding limits of previous steps; able to walk without aid or rest some 300 meters
5.0 Ambulatory without aid or rest for about 200 meters; disability severe enough to impair full daily activities (e.g., to work a full day without special provisions)

---

* Excludes cerebral function grade 1.

(usual FS equivalents are one grade 5 alone, others 0 or 1; or combinations of lesser grades, usually exceeding specifications for step 4.0)

5.5 Ambulatory without aid or rest for about 100 meters; disability severe enough to preclude full daily activities (usual FS equivalents are one grade 5 alone, others 0 or 1; or combination of lesser grades, usually exceeding those for step 4.0)

6.0 Intermittent or unilateral constant assistance (cane, crutch, brace) required to walk about 100 meters with or without resting (usual FS equivalents are combinations with more than two FS grade 3+)

6.5 Constant bilateral assistance (canes, crutches, braces) required to walk about 20 meters without resting (usual FS equivalents are combinations with more than two FS grade 3+)

7.0 Unable to walk beyond approximately 5 meters even with aid, essentially restricted to wheelchair; wheels self in standard wheelchair and transfers alone; up and about in wheelchair some 12 hours a day (usual FS equivalents are combinations with more than one FS grade 4+; very rarely pyramidal grade 5 alone)

7.5 Unable to take more than a few steps; restricted to wheelchair; may need aid in transfer; wheels self but cannot carry on in standard wheelchair a full day; may require motorized wheelchair (usual FS equivalents are combinations, with more than one FS grade 4+)

8.0 Essentially restricted to bed or chair or perambulated in wheelchair, but may be out of bed itself much of the day; retains many self-care functions; generally has effective use of arms (usual FS equivalents are combinations, generally grade 4+ in several systems)

8.5 Essentially restricted to bed much of day; has some effective use of arm(s); retains some self-care functions (usual FS equivalents are combinations, generally 4+ in several systems)

9.0 Helpless bed patient; can communicate and eat (usual FS equivalents are combinations, mostly grade 4+)

9.5 Totally helpless bed patient; unable to communicate effectively or eat/swallow

(usual FS equivalents are combinations, almost all grade 4+)

10.0 Death due to MS

INCAPACITY STATUS SCALE (ISS)

1. **Stair climbing:** refers to ascending and descending a flight of 12 steps. The 'mechanical devices' referred to include the use of a banister, since the individual without disability can navigate stairs if a railing is not available. Climbing stairs by sitting on each successive step does not satisfy the criteria for 'climbing.' Use of a mechanical chair lift also does not constitute 'climbing.' In this instance, the individual would be scored a 4.

   0 Normal
   1 Some difficulty but performed without aid
   2 Need for canes, braces, prostheses, or dependent upon banister to perform
   3 Need human assistance to perform
   4 Unable to perform; includes mechanical lifts

2. **Ambulation:** is the ability to walk 50 meters (approximately 160 feet) without rest on level ground or indoors. Anyone who needs to use a cane intermittently in order to walk 50 meters without rest would be scored a 2. Likewise, individuals who need to use a cane owing to poor eyesight would also receive a score of 2. The difference between a 3 and a 4 depends on whether the individual can use a wheelchair independently. As a result, anyone who is independent only if using a motorized wheelchair (e.g., with electric 'joystick' control) would be rated a 4.

   0 Normal
   1 Some difficulty but performed without aid
   2 Need for canes, braces, prostheses to perform
   3 Need for human assistance or use of manual wheelchair which patient enters, leaves, and maneuvers without aid
   4 Unable to perform; includes perambulation in a wheelchair and motorized wheelchair

3. **Toilet/chair/bed transfer:** takes into account the ability to position oneself and arise from a regular toilet, chair, bed, and

wheelchair. The *worst* transfer determines the grade. Special chairs, such as those with mechanical lift mechanisms, are mechanical aids. *Needing* to hold onto adjacent structures such as a sink or bars would constitute using a mechanical aid and would be rated a 2. Use of the arms on an armchair is *not*, however, considered using a mechanical aid since pushing up on a chair's arms is an integral part of elevating oneself from a regular chair under normal circumstances.

0 Normal
1 Some difficulty but performed without aid
2 Need for adaptive or assistive devices such as trapeze, sling, bars, lift, sliding board to perform
3 Requires human aid to perform
4 Must be lifted or moved about completely by another person

4. **Bowel function:** among the most complex of the items in the MRD, bowel function requires the evaluator carefully to weigh a number of alternatives. Self-management of constipation is rated 1 or 2, depending on whether treatment is required *occasionally* or *frequently* (more often than once per week). Constipation managed by others is rated 3. Occasional loss of bowel control or a self-managed colostomy would also be rated 3. Frequent loss of control or a colostomy managed by others is rated 4.

0 Normal
1 Bowel retention not requiring more than high fiber diets, laxatives, occasional enemas or suppositories, self-administered
2 Bowel retention requiring regular laxatives, enemas, or suppositories, self-administered, in order to induce evacuation; cleanses and disimpacts self
3 Bowel retention requiring enemas or suppositories administered by another; and/or disimpacted by another; and/or needs assistance in cleansing; and/or occasional incontinence; and/or presence of colostomy tended by self
4 Frequent soiling due either to incontinence or a poorly maintained ostomy device or an ostomy device which patient cannot maintain without assistance

5. **Bladder function:** also difficult to rate. An important consideration here is how to take into account the patient's use of bladder medication. This item is rated for the purpose of reflecting actual bladder function even if that level of function is maintained by drugs. Thus, a person with normal bladder function maintained by medication is rated a 0. The same applies to all the grades.

0 Normal (even if maintained by drugs)
1 Occasional hesitancy or urgency
2 Frequent hesitancy, urgency, or retention; and/or use of indwelling or external catheter applied and maintained by self; and/or intermittent self-catheterization or manual compression to evacuate bladder
3 Occasional incontinence; and/or use of indwelling or external catheter applied and maintained by others; and/or ileostomy or suprapubic cystostomy maintained by self; and/or intermittent catheterization by others
4 Frequent incontinence; or ostomy device which patient cannot maintain without assistance

6. **Bathing:** rated according to how independent the individual is when getting into or out of a tub or shower. The need to hold onto nearby structures such as a sink, towel rack, grab bar, or tub seat is rated a 2.

0 Normal
1 Some difficulty with washing and drying self, though performed without aid whether in tub or shower or by sponge-bathing, whichever is usual for the patient
2 Need for assistive devices (trapeze, sling, lift, shower or tub bar) in order to bathe self; or need to bathe self outside of tub or shower if that is the usual method
3 Need for human assistance in bathing parts of the body or in entry/exit/positioning in tub or shower
4 Bathing performed by others (aside from face and hands)

7. **Dressing:** difficulty in dressing is defined as having problems in putting on or taking off clothing, use of buttons, tying laces, pulling zippers, fastening catches, etc. Specially adapted clothing refers to that which has Velcro closures, snaps instead of buttons, or no closures. Those who *avoid* cer-

tain types of standard clothing should be rated a 2.

0 Normal

1 Some difficulty clothing self completely in standard garments, but accomplished by self

2 Specially adapted clothing (special closures, elastic-laced shoes, front-closing garments) or devices (long shoe horns, zipper extenders) required to dress self

3 Need for human aid to accomplish, but performs considerable portion him/herself

4 Need for almost complete assistance; unable to dress self

8. **Grooming:** this item refers to care of teeth or dentures, hair, shaving, or application of cosmetics. Adaptive devices may include electric razors or toothbrushes, only if these are actually required for function.

0 Normal

1 Some difficulty but all tasks performed without aid

2 Need for adaptive devices (electric razors or toothbrushes, special combs or brushes, arm rests or slings) but performed without aid

3 Need for human aid to perform some of the tasks

4 Almost all tasks performed by another person

9. **Feeding:** includes ingestion, mastication, swallowing of solids and liquids, and manipulation of the appropriate utensils. Individuals who need to have their food cut but can feed themselves are to be rated a 2. Those who actually need assistance to bring food to their mouths are rated a 3 or 4. Use of a liquid diet (e.g., a feeding tube) is considered a 3 if self-maintained, and a 4 if administered by others. Some people with MS have more trouble with liquids than with solids. These individuals should be rated according to the same criteria: e.g., needing to use jelled liquids would be rated at 2 since it constitutes 'special preparation.'

0 Normal

1 Some difficulty but performed without aid

2 Need for adaptive devices (special feeding utensils, straws) or special prepara-

tion (portions precut or minced, bread buttered) to feed self

3 Need for human aid in the delivery of food; or dysphagia preventing solid diet, e.g., esophagostomy or gastrostomy maintained and utilized by self, or tube-feeding performed by self

4 Unable to feed self or to manage ostomies

10. **Vision:** two factors are rated: visual acuity and double vision. The overall rating is based on the *worse* of the two. If there is a significant difference between the two eyes, the *better eye* is rated. All the criteria refer to vision *with* corrective lenses if they are needed. Visual problems unrelated to MS are treated the same as MS-related visual deficits.

0 Normal vision: can read print finer than standard newsprint with corrective lenses

1 Cannot read print finer than standard newsprint even with corrective lenses, or complains of double vision

2 Magnifying lenses or large print necessary for reading, or double vision interferes with function

3 Can only read very large print such as major newspaper headlines, or has constant double vision, or sees movement of objects

4 Legal blindness

11. **Speech and hearing:** includes verbal expression and reception for communication with others. The *worse* of either speech or hearing is rated. Speech problems are more common than hearing problems in MS and so the rating will usually be dependent upon speech. Speech and hearing difficulties not related to MS are rated in the same way as those that are due to the illness.

0 Normal: no subjective hearing loss; articulation and language appropriate to the culture

1 Impaired hearing or articulation not interfering with communication

2 Deafness sufficient to require hearing aid, and/or dysarthria interfering with communication, and/or needs communication aids such as special keyboards, etc.

3 Severe deafness compensated for by sign language or lip reading facility, and/or severe dysarthria compensated for by sign language or self-written communication

4 Severe deafness and/or dysarthria without effective compensation

12. **Medical problems:** defined as the presence of other medical disorders (e.g., diabetes, asthma), and/or complications of MS such as decubiti, contractures, and urinary tract infections. Semi-annual checkups unrelated to any specific disorder (e.g., dentist, optometrist, personal physician) are not rated, nor are psychotherapy or counseling. Only *medical* problems requiring intervention by a physician, nurse, or other medical professionals are rated

0 No significant disorder present

1 Disorder(s) not requiring active care; may be on maintenance medication; monitoring not required more often than every 3 months

2 Disorder(s) requiring occasional monitoring by physician or nurse, more often than every 3 months but less often than weekly

3 Disorder(s) requiring regular attention (at least weekly) by physician or nurse

4 Disorder(s) requiring essentially daily attention by physician or nurse, usually in a hospital

13. **Mood and thought disturbances:** includes anxiety, depression, mood swings, euphoria, delusions, hallucinations, and thought disorder. The rating should reflect current behavior even if the patient is maintained on medication. For instance, an individual whose mood swings are observable, but which are controlled by lithium so that they do not interfere with everyday life, would be rated a 1. A rating of 3 requires that psychotherapy or professional help, not 'rap' or discussion groups, is needed.

0 No observable problem

1 Disturbance is present at times, but does not interfere with day-to-day functioning

2 Disturbance does interfere with day-to-day functioning, but the person can manage without professional assistance except for occasional visits to maintain medication

3 Disturbance interferes with day-to-day functioning and consistently requires professional intervention beyond that required to maintain medication, e.g., requires psychotherapy or hospitalization

4 Despite medication and/or other intervention, disturbance is severe enough to preclude day-to-day functioning

14. **Mentation:** refers to disturbances in memory, reasoning, calculation, judgment, or orientation. Mood and thought disturbances (emotional functions) and mentation (intellectual functions) may be difficult to differentiate because of the limited objectivity of a self-report. Information garnered from family members and direct observation will be important in rating these items. It is hoped that brief scales will be added to the MRD in the future to enhance the testing of these functions. More research is needed, however, before the appropriate scales can be selected.

0 No observable problem

1 Disturbance is present but does not interfere with performance of everyday activities

2 Disturbance interferes with performance of everyday activities, e.g., the person may need to use lists or other prompting devices, but manages without the help of other people; the person is likely to be a poor historian

3 Disturbance is severe enough to require prompting or assistance from others for performance of everyday activities

4 Disturbance precludes the performance of most everyday activities; may include severe confusion, disorientation, or memory loss

15. **Fatiguability:** is a sense of overwhelming weakness or lassitude which may alter motor function, coordination, sensation, vision, and mentation. Frequency and duration are variable – frequency may be transient or it may persist for hours or even days. This item rates the extent to which fatigue interferes with function, and how frequently it occurs.

0 No fatiguability

1 Fatiguability present but does not notably interfere with baseline physical function

2 Fatiguability causing intermittent and generally transient impairment of baseline physical function

3 Fatiguability causing intermittent transient loss or frequent moderate impairment of baseline physical function

4 Fatiguability which generally prevents prolonged or sustained physical function

16. **Sexual function:** two important terms are used here. *Sexual activity* refers to engaging in acts (i.e., physical acts or fantasy) which may bring about a sexual response. *Sexual function* refers to the ability of the genitalia to respond to sexual activity, e.g., genital sensation, erection, lubrication, orgasm, and ejaculation. Individuals who are voluntarily celibate or who have no sexual experience pose a special problem because they might not know if their sexual function has changed. Such individuals would be rated a 0 unless there is evidence to suggest a loss of sexual function. Anyone who is using a sexual prosthesis, such as a penile implant, would be rated a 1 or higher. An individual who uses sexual aids such as a vibrator to compensate for loss of function would be rated a 1 or higher.

This item provides for a global rating of sexual dysfunction. Such a rating may be too general to be of much use to professionals. A more detailed section entitled 'Sexual concern inquiry' is provided for those professionals who wish to collect more specific information.

0 Sexually active as before, and/or not experiencing some sexual problems. (No changes in patient's usual pattern of sexual activity; for example, no changes in frequency and type of sexual activities; and no changes from previous genital sensation, erection, and ejaculation in men, or vaginal lubrication and orgasm in women. This includes persons without previous sexual experience or who are voluntarily celibate.)

1 Sexually less active than before, and/or now experiencing some sexual problem(s) but not concerned. (Less frequent or less varied sexual activity, and/or some changes in previous genital sensation, erection, and ejaculation in men, or vaginal lubrication and orgasm in women but does not consider this an issue. May be using a prosthesis or sexual aids.)

2 Sexually less active than before, and now experiencing some sexual problems and concerned. (Would like to regain former sexual activity pattern, and/or would like to regain previous genital sensation, erection, ejaculation, and/or orgasmic experience. May be using a prosthesis or sexual aids.)

3 Sexually inactive but still concerned. (Sexual activity has ceased for several months or years, but wishes to regain previous pattern and functional ability.)

4 Sexually inactive and not concerned. (Sexual activity has ceased for several months, or years, but does not consider this an issue.)

ENVIRONMENTAL STATUS SCALE (ESS)

1. **Actual work status:** refers to one's customary social role: employment, student, or homemaker, etc. It describes the overall situation and is not limited to MS-related problems. A dilemma arises in rating males. Should males ever be rated as homemakers? Very often men are not working but are *capable* of doing housework, and in some instances are actually performing housework. There is no simple solution to this problem. The evaluator needs to determine what would be the *customary role* for a given individual. For most men, it will be external employment. For women, it may be homemaking and/or external employment. For younger persons, education is likely. Individuals who *could* do housework but who can afford to hire help and thus do not actually do housework would be rated a 5.

People who retire early, e.g., from age 50, also present some problems. Many nondisabled individuals retire early. The rater must judge whether a given retirement was 'normal' or was accelerated due to MS or other problems.

People are considered as 'working' even if their job is as a volunteer. While there are many special cases where the rating will be ambiguous, the vast majority of individuals will be easy to rate.

0 Normal or retired for age, e.g., full-time worker, homemaker, or student

1 Works essentially full time but in less demanding position

2 Works more than half time at job, housework, or school

3 Works between one quarter and one half time at job, housework, or school

4 Works less than one quarter time at job, housework, or school

5 Unemployed, not doing any housework or attending school

2. **Financial/economic status:** is focused exclusively on MS-related financial problems. Financial standard could also be termed 'standard of living' and refers to how well a family lives in terms of housing, clothing, food, transportation, recreation, vacations, etc. While there are ratings for individuals who get 'some' outside financial assistance, most people are receiving all the benefits to which they are entitled. At times adverse financial changes may be only partly due to MS, e.g., loss of income due to divorce. If MS is a contributing factor, those changes should be related.

0 No MS related financial problems

1 Family maintains usual financial standard without external support despite some financial disadvantages resulting from MS

2 Family maintains usual financial standard with aid of some external financial support

3 Family maintains usual financial standard by receiving basic disability pension as defined in location of residence

4 Family maintains usual financial standard only because it is receiving all available financial assistance

5 Family is unable to maintain usual financial standard despite receipt of all available financial assistance

3. **Personal residence/home:** this item refers only to MS-related changes. Grading changes as minor, moderate, or major is best illustrated by examples. *Minor* modifications are made at relatively small expense and require little or no reconstruction. Examples are installing a room air conditioner or grab bars, moving furniture, or removing a door. *Moderate* modifications involve significant expense and/or structural changes. Examples are installing several air conditioners, replacing a number of doors, structurally renovating a room, installing simple ramps. *Major* modifications call for renovations costing

thousands of dollars and involving extensive structural changes. Examples are installing a central air conditioning system, renovating several rooms, building extensive masonry ramps, adding an electric chair lift or elevator.

0 No change necessary

1 Minor modification necessary

2 Moderate modification necessary

3 Major structural alteration or addition necessary

4 Must move to satisfactory personal home

5 Must live in facility for dependent care because unable to continue in any personal home (institutionalized)

4. **Personal assistance required:** this refers to any MS-related aid a person might require in order to carry out daily activities such as eating, dressing, bathing, toileting, cooking, cleaning, shopping, child care, etc. It does *not* refer to medical care, counseling, physical therapy, etc. The assistance may be rendered by a family member, home attendant, home health aide, homemaker, volunteer, friend, etc. Needing minor help is rated a 1 and entails such activities as being driven to the supermarket weekly, having a cleaner come in weekly, or occasional (not daily) help in cooking.

0 None

1 Minor help: relatives involved but personal independence is maintained.

2 Requires assistance for activities of daily living up to 1 hour per day from relatives or others in the home

3 Requires assistance with activities of daily living up to 3 hours per day from relatives or others in the home

4 Requires more than 3 hours of personal assistance per day but is able to live at home and does not need a constant attendant

5 Requires a constant attendant or care in an institution, i.e., cannot be left alone for more than short periods such as 2 to 3 hours

5. **Transportation:** refers to transportation problems that are attributable to MS and includes difficulties in both availability and accessibility of transportation. Both public transportation and driving are included. The *better* of the two is rated. Thus the person who cannot use any public transportation but

who drives using hand controls is rated a 2. The problems rated for public transportation may include accessibility, schedule, etc. For instance, if the nearest bus stop is several blocks away and the individual cannot walk there, this would affect the rating.

0 Uses public transportation with no problems, or drives
1 Uses all forms of transportation available despite minor difficulties, or drives with minor difficulty, e.g., needs handicapped parking
2 Uses some public transportation despite difficulties, or needs hand controls to drive
3 Cannot use public transportation but can use private transportation; cannot drive but may be driven by others
4 Requires community (public or private agency) transportation in a wheelchair
5 Requires ambulance

6. **Community services:** this item applies to all persons with MS whether they are living at home or in an institution. Community services is a very broad category and may include medical, social, household, personal assistance, or similar services whether administered at home or in an institution. Community services may include seeing a doctor, nurse, physical therapist, social worker, counselor, or assistance in cooking, housework, bathing, dressing, shopping, etc. Community services include, but are not limited to, the services mentioned in item #4, Personal assistance. Personal assistance is thus a subset of community services.

0 None required
1 Requires service once per month or less frequently
2 Requires not more than 1 hour per week
3 Requires not more than average of 1 hour per day
4 Requires 1 to 4 hours per day
5 Requires more than 4 hours per day, or institutionalized

7. **Social activity:** two dimensions are included in this item: the extent to which the pattern (type and frequency) of social activity is maintained, and the difficulty involved in maintaining that activity. An important consideration is how much social activity the person can initiate.

0 Socially active as before, with no changes in the usual pattern of social activity, and no difficulty in maintaining this pattern
1 Maintains usual pattern of social activity despite some difficulties
2 Some restrictions on social activity such as change in type or frequency of some activities or increased dependence on others
3 Significant restriction of social activity; largely dependent on actions of others but still able to initiate some activity
4 Socially inactive except for the initiative of others
5 No social activity; does not see friends or family; social contact is limited to that provided by community service providers, e.g., visiting nurse

MINIMAL RECORD OF DISABILITY SUMMARY RECORD OF CLINICAL SCORES AND NOTES

Demographic information

1. Patient code

2. Today's date

3. Date of onset (month, year)

4. Date of diagnosis (month, year)

5. Sex

6. Date of birth

7. Total number of years of education
   Elementary 1–8
   High School 9–12
   College 13–16
   Masters 17–18
   Doctorate 19–20

8. What is your marital status?
   1 Married
   2 Cohabiting
   3 Separated
   4 Divorced
   5 Widowed
   6 Single (never married)
   7 Other: _____

9. Who lives with you at the present time?
   A) Spouse
   B) Children
   C) Parent(s)
   D) Brother(s) and/or sister(s)
   E) Other relative(s)
   F) Friend(s)
   G) Live alone

10. Have you ever held a job?

11. What is your current employment status?
   1 Employed outside the home
   2 Homebound employment
   3 Homemaker
   4 Sheltered workshop
   5 Volunteer work
   6 Retired
   7 Unemployed
   8 Student or trainee

12. (If employed) What kind of work do you do?

Neurological assessment (Kurtzke) functional systems

1. Pyramidal

2. Cerebellar

3. Brainstem

4. Sensory

5. Bowel & bladder

6. Visual

7. Mental

8. Other functions
   a) Spasticity
   b) Other _____

Disability Status Scale

Expanded Disability Status Scale

Incapacity Status Scale
1. Stair climbing
2. Ambulation
3. Transfers
4. Bowel function
5. Bladder function
6. Bathing
7. Dressing
8. Grooming
9. Feeding
10. Vision
11. Speech and hearing
12. Medical problems
13. Mood and thought
14. Mentation
15. Fatiguability
16. Sexual function

Sexual Concern Inquiry
1. Does not feel like sex
2. Can't find partner
3. Can't keep partner
4. Can't satisfy partner (sexual problems)
5. Can't satisfy partner (physical problems)
6. Can't satisfy self (sexual problems)
7. Can't satisfy self (physical problems)
8. Can't become a father or mother
9. Can't be like a man or a woman
10. Partner doesn't feel like sex
11. Genitourinary hygiene
12. Lack of privacy
13. Other concerns, specify _____

Which is the area of greatest concern?

Environmental Status Scale
1. Work
2. Financial
3. Home
4. Personal assistance
5. Transportation
6. Community assistance
7. Social activity

Clinical comments

Signature

References

Abbruzzese G, Gandolfo C, Loeb C. (1983) Bolus methylprednisolone versus ACTH in the treatment of multiple sclerosis. *Ital J Neurol Sci 4*:169–172.

Achiron A, Pras E, Gilad R et al. (1992) Open controlled therapeutic trial of intravenous immune globulin in relapsing-remitting multiple sclerosis. *Arch Neurol 49*:1233–1236.

Adams JM, Imagawa DT. (1962) Measles antibody in multiple sclerosis. *Proc Soc Exp Biol 111*:562–566.

Adams RD, Kubik CS. (1952) The morbid anatomy of demyelinating diseases. *Am J Med 12*:510–546.

Adolf GR. (1995) Human interferon omega, a review. *Multiple Sclerosis 1*(Suppl. 1):S44–S47.

Aimard G, Girard P-F, Raveau J. (1966) Sclerose en plaques et processus d'autoimmunisation. Traitement par le antimitotiques. *Lyon Med 215*:345–353.

Aisen ML, Holzer M, Rosen M, Dietz M, McDowell F. (1991) Glutethimide treatment of disabling action tremor in patients with multiple sclerosis and traumatic brain injury. *Arch Neurol 48*:513–515.

Alam SM, Kyriakides T, Lawden M, Newman PK. (1993) Methylprednisolone in multiple sclerosis: a comparison of oral with intravenous therapy at equivalent high dose. *J Neurol Neurosurg Psychiatry 56*:1219–1220.

Albers JW, Bastron JA. (1981) Limb myokymia. *Muscle and Nerve 4*:494–504.

Alexander EL, Malinow K, Lejewski JE, Jerdan MS, Provost TT, Alexander GE. (1986) Primary Sjögren's syndrome with central nervous system disease mimicking multiple sclerosis. *Ann Intern Med 104*:323–330.

Allen IV. (1981) The pathology of multiple sclerosis. *Neuropathol Appl Neurobiol 7*:169–182.

Allen IV. (1983) Hydrolytic enzymes in multiple sclerosis. *Prog Neuropathol 5*:1–17.

Allen IV, McKeown SR. (1979) A histological, histochemical and biochemical study of the macroscopically normal white matter in multiple sclerosis. *J Neurol Sci 41*:81–91.

Allen IV, Millar JHD, Hutchinson MJ. (1978) General disease in nectropsy-proven cases of multiple sclerosis. *Neuropathol Appl Neurobiol 4*:279–284.

Allen IV, Miller JHD, Kirk J, Shillington RKA. (1979) Systemic lupus erythematosus clinically resembling multiple sclerosis and with unusual pathological and ultrastructural features. *J Neurol Neurosurg Psychiat 42*:392–401.

Alter M. (1981) Multiple sclerosis, herpes viruses, and immunity. *Lancet ii*:1224–1225.

Alvord EC. (1970) Acute disseminated encephalomyelitis and allergic neuroencephalopathies. In: Vinken PI, Bruyn GW, eds. *Handbook of Clinical Neurology*. New York, NY: Elsevier; 9:500–571.

Alvord EC. (1984) Species-restricted encephalitogenic determinants. In: Alvord EC, Kies MW, Suckling AJ, eds. *Experimental Allergic Encephalomyelitis*. New York, NY: Alan Liss; 523–537.

Alvord EC. (1986) Disseminated encephalomyelitis: its variations in form and their relationships to other diseases of the nervous system. In: Koetster JC, ed. *Handbook of Clinical Neurology*. New York, NY: Elsevier; 3, 47:467–502.

Alvord EC Jr, Jahnke U, Fischer EH, Kies MW, Driscoll BF, Compston DAS. (1987) The multiple causes of multiple sclerosis: the importance of age of infections in childhood. *J Child Neurol 2*:313–321.

Amato MP, Fratiglioni L, Groppi C et al. (1988) Interrater reliability in assessing functional systems and disability on the Kurtzke scale in multiple sclerosis. *Arch Neurol 45*:746–748.

Anderman F, Cosgrove JBR, Lloyd-Smith DL, Gloor P, McNaughton FL. (1961) Facial myokymia in multiple sclerosis. *Brain 84*:31–44.

Andersson M, Alvarez-Cermeno J, Bernardi G et al. (1994) Cerebrospinal fluid in the diagnosis of multiple sclerosis: a consensus report. *J Neurol Neurosurg Psychiatry 57*:897–902.

Angelé KH. (1980) *Your Daily Health Care*. Bad Wörishafen, Germany: Kneipp Verlag.

Arnason BGW, Chelmicka-Szave E. (1974) Peripheral nerve segmental demyelination induced by intraneural diphtheria toxin injection. I. Effect of hydrocortisone as measured by muscle twitch tension. *Arch Neurol 30*:157–162.

Arnason BGW, Reder AT. (1994) Interferons and multiple sclerosis. *Clinical Neuropharmacology 17*:495–547.

Arnold DL, Mattews PM, Francis G, Antel J. (1990) Proton magnetic resonance spectroscopy of human brain in vivo in the evaluation of multiple sclerosis: assessment of the load of disease. *Magn Reson Med 14*:154–159.

Aschoff JC, Conrad B, Kornhuber HH. (1974) Acquired pendular nystagmus with oscillopsia in multiple sclerosis. *J Neurol Neurosurg Psychiat 37*:570–577.

Asselmann P, Chadwick DW, Marsden CD. (1975) Visual evoked responses in the diagnosis and management of patients suspected of multiple sclerosis. *Brain* 98:261–282.

Auphan N, Didonato JA, Rosette C et al. (1995) Immunosuppression by glucocorticoids: inhibition of NF-kappaB activity through induction of I-kappaB synthesis. *Science* 270:286–290.

Awad SA, Gajewski JB, Sogbein SK, Murray TJ, Field CA. (1984) Relationship between neurological and urological status in patients with multiple sclerosis. *J Urol* 132:499–502.

Baasch E. (1966) Theoretische Überlegungen zur Aetiologie der Sclerosis multiplex. *Schweiz Arch Neurol Neurochir Psychiat* 98:1–19.

Babinski J. (1885) Recherches sur l'anatomie pathologique de la sclérose en plaques et étude comparative des diverses varietées de sclérose de la moëlle. *Arch Physiol* (Paris) 5–6 (séries 3). 186–207.

Bach MA, Phan-Dinh-Tuy F, Tournier E, Chatenoud L, Bach JF, Martin C, Degos JD. (1980) Deficit of suppressor T-cells in active multiple sclerosis. *Lancet* ii:1221–1223.

Bakker DA, Ludwin SK. (1987) Blood-brain barrier permeability during cuprizone-induced demyelination: implications for the pathogenesis of immune mediated demyelinating diseases. *J Neurol Sci* 87:125–137.

Balo J. (1928) Encephalitis periaxialis concentrica. *Arch Neurol* 19:242–264.

Baltus JA, Boersma JW, Hartman AP, Vandenbroucke JP. The occurrence of malignancies in patients with rheumatoid arthritis–treated with cyclophosphamide: a controlled retrospective follow-up. *Ann Rheum Dis* 42:368–373.

Bamford CR, Sibley WA, Thies C. (1983) Seasonal variation of multiple sclerosis exacerbations in Arizona. *Neurology* 33:697–701.

Bamford CR, Sibley WA, Thies C, Laguna JF, Smith MS, Clark K. (1981) Trauma as an aetiologic and aggravating factor in multiple sclerosis. *Neurology* 31:1229–1234.

Baradelli A, Sabra AG, Hallet M, Berenberg W, Simon SR. (1984) Stretch reflexes of triceps surae in patients with upper motor neuron syndromes. *J Neurol Neurosurg Psychiat* 46:54–60.

Barker AT, Jalinous R, Freeston IL. (1985) Non-invasive magnetic stimulation of the human motor cortex. *Lancet* i:1106–1107.

Barkhof F, Frequin ST, Hommes OR, Laners K, Scheltens P. (1992) A correlative trial of gadolinium – DTPA MRI, EDSS, and CSF–MBP in relapsing multiple sclerosis patients treated with high dose intravenous methylprednisolone. *Neurology* 42:63–67.

Barkhof F, Hommes OR, Scheltens P, Valk J. (1991) Quantitative MRI changes in gadolinium – DTPA enhancement after high dose intravenous methylprednisolone in multiple sclerosis. *Neurology* 41:1219–1222.

Barkhof F, Scheltens P, Frequin ST et al. (1992) Relapsing-remitting multiple sclerosis: sequential enhanced MR imaging vs clinical findings in determining disease activity. *Am J Roentgenol* 159:1041–1047.

Barkhof F, Tas MW, Frequin STFM et al. (1994) Limited duration of the effect of methylprednisolone on changes on MRI in multiple sclerosis. *Neuroradiology* 36:382–387.

Barnes D, McDonald WI. (1992) The ocular manifestations of multiple sclerosis. 2. Abnormalities of eye movements. *J Neurol Neurosurg Psychiat* 55:863–868.

Barnes D, McDonald WI, Johnson G, Landon DN. (1988) Characterisation of experimental gliosis by quantitative nuclear magnetic resonance imaging. *Brain* 111:83–94.

Barnes D, McDonald WI, Johnson G, Tofts PS, Landon DN. (1987) Quantitative nuclear magnetic resonance imaging. Characterisation of experimental brain oedema. *J Neurol Neurosurg Psychiat* 50:125–133.

Barnes D, McDonald WI, Tofts PS, Johnson G, Landon DN. (1986) Magnetic resonance imaging of experimental cerebral oedema. *J Neurol Neurosurg Psychiat* 49:1341–1347.

Barnes MP, Bateman DE, Cleland PG et al. (1985) Intravenous methylprednisolone for multiple sclerosis in relapse. *J Neurol Neurosurg Psychiatry* 48:157–159.

Bates D, French J, Hawkins SA, Millar JHD, Smith AD, Thompson RHS, Zilkha K. (1987) Dietary supplementation with omega-3 polyunsaturated fatty acids in multiple sclerosis: Results of a controlled double blind trial. *Proceedings of the ECTRIMS Meeting on Multiple Sclerosis*, Lyon. 387–392.

Bauer HJ. (1983) Umstrittene Multiple Sklerose-Therapie. *Nervenarzt* 54:400–405.

Bauer HJ. (1985) *Multiple Sklerose – Ratgeber: praktische Probleme der Multiplen Sklerose*. New York, NY: Gustav-Fischer Verlag; 3. Auflage.

Bauer HJ, Firnhaber W. (1963) Zur Leistungsprognose Multiple Sklerose Kranker. *DMW* 88:1357–1364.

Bauer HJ, Hanefeld IA. (1993) *Multiple Sclerosis – Its Impact from Childhood to Old Age*. Philadelphia, PA: WB Saunders Co.

Bauer HJ, Orthner H, Poser S. (1975) Neurological aspects of false diagnosis and failure to diagnose multiple sclerosis. *Adv Neurosurg* 2:145–151.

Baum HM, Rothschild BB. (1981) The incidence and prevalence of reported multiple sclerosis. *Ann Neurol* 10:420–428.

Beatty WW, Paul RH, Wilbanks SL et al. (1995) Identifying multiple sclerosis paients with mild or global cognitive impairment using the screening examination for cognitive impairment (SEFCI). *Neurology* 45:718–723.

Beck DW, Vinters HV, Hart MN, Cancilla PA. (1984) Glial cells influence polarity of the blood-brain barrier. *J Neuropathology Exp Neurology* 43:219–224.

Beck J, Rondot P, Catinot L, Falcoff E, Kirchner H, Wietzerbin J. (1988) Increased production of interferon gamma and tumor necrosis factor precede clinical manifestations in multiple sclerosis: Do cytokines trigger off exacerbations? *Acta Neurol Scand* 78:318–323.

Beck RW. (1995) The optic neuritis treatment trial: three-year follow-up results. *Arch Ophthalmol* 113:136–137.

Beck RW, Cleary PA, Anderson MM, JR et al. (1992) A randomized, controlled trial of corticosteroids in the treatment of acute optic neuritis. *New Engl J Med* 326:581–588.

Beck RW, Cleary PA, Trobe JD et al. (1993) The effect of corticosteroids for acute optic neuritis on the subsequent development of multiple sclerosis. *N Engl J Med* 329:1764–1769.

Bednarik J, Kandanka Z. (1992) Multimodal sensory and motor evoked potentials in a two-year follow-up study of MS patients with relapsing course. *Acta Neurol Scand* 86:15–18.

Beer, S, Kesselring J. (1988) Die Multiple Sklerose im Kanton Bern. *Fortschr Neurol Psychiat* 56:390–397.

Beer S, Kesselring J. (1991) Steroidtherapie bei Multipler Sklerose. *Schweiz Med Wschr* 121:961–969.

Beer S, Kesselring J. (1994) High prevalence of multiple sclerosis in Switzerland. *Neuroepidemiology* 13:11–18.

Bellamy AS, Calder VL, Feldmann M, Davison AN. (1985) The distribution of interleukin-2 receptor bearing lymphocytes in multiple sclerosis: evidence for a key role of activated lymphocytes. *Clin Exp Immunol* 61:248–255.

Bemelmans BL, Hommes OR, van Kerrebroeck PE, Lemmens WA, Doesburg WH, Debruyne FM. (1991) Evidence for early lower urinary tract dysfunction in clinically silent multiple sclerosis. *J Urol* 145:1219–1224.

Benecke R, Conrad B, Meinek HM. (1984) Neue Erkenntnisse zur Pathophysiologie der Spastizität. In: Conrad B, Benecke R, Bauer HJ. *Die klinische Wertung der Spastizität.* New York, NY: FK Schattauer Verlag; 17–30.

Benecke R, Emre M, Davidoff RA (Eds). (1990) *The Origin and Treatment of Spasticity.* Carnforth: The Parthenon Publ. Group Ltd.

Ben Nun A, Wekerle H, Cohen IR. (1981) The rapid isolation of clonable antigen specific T lymphocyte line capable of mediating autoimmune encephalomyelitis. *Eur J Immunol* 11:195–199.

Beraud E, Reshef T, Vanderbark AA, et al. (1986) Experimental autoimmune encephalomyelitis mediated by T lymphocyte lines: Genotype of antigen-presenting cells influences immunodominant epitope of basic protein. *J Immunology* 136:511–515.

Berger JR, Sheremata WA, Mekamed E. (1984) Paroxysmal dystonia as the initial manifestation of multiple sclerosis. *Arch Neurol* 41:747–750.

Bernat JL. (1981) Intraspinal steroid therapy. *Neurology* 31:168–171.

Bernstein JJ, Bernstein ME. (1973) Neuronal regeneration and alteration and reinnervation following axonal regeneration and sprouting in mammalian spinal cord. *Brain Behav Evol* 8:135–161.

Betts CD, Mellow MT, Fowler CJ. (1993) Urinary symptoms and the neurological features of bladder dysfunction in multiple sclerosis. *J Neurol Neurosurg Psychiat* 56:245–250.

Beutler E. (1992) Cladribine (2-chlorodeoxyadenosine). *Lancet* 340:952–956.

Beutler E, Koziol JA, McMillan R et al. (1994) Marrow suppression produced by repeated doses of cladribine. *Acta Haematol* 91:10–15.

Bever CTJ, Young D, Anderson PA et al. (1994) The effects of 4-aminopyridine in multiple sclerosis patients. *Neurology* 44:1054–1059.

Bever CTJ, Young D, Tierney D et al. (1995) The pharmacokinetics and tolerability of slow-release formulation of 4-aminopyridine in multiple sclerosis patients. *Neurology* 45(Suppl 4):A351 (Abstract).

Bindoff L. (1988) Methylprednisolone in multiple sclerosis: a comparative dose study. *J Neurol Neurosurg Psychiatry* 51:1108–1109.

Bing R, Reese H. (1926) Die Multiple Sklerose in der Nord-Westschweiz. *Schweiz Med Wschr* 56:30–34.

Birk K, Rudick R. (1986) Pregnancy and multiple sclerosis. *Arch Neurol* 43:719–726.

Blaivas JG. (1984) Evaluation of urinary bladder symptoms in multiple sclerosis. In: Poser CM, et al., eds. *The Diagnosis of Multiple Sclerosis.* New York, NY: Thieme Stratton Inc; 76–93.

Blaivas JG, Barballias GA. (1984) Detrusor-external sphincter dyssynergia in men with multiple sclerosis: an ominous urologic condition. *J Urol* 131:91–94.

Blakemore WF. (1976) Invasion of Schwann cells into the spinal cord of the rat following local injections of lysolecithin. *Neuropath Appl Neurobiol* 2:21–39.

Bobath B. (1990) *Adult Hemiplegia. Evaluation and Treatment.* 3rd Edition. Oxford: Butterworth/Heinemann.

Bolton C. (1992) The efficacy of Cyclosporin A, FK-506 and prednisolone to modify the adoptive transfer of experimental allergic encephalomyelitis (EAE). *Agents Actions* 35:79–84.

Bonduelle M, Bouyges P, Degos CF, Gauthier C. (1979) Les formes bénignes de la sclérose en plaques. *Réévaluation Rev Neurol* 135:593–604.

Booss J, Esiri MM, Tourtellotte WW, Mason DY. (1983) Immunological analysis of T-lymphocyte subsets in the central nervous system in chronic progressive multiple sclerosis. *J Neurol Sci* 62:219–232.

Bornstein MB, Johnson KP. (1992) Treatment of multiple sclerosis with copolymer I. In: Rudick RA, Goodkin DE, eds. *Treatment of Multiple Sclerosis.* New York: Springer-Verlag. 173–198.

Bornstein MB, Miller A, Slagle S, et al. (1987) A pilot trial of Cop 1 in exacerbating-remitting multiple sclerosis. *New Eng J Med* 317:408–414.

Bornstein MB, Miller A, Slagle S, et al. (1991) A placebo-controlled, double-blind, randomized, two-center, pilot trial of Cop-1 in chronic progressive multiple sclerosis. *Neurology* 41:533–539.

Bostock H, Sears TA. (1978) The internodal axon membrane: electrical excitability and continuous conduction in segmental demyelination. *J Physiol (London)* 280:273–301.

Bourdette DN, Whitham RH, Chou YK et al. (1994) Immunity to TCR peptides in multiple sclerosis. I. Successful immunization of patients with synthetic Vbeta5.2 and Vbeta6.1 CDR2 peptides. *J Immunol* 152:2510–2519.

Bourneville DM, Guérard I. (1869) *De la Sclérose en Plaques disséminées.* Paris, France: A. Delahaye.

Boutin B, Esquivel E, Mayer M, Chaumet S, Ponsot

G, Arthuis M. (1988) Multiple sclerosis in children: report of clinical and paraclinical features of 19 cases. *Neuropediatrics* 19:118–123.

Brain WR. (1930) Critical review: disseminated sclerosis. *Quart J Med* 23:343–391.

Brain WR, Wilkinson M. (1957) The association of cervical spondylosis and multiple sclerosis. *Brain* 80:456–478.

Bramwell B. (1917) The prognosis of disseminated sclerosis: duration of 200 cases of disseminated sclerosis. *Edinburgh Med J* 18:16–23.

Brandt S, Gyldensted C, Offner H, Melchior JC. (1981) Multiple sclerosis with onset in a two-year-old boy. *Neuropediatrics* 12:75–82.

Brant-Zawadzki M, Norman D, eds. (1987) *Magnetic Resonance Imaging of the Central Nervous System.* New York, NY: Raven Press.

British and Dutch Multiple Sclerosis Azathioprine Trial Group. (1988) Double-masked trial of azathioprine in multiple sclerosis. *Lancet* ii:179–183.

Brochet B, Guinot P, Orgogozo JM et al. and the Ginkgolide Study Group in Multiple Sclerosis. (1995) Double blind placebo controlled multicenter study of ginkgolide B in treatment of acute exacerbations of multiple sclerosis: short report. *J Neurol Neurosurg Psychiat* 58:360–362.

Broadwell RD. (1989) Transcytosis of macromolecules through the blood brain barrier: a cell biological perspective and clinical appraisal. *Acta Neuropathol* (Berl). 79:177–128.

Brocke S, Gijbels K, Allegretta M et al. (1996) Treatment of experimental encephalomyelitis with peptide analogue of myelin basic protein. *Nature* 379:343–346.

Brod SA, Al-Sabbagh A, Sobel RA et al. (1991) Suppression of experimental autoimmune encephalomyelitis by oral administration of myelin antigens: IV. Suppression of chronic relapsing disease in the Lewis rat and strain 13 guinea pig. *Ann Neurol* 29:615–622.

Brod SA, Burns DK. (1994) Suppression of relapsing experimental autoimmune encephalomyelitis in the SJL/J mouse by oral administration of type I interferons. *Neurology* 44:1144–1148.

Brooks VB. (1986) *The Neural Basis of Motor Control.* New York: Oxford University Press.

Brostoff S, Burnett P, Lampert P, Eylar EH. (1972) Isolation and characterization of a protein from sciatic nerve myelin responsible for experimental allergic neuritis. *Nature* 235:210–212.

Brown AM, McFarlin DE, Raine CS. (1982) Chronologic neuropathology of relapsing experimental allergic encephalomyelitis in the mouse. *Lab Invest* 46:171–185.

Brown WJ. (1978) The capillaries in acute and subacute multiple sclerosis plaques: a morphometric analysis. *Neurology* 28:84–92.

Brück W, Schmied M, Suchanek G, et al. (1994) Oligodendrocytes in early course of multiple sclerosis. *Ann Neurol* 35:65–73.

Budka H, Bernheimer H, Haaijman JJ, Radl J. (1985) Occurrence of IgA subclasses (Iga1 and Iga2) in human nervous system. Correlation with disease. *Int Arch Allergy Appl Immun* 76:107–115.

Bunge MB, Bunge RP, Ris H. (1961) Ultrastructural study of remyelination in an experimental lesion

in adult cat spinal cord. *J Biophys Biochem Cytol* 10:67–74.

Burnfield A. (1984) Doctor – patient dilemmas in multiple sclerosis. *J Med Ethics* 1:21–26.

Burnfield A, Burnfield P. (1978) Common psychological problems in multiple sclerosis. *Br Med J* i:1193–1194.

Bürge T, Griot C, Vandevelde M, Peterhans E. (1989) Antiviral antibodies stimulate production of oxygen species in cultured canine brain cells infected with canine distemper virus. *J Virol* 63:2790–2797.

Burgerman R, Rigamonti D, Randle JM, Fishman P, Panitch HS, Johnson KP. (1992) The association of cervical spondylosis and multiple sclerosis. *Surg Neurol* 38:265–270.

Burnham JA, Wright RR, Dreisbach J, Murray RS. (1991) The effect of high-dose steroids on MRI gadolinium enhancement in acute demyelinating lesions. *Neurology* 41:1349–1354.

Bye AME, Kendall B, Wilson J. (1985) Multiple sclerosis in childhood: a new look. *Dev Med Child Neurol* 27:215–222.

Calabresi PA, Hanham A, Carlino J et al. (1995) Report of an ongoing phase I trial of recombinant transforming growth factor-beta 2 (TGF-beta2) in chronic progressive multiple sclerosis. *Neurology* 45(Suppl 4):A417(Abstract).

Cambi F, Lees MB, Williams RM, Macklin WB. (1983) Chronic experimental allergic encephalomyelitis produced by bovine proteolipid apoprotein: Immunological studies in rabbits. *Ann Neurol* 13:303–308.

Canadian Cooperative Multiple Sclerosis Study Group. (1991) The Canadian cooperative trial of cyclophosphamide and plasma exchange in progressive multiple sclerosis. *Lancet* 337:441–446.

Cannella B, Raine CS. (1995) The adhesion molecule and cytokine profile of multiple sclerosis lesions. *Ann Neurol* 37:424–435.

Capra R, Mattioli F, Vignolo LA et al. (1989) Lesion detection in MS patients with and without clinical brainstem disorders: magnetic resonance imaging and brainstem auditory evoked potentials compared. *Eur Neurol* 29:317–322.

Carroll M, Gates R, Roldan F. (1984) Memory impairment in multiple sclerosis. *Neuropsychologia* 22:297–302.

Carswell R. (1838) *Pathological Anatomy: Illustrations on Elementary Forms of Disease.* London, England: Longman.

Carter J, Sciarra D, Merrit HH. (1950) The course of multiple sclerosis as determined by autopsy proven cases. *Ass Res Nerv Dis Proc* 28:471–511.

Cartlidge NEF. (1972) Autonomic function in multiple sclerosis. *Brain* 95:661–664.

Castaigne P, Cambier J, Masson M, et al. (1979) Les manifestations motrices paroxystiques de la sclérose en plaques. *Presse Méd* 78:1921–1924.

Castillo Morales R. (1991) Die orofaciale Regulationstherapie. Munich, Germany: Pflaum Verlag.

Charcot JM. (1868) Histologie de la sclérose en plaques. *Gaz Hôp* 41:554–555, 557–558, 566.

Charcot JM. (1872–1873) *Lessons sur les Maladies du Systeme Nerveux faites à la Salpetrière.* Paris, France: A. Delahaye.

Charcot JM. (1879) Diagnostic des formes frustes de la sclérose en plaques. *Progr Med* 7:97–99.

Chiappa KH. (1980) Pattern shift visual brainstem auditory and short latency somatosensory evoked potentials in multiple sclerosis. *Neurology* 30:110–130.

Chofflon M, Juillard C, Juillard P, Gauthier G, Grau GE. (1992) Tumor necrosis factor alpha production as a possible predictor of relapse in patients with multiple sclerosis. *Euro Cytokine Netw* 3:523–531.

Chung IY, Norris JG, Benveniste EN. (1991) Differential tumor necrosis factor α expression by astrocytes from experimental allergic encephalomyelitis-susceptible and resistant rat strains. *J Exp Med* 173:801–812.

Claus D, Harding AE, Hess CW, Mills KR, Murray NMF, Thomas PK. (1988) Central motor conduction in degenerative ataxic disorders: a magnetic stimulation study. *J Neurol Neurosurg Psychiat* 51:790–795.

Clifford DB, Trotter JL. (1984) Pain in multiple sclerosis. *Arch Neurol* 41:1270–1272.

Cohen O, Sela BA, Schwartz M, Eshhar N, Cohen IR. (1981) Multiple sclerosis like disease induced in rabbits by immunization with brain gangliosides. *Isr J Med Sci* 17:711–714.

Cohen RA, Kessler HR, Fischer M. (1993) The Extended Disability Status Scale (EDSS) as a predictor of impairments of functional activities of daily living in multiple sclerosis. *J Neurol Sci* 115:132–135.

Comi G, Barkhof F, Durelli L et al. (1995) Early treatment of multiple sclerosis with Rebif (recombinant human interferon beta): design of the study. *Multiple Sclerosis* 1(Suppl. 1):S24–S27.

Comi G, Filippi M, Martinelli V et al. (1993) Brain magnetic resonance imaging correlates of cognitive impairment in multiple sclerosis. *J Neurol Sci* 115(Suppl):66–73.

Compston A. (1983) Lymphocyte subpopulations in patients with multiple sclerosis. *J Neurol Neurosurg Psychiat* 46:105–114.

Compston A, Scolding N, Wren D, Noble M. (1991) The pathogenesis of demyelinating disease: insights from cell biology. *Trends Neurosci* 14:175–181.

Compston DA, Batchelor JR, Earl CJ, McDonald WI. (1978) Factors influencing the risk of multiple sclerosis developing in patients with optic neuritis. *Brain* 101:495–511.

Compston DAS. (1982) Multiple sclerosis in the Orkneys. *Lancet* ii:98.

Compston DAS. (1988) The 150th anniversary of the first depiction of the lesions of multiple sclerosis. *J Neurol Neurosurg Psychiat* 51:1249–1252.

Compston DAS, Vakarelis BN, Paul E, McDonald WI, Batchelor JR, Meins CA. (1986) Viral infection in patients with multiple sclerosis and HLA-DR matched controls. *Brain* 109:325–344.

Confavreux C, Aimard G, Devic M. (1980) Course and prognosis of multiple sclerosis assessed by the computerized data processing of 349 patients. *Brain* 103:281–300.

Cook SD, Cromarty MB, Tapp W, Poskanzner D, Walker JD, Dowling PC. (1985) Declining incidence of multiple sclerosis in the Orkney Islands. *Neurology* 35:545–551.

Cook SD, Devereux C, Troiano R et al. (1987) Total lymphoid irradiation in multiple sclerosis: blood lymphocytes and clinical course. *Ann Neurol* 22:634–638.

Cook SD, MacDonald J, Tapp W, Poskanzner D, Dowling PC. (1988) Multiple sclerosis in the Shetlands: an update. *Acta Neurol Scand* 77:148–151.

Coombes K. (1992) *The Oro-facial Therapy*. New York, NY: Springer Verlag.

Cottrell SS, Wilson SAK. (1926) The effective symptomatology of disseminated sclerosis. A study of 100 cases. *J Neurol Psychopathol* 25:1–30.

Courrier RD, Haerer AF, Meydrech EF. (1993) Low dose oral methotrexate treatment of multiple sclerosis: a pilot study. *J Neurol Neurosurg Psychiatry* 56:1217–1218.

Courville CB. (1970) Concentric sclerosis. In: Vinken PJ, Bruyn GW, eds. *Handbook of Clinical Neurology*. NewYork, NY: Elsevier; 9:437–451.

Cowan JMA, Dick JPR, Day BL, Rothwell JC, Thompson PD, Marsden DC. (1984) Abnormalities in central motor pathway conduction in multiple sclerosis. *Lancet* ii:304–307.

Cox TA, Thompson HS, Corbett JJ. (1981) Relative afferent pupillary defects in optic neuritis. *Am J Ophthalmol* 92:685.

Coyle PK, Krupp LB, Doscher C. (1993) Significance of reactive Lyme serology in multiple sclerosis. *Ann Neurol* 34:745–747.

Cruveilhier J. (1829–1842) *Anatomie Pathologique du Corps Humain*. Paris, France: JB Bailliére.

Currier R, Eldridge R. (1982) Possible risk factors in multiple sclerosis as found in a national twin study. *Arch Neurol* 39:140–144.

Cyong JC, Witkin SS, Rieger B, Barbarese E, Good RA, Day NK. (1982) Antibody-independent complement activation by myelin via the classical complement pathway. *J Exp Med* 155:587–598.

Dalakas M, Wright RG, Prineas JW. (1980) Nature of the reversible white matter lesion in multiple sclerosis: effects of acute inflammation on myelinated tissue studied in rabbit eye. *Brain* 103:515–524.

Dal Canto MC, Barbano RL. (1985) Immunocytochemical localization of MAG, MBP and PO protein in acute and relapsing demyelinating lesions of Theiler's virus infection. *J Neuroimmunol* 10:129–140.

Dal Canto MC, Lipton HL. (1975) Primary demyelination in Theiler's virus infection: an ultrastructural study. *Lab Invest* 33:626–637.

Dal Canto MC, Rabinowitz SG. (1982) Experimental models of virus induced demyelination of the central nervous system. *Ann Neurol* 11:109–127.

Davies PM, Mertin J. (1989) *Hometraining for Patients with Multiple Sclerosis*. Video films A and B. Zurich: Media Productions/Swiss Multiple Sclerosis Society.

Davis FA, Becker FO, Michael JA, Sorensen E. (1970) Effect of intravenous sodium bicarbonate, disodium edetate (Na2EDTA), and hyperventilation on visual and oculomotor signs in multiple sclerosis. *J Neurol Neurosurg Psychiat* 33:723–732.

Davis FA, Bergen D, Schauf C, McDonald WI. (1976) Movement phosphenes in optic neuritis: a new clinical sign. *Neurology* 26:1100–1104.

Davis FA, Jacobson S. (1971) Altered thermal sensitivity in injured and demyelinated nerve: a possible model of temperature effects in multiple sclerosis. *J Neurol Neurosurg Psychiat* 34:551–561.

Davis SEC, Newcombe J, Williams SR et al. (1995) High resolution proton NMR spectroscopy of multiple sclerosis lesions. *Neurochemistry* 64:742–748.

Dawson GD. (1951) A summation technique for the detection of small signals in a large irregular background. *J Physiol* 115:2–3.

Dawson JW. (1916) The histology of disseminated sclerosis. *Trans R Soc* 50:517–740.

Dean G. (1984) Epidemiology of multiple sclerosis. *Neuroepidemiology* 3:58–73.

Dean G, Kurtzke JF. (1971) On the risk of multiple sclerosis according to age at immigration to South Africa. *Br Med J* ii:725–729.

Dean G, McLoughlin H, Brady R, Adelstein AM, Tallett-Williams J. (1976) Multiple sclerosis among immigrants in Greater London. *Br Med J* i:861–864.

Debets R, Savelkoul HFJ. (1994) Cytokine antagonists and their potential therapeutic use. *Immunol Tod* 15:455–458.

DeFreitas EC, Sandberg-Wollheim M, Schonely K, Boufal M, Koprowski H. (1986) Regulation of interleukin 2 receptors on T-cells from multiple sclerosis patients. *Immunology* 83:2637–2641.

Desmedt JE, Cheron G. (1981) Prevertebral (oesophageal) recording of subcortical SEPs in man: the spinal N13 component and the dual nature of spinal generators. *Electroencephalogr Clin Neurophysiol* 52:257–276.

Deuschl G, Strahl K, Schenck E, Lücking CH. (1988) The diagnostic significance of longlatency reflexes in multiple sclerosis. *Electroenceph Clin Neurophysiol* 70:56–61.

Dimitrijevic MR, Nathan PW. (1967a) Studies on spasticity in man: 1: some features of spasticity. *Brain* 90:1–30.

Dimitrijevic MR, Nathan PW. (1967b) Studies on spasticity in man: 2: analysis of stretch reflexes in spasticity. *Brain* 90:333–358.

Dousset V, Grossman RI, Ramer KN et al. (1992) Experimental allergic encephalomyelitis and multiple sclerosis: Lesion characterization with magnetization transfer imaging. *Radiology* 182:483–491.

Drews J. (1990) Glucocorticoids. In: Drews J, ed. *Immunopharmacology*. New York: Springer-Verlag. 140–145.

Dubois-Dalq M, Niedieck B, Buyse M. (1970) Action of anticerebroside sera on myelinated nervous tissue cultures. *Pathologica* 5:331–347.

Duckett JW, Raezer DM. (1976) Neuromuscular dysfunction of the lower urinary tract. In: Kelalis PP, King LR, eds. *Clinical Pediatric Urology*. Philadelphia, Pa: WB Saunders; 1:401–426.

Durelli L, Bongioanni MR, Cavallo R et al. (1994) Chronic systemic high-dose recombinant interferon alpha-2a reduces exacerbation rate, MRI signs of disease activity, and lymphocyte interferon gamma production in relapsing-remitting multiple sclerosis. *Neurology* 44:406–413.

Durelli L, Cocito D, Riccio A et al. (1986) High-dose intravenous methylprednisolone in the treatment of multiple sclerosis: clinical-immunologic correlations. *Neurology* 36:238–243.

Dworkin RH. (1984) Linoleic acid and multiple sclerosis. *Neurology* 34:1441–1445.

Ebers GC. (1983) Genetic factors in multiple sclerosis. *Neurol Clin* 87:336–345.

Ebers GC. (1984) Cerebrospinal fluid electrophoresis in multiple sclerosis. In: Poser CM, ed. *The Diagnosis of Multiple Sclerosis*. New York, NY: Thieme Stratton Inc; 179–184.

Ebers GC. (1985) Optic neuritis and multiple sclerosis. *Arch Neurol* 42:702–704.

Ebers GC. (1994) Treatment of multiple sclerosis. *Lancet* 343:275–279.

Ebers GC, Bulman DE, Sadovnick AD, et al. (1986) A population-based study of multiple sclerosis in twins. *N Engl J Med* 315:1638–1642.

Eccles RM, Lundberg A. (1959) Supraspinal control of interneurons mediating spinal reflexes. *J Physiol* 147:565–584.

Edan G, Miller D, Confavreux C et al. (1995) Evaluation of the efficacy of mitoxantrone by use of MRI: a multicenter randomised study in multiple sclerosis. *Neurology* 242(Suppl. 2):S38(Abstract).

Edwards MK, Farlow MR, Stevens JC. (1986) Multiple sclerosis: MRI and clinical correlation. *AJR* 147:571–574.

Eisen A, Shytbel W, Murphy K, Hoirch M. (1990) Cortical magnetic stimulation in amyotrophic lateral sclerosis. *Muscle & Nerve* 13:146–151.

Elion GB, Hitchings GH. (1990) Azathioprine. In: Eichler O , Farrah A, Heiken H, Wech AD, eds. *Handbook of experimental pharmacology Vol. 38 No 2*. New York: Springer. 404–425.

Elien M, Dean G. (1985) To tell or not to tell the diagnosis of multiple sclerosis. *Lancet* ii:27–28.

Elliot MJ, Maini RN, Feldmann M et al. (1994a) Randomised double-blind comparison of chimeric monoclonal antibody to tumour necrosis factor alpha (cA2) versus placebo in rheumatoid arthritis. *Lancet* 344:1105–1110.

Elliott MJ, Maini RN, Feldmann M et al. (1994b) Repeated therapy with monoclonal antibody to tumour necrosis factor alpha (cA2) in patients with rheumatoid arthritis. *Lancet* 344:1125–1127.

Engell T. (1986) Neurological disease activity in multiple sclerosis patients with periphlebitis retinae. *Acta Neurol Scand* 73:168–172.

Esiri M. (1977) Immunoglobulin containing cells in multiple sclerosis plaques. *Lancet* i:478–480.

Espir MLE, Watkins S, Smith HV. (1966) Paroxysmal dysarthria and other transient neurological disturbances in disseminated sclerosis. *J Neurol Neurosurg Psychiat* 29:323–330.

Fallis RJ, Powers ML, Sy M, Weiner HL. (1987) Adoptive transfer of murine chronic relapsing autoimmune encephalomyelitis: Analysis of basic protein reactive cells in lymphoid organs and nervous system of donor and recipient animals. *J Neuroimmunol* 14:205–220.

Farrar MA, Schreiber RD. (1993) The molecular cell biology of interferon-gamma and its receptor. *Ann Rev Immunol* 11:571–611.

Faulds D, Balfour JA, Chrisp P, Langtry HD. (1991) Mitoxantrone. *Drugs* 41:400–449.

Feigin I, Ogata J. (1971) Schwann cells and peripheral myelin within human central nervous tissues: the mesenchymal character of Schwann cells. *J Neuropathol Exp Neurol* 30:603–612.

Feinstein A, Ron M, Thompson A. (1993) A serial study of psychometric and magnetic resonance imaging changes in multiple sclerosis. *Brain* 116:569–602.

Felgenhauer K, Schädlich JH, Nekic M, Ackermann R. (1985) Cerebrospinal fluid virus antibodies. A diagnostic indicator for multiple sclerosis? *J Neurol Sci* 71:291–299.

Fernandez O, Antiquedad A, Arbizu T et al. (1995) Treatment of relapsing-remitting multiple sclerosis with natural interferon beta: a multicenter, randomized clinical trial. *Multiple Sclerosis* 1(Suppl. 1):S67–S69.

Fernell EB, Smith MC. (1990) Neuropsychological assessment. In: Rao SM, ed. *Neurobehavioral aspects of multiple sclerosis.* New York Oxford: Oxford University Press. 63–81.

Feurer C, Prentice DE, Cammisuli S. (1985) Chronic relapsing experimental allergic encephalomyelitis in the Lewis rat. *J Neuroimmunol* 10:159–166.

Fidler JM, Dejoy SQ, Gibbons JJJ. (1986a) Selective immunomodulation by the antineoplastic agent mitoxantrone. I Suppression of B lymphocyte function. *J Immunol* 137:727–732.

Fidler JM, Dejoy SQ, Smith FRD, Gibbons JJJ. (1986b) Selective immunomodulation by the antineoplastic agent mitoxantrone. II Nonspecific adherent suppressor cells derived from mitoxantrone-treated mice. *J Immunol* 136:2747–2754.

Field EJ, Miller H, Russel DS. (1962) Observations on glial inclusion bodies in a case of acute disseminated sclerosis. *J Clin Pathol* 15:278–284.

Fierz W, Dommasch D, Niederwieser A. (1987) Neopterin in cerebro-spinal fluid as a parameter of local cellular immune reactions in the central nervous system. In: A Lowenthal, J. Raus, eds. *Cellular and Humoral Immunological Components of Cerebrospinal Fluid in Multiple Sclerosis.* New York, NY: Plenum Press; 369–379.

Fierz W, Endler B, Reske K, Wekerle H, Fontana A. (1985) Astrocytes as antigen-presenting cells. I. induction of Ia antigen expression on astrocytes by T-cells via immune interferon and its effect on antigen presentation. *J Immunol* 134:3785–3793.

Fierz W, Fontana A. (1986) The role of astrocytes in the interaction between the immune and nervous system. In: Fedoroff S, Vernadakis A, eds. *Astrocytes: Cell Biology and Pathology of Astrocytes.* London, England: Academic Press; 3:203–229.

Fieschi C, Pozzilli C, Bastianello S et al. (1995) Human recombinant interferon beta in the treatment of relapsing-remitting multiple sclerosis: preliminary observations. *Multiple Sclerosis* 1(Suppl. 1):S28–S31.

Filippi M, Horsfield MA, Bressi S et al. (1995a) Intra- and inter-observer agreement of brain MRI lesion volume measurements in multiple sclerosis. A comparison of techniques. *Brain* 118:1593–1600.

Filippi M, Horsfield MA, Tofts PS et al. (1995b) Quantitative assessment of MRI lesion load in monitoring the evolution of multiple sclerosis. *Brain* 118:1601–1612.

Filippi M, Paty DW, Kappos L et al. (1995c) Correlations between changes in disability and T2-weighted brain MRI activity in multiple sclerosis: a follow up study. *Neurology* 45:255–260.

Firth D. (1948) *The Case of Augustus d'Este.* At the University Press, Cambridge, England.

Fishman HR. (1982) Multiple sclerosis: a new perspective on epidemiological patterns. *Neurology* 32:864–870.

Fleischer B, Marquardt P, Poser S, Kreth HW. (1984) Phenotypic markers and functional characteristics of T lymphocyte clones from cerebrospinal fluid in multiple sclerosis. *J Neuroimmun* 7:151–162.

Fog T. (1950) Topographic distribution of plaques in the spinal cord in multiple sclerosis. *Arch Neurol* 63:382–414.

Fontana A, Fierz W, Wekerle H. (1984) Astrocytes present myelin basic protein to encephalitogenic T-cell lines. *Nature* 307:273–276.

Fontana A, Grieder A, Arrenbrecht ST, Grob P. (1980) In vitro stimulation of glia cells by a lymphocyte produced factor. *J Neurol Sci* 46:55–62.

Foster DH, Snelgar RS, Heron JR. (1985) Nonselective losses in foveal chromatic and luminance sensitivity in multiple sclerosis. *Invest Ophthalmol Vis Sci* 26:1431–1441.

Fowler CJ, van Kerrebroeck Ph EV, Nordenbo A, van Poppel H. (1992) Treatment of lower urinary tract dysfunction in patients with multiple sclerosis. *J Neurol Neurosurg Psychiat* 55:986–989.

Fraenkel M, Jakob A. (1913) Zur Pathologie der Multiplen Sklerose mit besonderer Berücksichtigung der akuten Formen. *Z Neurol* 14:565–603.

Francis DA, Bain P, Swan AV, Hughes RAC. (1991) An assessment of disability rating scales used in multiple sclerosis. *Arch Neurol* 48:299–301.

Francis DA, Batchelor JR, McDonald WI. (1987a) HLA-determinants in familial multiple sclerosis: a study from the Grampian region of Scotland. *Tissue Antigens* 29:7–12.

Francis DA, Compston DA, Batchelor JR, McDonald WI. (1987b) A reassessment of the risk of multiple sclerosis developing in patients with optic neuritis after extended follow-up. *J Neurol Neurosurg Psychiat* 50:758–765.

Francis DA, Thompson AJ, Brooks P, et al. (1991) Multiple sclerosis and HLA: Is the susceptibility gene really HLA-DR or DQ? *Hum Immunol* 32:119–124.

Freal JE, Kraft GH, Coryell JK. (1984) Symptomatic fatigue in multiple sclerosis. *Arch Phys Med Rehabil* 65:135–138.

Freedman MS, Ruijs TC, Selin LK, Antel JP (1991) Peripheral blood gamma/delta T-cells lyse fresh human brain derived oligodendrocytes. *Ann Neurol* 30:794–800.

Frei K, Siepl Ch, Groscurth P, Bodmer S, Schwerdel C, Fontana A. (1987) Antigen presentation and tumor cytotoxicity by interferon-gamma-treated microglial cells. *Eur J Immunol* 17:1271–1278.

Frequin STFM, Lamers KJB, Barkhof F, Borm GF, Hommes OR. (1994) Follow-up study of MS patients treated with high-dose intravenous methylprednisolone. *Acta Neurol Scand* 90:105–110.

Frerichs FT. (1849) Über Hirnsklerose. *Arch Ges Med* 10:334–337.

Friedmann A, Frankel G, Lorch Y, Steinman L. (1987) Monoclonal anti-Ia antibody reverses chronic paralysis and demyelination in Theiler's virus infected mice: Critical importance of timing of treatment. *J Virol* 61:898–903.

Frisén L, Hoyt WF. (1974) Insidious atrophy of retinal nerve fibres in multiple sclerosis. *Arch Ophthalmology* 92:91–97.

Fromm GH, Terrence CF. (1987) Comparison of L-baclofen and racemic baclofen in trigeminal neuralgia. *Neurology* 37:1725–1728.

Funder JW, Sheppard K. (1987) Adrenocortical steroids and the brain. *Annu Rev Physiol* 49:397–411.

Futrell N, Schultz LR, Millikan C. (1992) Central nervous system disease in patients with systemic lupus erythematosus. *Neurology* 42:1549–1657.

Ganrot K, Laurell CB. (1974) Measurement of IgG and albumin content of cerebrospinal fluid, and its interpretation. *Clin Chem* 20:571–573.

Garcin R, Lapresle J, Fardeau M. (1962) Documents pour servir a l'étude des amyotrophies et des abolitions durables des reflexes tendineux observées dans la sclérose en plaques. *Rev Neurol* 107:417–431.

Gass A, Barker GJ, Kidd D, et al. (1994) Correlation of magnetization transfer ratio with clinical disability in multiple sclerosis. *Ann Neurol* 36:62–67.

Gauthier-Smith PC. (1973) Lhermitte's sign in subacute combined degeneration of the spinal cord. *J Neurol Neurosurg Psychiat* 36:861–863.

Gay D, Dick G. (1986) Is multiple sclerosis caused by an oral spirochaete? *Lancet* ii:75–77.

Gean Marton AD, Vezina LG, Marton KI, et al. (1991) Abnormal corpus callosum: a sensitive and specific indicator of multiple sclerosis. *Radiology* 180:215–221.

Georgi F. (1961) Multiple Sklerose: Pathologisch-anatomischer Befund multipler Sklerose bei klinisch nicht diagnostizierten Krankheiten. *Schweiz Med Wschr* 91:605–607.

Georgi F, Hall P, Müller HR. (1961) Zur Problematik der Multiplen Sklerose. Geomedizinische Studien in der Schweiz und in Ostafrika und ihre Bedeutung für Aetiologie und Pathogenese. *Bibl Psychiatr Neurol* 114:1–123.

Ghatak NR, Hirano A, Lijtmaer H, Zimmermann HM. (1974) Asymptomatic demyelinated plaque in the spinal cord. *Arch Neurol* 30:484–486.

Giesser BS, Kurtzberg D, Vaughan HG, et al. (1987) Trimodal evoked potentials compared with magnetic resonance imaging in the diagnosis of multiple sclerosis. *Arch Neurol* 44:281–284.

Gilbert JJ, Sadler M. (1983) Unsuspected multiple sclerosis. *Arch Neurol* 40:533–536.

Gill TM, Feinstein R. (1994) A critical appraisal of the quality of life measurements. *JAMA* 272:619–626.

Gilliatt RW. (1982) Electrophysiology of peripheral neuropathies – an overview. *Muscle & Nerve* 5:108–116.

Giovannoni G, Lai M, Kidd D et al. (in press) Serial urinary neopterin excretion as an immunological marker of disease activity in multiple sclerosis. *Lancet*.

Golaz J, Steck A, Moretta L. (1983) Activated T lymphocytes in patients with multiple sclerosis. *Neurology* 33:1371–1373.

Goldstein I, Siroky MB, Sax DS, Krane RJ. (1982) Neurologic abnormalities in multiple sclerosis. *J Urol* 128:541–545.

Goldstein JL, Anderson RGW, Brown MS. (1979) Coated pits, coated vesicles and receptor mediated endocytosis. *Nature* 279:679–685.

Gonsette RE, Demonty L. (1989) Mitoxantrone, a new immunosuppressive agent in multiple sclerosis. In: Gonsette RE, Delmontle P, eds. *Recent Advances in MS Therapy*. Amsterdam: Elsevier. 161–164.

Gonsette RE, Demonty L, Delmotte P. (1977) Intensive immunosuppression with cyclophosphamide in multiple sclerosis. Follow up of 110 patients for 2–6 years. *J Neurol* 214:173–181.

Gonzalez-Scarano F, Grossman RI, Galetta S, Atlas SW, Silberberg DH. (1987) Multiple sclerosis disease activity correlates with gadolinium-enhanced magnetic resonance imaging. *Ann Neurol* 21:300–306.

Good K, Clark CM, Oger J, Paty D, Klonoff H. (1992) Cognitive impairment and depression in mild multiple sclerosis. *J Nerv Ment Dis* 180:730–732.

Goodkin DE. (1991) EDSS reliability. *Neurology* 41:332.

Goodkin DE. (1994) Interferon beta-1b. *Lancet* 344:1057–1060.

Goodkin DE, Rudick RA, Vanderbrug-Medendorp S et al. (1995) Low-dose (7.5 mg) oral methotrexate reduces the rate of progression in chronic progressive multiple sclerosis. *Ann Neurol* 37:30–40.

Goodman AD, Giang D, Mattson DH et al. (1990) Minimal toxicity associated with monthly pulses of cyclophosphamide in the treatment of chronic progressive multiple sclerosis: preliminary observations. *Ann Neurol* 28:245.

Gorman E, Rudd A, Ebers GC. (1984) Giving the diagnosis of multiple sclerosis. In: Poser C et al., eds. *The Diagnosis of Multiple Sclerosis*. New York, NY: Thieme Stratton Inc; 216–222.

Granger CV, Cotter AC, Hamilton BB, Fiedler RC, Hens MM. (1990) Functional assessment scales: a study of persons with multiple sclerosis. *Arch Phys Med Rehabil* 71:870–875.

Grant I. (1986) Neuropsychological and psychiatric disturbances in multiple sclerosis. In: McDonald WI, Silberberg DH, eds. (1986) *Multiple Sclerosis*. London: Butterworths; 134–152.

Grant I, McDonald WI, Trimble MR, Smith E, Reed R. (1984) Deficient learning and memory in early and middle phases of multiple sclerosis. *J Neurol Neurosurg Psychiat* 47:250–255.

Griffin JW, Goren E, Schaumburg H, King Engel W, Loriaux L. (1977) Adrenomyeloneuropathy: A probable variant of adrenoleukodystrophy. *Neurology* 27:1107–1113.

Grigoresco D. (1932) Contribution à l'étude des troubles dus à des lésions des noyaux gris centraux dans la sclérose en plaques. *Rev Neurol* 58:27–45.

Griot C, Bürge T, Vandevelde M, Peterhans E. (1989) Antibody induced generation of reactive oxygen radicals by brain macrophages in canine distemper: a mechanism for bystander demyelination. *Acta Neuropathol (Berl)* 78:396–403.

Groebke-Lorenz W, Balint S, Frey UP, et al. (1992) Die Multiple Sklerose in der Nordwestschweiz. *Schweiz Med Wschr* 122:582–587.

Grossman RI, Lenkinski RE, Ramer KN, Gonzalez Scarano F, Cohen JA. (1992) MR proton spectroscopy in multiple sclerosis. *Am J Neuroradiol* 13:1535–1543.

Guseo A, Jellinger K. (1975) The significance of perivascular infiltrations in multiple sclerosis. *Neurol* 211:51–60.

Haas J, Patzold U. (1982) Über die Blutbildveränderungen bei langfristiger Behandlung der Multiplen Sklerose und Myasthenie mit Azathioprin. *Nervenarzt* 53:105–109.

Haase AT, Ventura P, Gibbs CJ, Tourtellottee WW. (1981) Measles virus nucleotide sequences: detection by hybridization in situ. *Science* 212:672–675.

Hafler DA, Cohen I, Benjamin DS, Weiner HL. (1992) T cell vaccination in multiple sclerosis: a preliminary report. *Clin Immunol Immunopathol* 62:307–313.

Hafler DA, Fox DA, Manning ME, Schlossman SF, Reinherz EL, Weiner HL. (1985) In vivo activated T lymphocytes in the peripheral blood and cerebrospinal fluid of patients with multiple sclerosis. *N Engl J Med* 312:1405–1411.

Hafler DA, Ritz J, Schlossman SF, Weiner HL. (1988) Anti-CD4 and anti-CD2 monoclonal antibody infusions in subjects with multiple sclerosis: immunosuppressive effects and human antimouse responses. *J Immunol* 141:131–138.

Hall WW, Lamb RA, Choppin PW. (1980) The polypeptides of canine distemper virus: Synthesis in infected cells and relatedness to the polypeptides of other morbilliviruses. *Virology* 100:433–449.

Hallervorden J. (1940) Die zentralen Entmarkungserkrankungen. *Dtsch Z Nervenheilk* 150:?201–239.

Hallervorden J, Spatz H. (1933) Über die konzentrische Sklerose und die physikalisch-chemischen Faktoren bei der Ausbreitung von Entmarkungsprozessen. *Arch Psychiat Nervenkr* 98:641–701.

Halliday AM, ed. (1982) *Evoked Potentials in Clinical Testing*. Edinburgh, Scotland: Churchill Livingstone.

Halliday AM, McDonald WI, Mushin J. (1972) Delayed visual evoked response in optic neuritis. *Lancet* i:982–985.

Hallpike JF. (1983) Clinical aspects of multiple sclerosis. In: Hallpike JF, Adams CWM, Tourtellotte WW, eds. *Multiple Sclerosis. Pathogy, Diagnosis and Management*. London, England: Chapman and Hall; 129–161.

Hallpike JF, Adams CWM. (1969) Proteolysis and myelin breakdown, a review of recent histological and biochemical studies. *Histochem J* 1:559–578.

Hammond SR, English D, Dewytt C, et al. (1988) The clinical profile of multiple sklerose in Australia – a comparison between medium frequency and high-frequency prevalence zones. *Neurology* 38:980–986.

Hankins RW, Black FL. (1986) Western blot analysis of measles virus antibody in normal persons and in patients with multiple sclerosis, subacute sclerosing panencephalitis, or atypical measles. *J Clin Microbiol* 24:324–329.

Harding AE. (1984) *The Hereditary Ataxias and Related Disorders*. London, England: Churchill Livingstone.

Hartung H-P, Michels M, Reiners K et al. (1993) Soluble ICAM-1 serum levels in multiple sclerosis and viral encephalitis. *Neurology* 43:2331–2335.

Hartung HP, Will RG, Francis D, et al. (1988) Familial multiple sclerosis. *J Neurol Sci* 83:259–268.

Hassler R, Bronisch F, Mundinger F, Riechert T. (1975) Intention myoclonus of multiple sclerosis, its patho-anatomical basis and its stereotactic relief. *Neurochirurgia* 18:90–106.

Hasson J, Terry RD, Zimmermann HM. (1958) Peripheral neuropathy in multiple sclerosis. *Neurology* 8:503–510.

Hauser SL, Bresnan MJ, Reinherz EL, Weiner HL. (1982) Childhood multiple sclerosis: clinical features and demonstration of changes in T-cell subsets with disease activity. *Ann Neurol* 11:463–468.

Hauser SL, Dawson DM, Lehrich JR, et al. (1983a) Intensive immunosuppression in progressive multiple sclerosis. A randomized, three-arm study of high-dose intravenous cyclophosphamide, plama exchange and ACTH. *N Engl J Med* 308:173–180.

Hauser SL, Reinherz EL, Hoban CJ, Schlossman SF, Weiner HL. (1983b) Immunoregulatory T-cells and lymphocytotoxic antibodies in active multiple sclerosis: weekly analysis over a six-months period. *Ann Neurol* 13:418–425.

Hawkins CP, Munro PMG, MacKenzie F, et al. (1990) Duration and selectivity of blood-brain barrier breakdown in chronic relapsing experimental allergic encephalomyelitis studied by gadolinium-DTPA and protein markers. *Brain* 113:365–378.

Hawkins CP, Williams SCR, Barker GJ, et al. (1991) Lipid imaging to detect myelin breakdown in multiple sclerosis. *Neuroradiology* 33(suppl):404–405.

Hazleton RA, Reid AC, Rooney PJ. (1980) Cerebral systemic lupus erythematosus: a case report and evaluation of diagnostic tests. *J Neurol Neurosurg Psychiat* 49:357–359.

Heltberg A. (1986) Twin studies in multiple sclerosis. In: Hommes, OR, ed. *Multiple Sclerosis Research in Europe*. Lancaster, England: MTP Press; 337–341.

Hely MA, McManis PG, Doran TJ, Walsh JC, McLeod JG. (1986) Acute optic neuritis: a prospective study of risk factors for multiple sclerosis. *J Neurol Neurosurg Psychiat* 49:1125–1130.

Henderson IC, Allegra JC, Woodcock T et al. (1989) Randomized clinical trial comparing mitoxantrone with doxorubicin in previously treated patients with metastatic breast cancer. *J Clin Oncol* 7:560–571.

Hengst JCD, Kempf RA. (1984) Immunomodulation by cyclophosphamide. *Clin Immunol All* 4:199–216.

Herndon RM, Brooks B. (1985) Misdiagnosis of multiple sclerosis. *Sem Neurol* 5:94–98.

Herndon RM, Rudick RA. (1983) Multiple sclerosis: the spectrum of severity. *Arch Neurol* 40:531–532.

Hess CW, Mills KR, Murray NMF. (1986a) Measurement of central motor conduction in multiple sclerosis by magnetic brain stimulation. *Lancet* ii:355–358.

Hess CW, Mills KR, Murray NMF. (1987a) Extreme prolongation of central motor conduction in multiple sclerosis: A magnetic stimulation study. *J Electroenceph Clin Neurophysiol* 66:7.

Hess CW, Mills KR, Murray NMF. (1987b) Central motor conduction in hereditary motor and sensory neuropathy. *J Electroenceph Clin Neurophysiol* 66:46.

Hess CW, Mills KR, Murray NMF. (1987c) Responses in small hand muscles from magnetic stimulation of the human brain. *J Physiol* 388:397–419.

Hess CW, Mills KR, Murray NMF, Schriefer T. (1987d) Magnetic brain stimulation: central motor conduction studies in multiple sclerosis. *Ann Neurol* 22:744–752.

Hess CW, Müri R, Meienberg O. (1986b) Recording of horizontal saccadic eye movements: Methodological comparison between electro-oculography and infrared reflection oculography. *Neuroophthalmology* 6:189–198.

Hess K. (1979) Stapedius reflex in multiple sclerosis. *J Neurol Neurosurg Psychiat* 42:331–337.

Heun R, Sliwka U, Rüttinger H, Schimrigk K. (1992) Intrathecal versus systemic corticosteroids in the treatment of multiple sclerosis: results of a pilot study. *J Neurol* 239:31–35.

Hickey WF. (1991) Migration of hematogenous cells through the blood brain barrier and the initiation of CNS inflammation. *Brain Pathol* 1:97–105.

Hickey WF, Hsu BL, Kimura H. (1991) T-lymphocyte entry into the central nervous system. *J Neurosci Res* 28:254–260.

Hickey WF, Kimura H. (1987) Graft-vs.-host disease elicits expression of Class I and class II histocompatibility antigens and the presence of scattered T lymphocytes in rat central nervous system. *Neurobiology* 84:2082–2086.

Hickey WF, Kimura H. (1988) perivascular microglia are bone marrow derived and present antigen in vivo. *Science* 239:290–292.

Hickey WF, Vass K, Lassmann H. (1992) Bone marrow derived elements in the central nervous system: an immunohistochemical and ultrastructural survey of rat chimeras. *J Neuropath Exp Neurol* 51:246–256.

Hiele JFJ, Grossman RI, Ramer KN et al. (1995) Magnetization transfer effects in Mr-detected multiple sclerosis lesions: comparison with gadolinium-enhanced spin-echo images and non-enhanced &1-weighted images. *Am J Neuroradiol* 16:69–77.

Hilton P, Hertogs K, Stanton SL. (1983) The use of desmopressin (DDAVP) for nocturia in women with multiple sclerosis. *J Neurol Neurosurg Psychiat* 46:854–855.

Ho HZ, Tiwari JL, Haile RW, Teraski PI, Morton NE. (1982) HLA-linked and unlinked determinants of multiple sclerosis. *Immunogenetics* 15:509–517.

Hofman FM, von Hanwehr RI, Dinarello CA, Mizel SD, Hinton D, Merrill JE. (1986) Immunoregulatory molecules and IL2 receptors identified in multiple sclerosis brain. *J Immunol* 136:3239–3245.

Hohlbrugger G. (1991) The pathophysiological significance of the bladder mucosa in urodynamic problems following MS. In: Wiethölter H, Dichgans J, Mertin J, eds. *Current Concepts in Multiple Sclerosis*. New York, NY: Excerpta Medica; 231–236.

Hohlbrugger G. (In press) The vesical blood-urine barrier: a relevant and dynamic interface between renal function and nervous bladder control. *J Urol.*

Hommes OR, Prick JJ, Lamers KJ. (1975) Treatment of the chronic progressive form of multiple sclerosis with a combination of cyclophosphamide and prednisone. *Clin Neurol Neurosurg* 78:59–72.

Hooge JP, Redekop WK. (1992) Multiple sclerosis with very late onset. *Neurology* 42:1907–1910.

Hooper R. (1828) *The Morbid Anatomy of the Human Brain, Illustrated by Colored Engravings of the Most Frequent and Important Organic Diseases to which that Viscus is Subject.* London, England: Longman, Orme, Brown & Green.

Hopf HC, Stamatovic AM, Wahren W. (1970) Die cerebralen Anfälle bei der multiplen Sklerose. *Z Neurol* 198:256–279.

Howell MD, Winters ST, Olee T et al. (1989) Vaccination against experimental allergic encephalomyelitis with T cell receptor peptides. *Science* 246:668–670.

Hughes GRV. (1980) Central nervous system lupus: diagnosis and treatment. *J Rheumatol* 3:405–411.

Hughes R. (1994) Editorial: Immunotherapy for multiple sclerosis. *J Neurol Neurosurg Psychiatry* 57:3–6.

Hughes RAC. (1991) Editorial. *J Roy Soc Med* 84:63–64.

Hughes RAC (1992) Treatment of multiple sclerosis with azathioprine. In: Rudick RA, Goodkin DE, eds. *Treatment of Multiple Sclerosis.* New York: Springer-Verlag, 157–172.

Hutchinson M, Bresnihan B. (1983) Neurological lupus erythematosus with tonic seizures simulating multiple sclerosis. *J Neurol Neurosurg Psychiat* 46:583–585.

Hutchinson WM. (1976) Acute optic neuritis and the prognosis for multiple sclerosis. *J Neurol Neurosurg Psychiat* 39:283–289.

IFNB Multiple Sclerosis Study Group. (1993) Interferon beta-1b is effective in relapsing-remitting multiple sclerosis. I. Clilnical results of a multicenter, randomized, double-blind, placebo-controlled trial. *Neurology* 43:655–661.

Iivanainen MV. (1981) The significance of abnormal immune response in patients with multiple sclerosis. *J Neuroimmunol* 1:141–172.

Ingram DA, Thompson AJ, Swash M. (1988) Central motor conduction in multiple sclerosis: evaluation of abnormalities revealed by transcutaneous magnetic stimulation of the brain. *J Neurol Neurosurg Psychiat* 51:487–494.

Ipsen J. (1950) Life expectancy and probable disability in multiple sclerosis. *N Engl J Med* 243:909–913.

Izquierdo G, Hauw, JJ, Lyon-Caen O, et al. (1985) Value of multiple sclerosis diagnostic criteria. *Arch Neurol* 42:848–850.

Itoyama Y, Ohnishi A, Tateishi J, Kuroiwa Y, Webster HdeF. (1985) Spinal cord multiple sclerosis lesions in Japanese patients: Schwann cell remyelination occurs in areas that lack glial fibrillary acidic protein (GFAP). *Acta Neuropathol* 65:217–223.

Itoyama Y, Sternberger NH, Webster HdeF, Quarles RH, Cohen SR, Richardson EP. (1980) Immunocytochemical observations on the distribution of myelin associated glycoprotein and myelin basic protein in multiple sclerosis lesions. *Ann Neurol* 7:167–177.

Jacobs L, Cookfair D, Rudick R et al. (1994) Results of a phase III trial of intramuscular recombinant beta interferon as treatment for multiple sclerosis. *Ann Neurol* 36:259(Abstract).

Jacobs L, Johnson KP (1994). A brief history of the use of interferons as treatment of multiple sclerosis. *Arch Neurol* 51:1245–1252.

Jacobs L, Kinkel WR, Polachini I, Kinkel RP. (1986) Correlation of nuclear magnetic resonance imaging, computerized tomography and clinical profiles in multiple sclerosis. *Neurology* 36:27–34.

Jacobs L, O'Malley JA, Freeman A, Ekes R. (1982) Intrathecal interferon reduces exacerbations of multiple sclerosis. *Science* 214:1026–1028.

Jacobs LD, Cookfair DL, Rudick RA et al. (1995) A phase III trial of intramuscular recombinant interferon beta as treatment for exacerbating-remitting multiple sclerosis: design and conduct of study and baseline characteristics of patients. *Multiple Sclerosis* 1:118–135.

Jacobs LD, Cookfair DL, Rudick RA et al. (1996) Intramuscular interferon beta-1a for disease progression in relapsing multiple sclerosis: expedited publication. *Ann Neurol* 39:285–294.

Jacobson S, Flerlage ML, McFarland HF. (1985) Impaired measles virus-specific cytotoxic T-cell responses in multiple sclerosis. *J Exp Med* 162:839–850.

Jacobson SG, Eames RA, McDonald WI. (1979) Optic nerve fibre lesions in adult cats: pattern of recovery of spatial vision. *Exp Brain Res* 36:491–508.

James WH. (1984) Multiple sclerosis and birth order. *J Epidemiol Community Health* 38:21–22.

James WH. (1988) Further evidence in support of the hypothesis that one cause of multiple sclerosis is childhood infection. *Neuroepidemiology* 7:130–133.

Janmohammed R, Milligan DW. (1989) Mitoxantrone induced congestive heart failure in patients previously treated with anthracyclines. *Br J Haematol* 71:292–293.

Janzer RC, Raff MC. (1987) Astrocytes induce blood-brain barrier properties in endothelial cells. *Nature* 325:253–257.

Jellinek EH. (1990) Heine's illness: the case for multiple sclerosis. *JR Soc Med* 83:516–519.

Jellinger K. (1969) Einige morphologische Aspekte der multiplen Sklerose. *Wien Z Nervenheilk*. Suppl II:12–37.

Joffe RT, Lippert GP, Gray TA, Sawa G, Horvath Z. (1987) Mood disorder and multiple sclerosis. *Arch Neurol* 44:376–378.

Johns LD, Flanders KC, Ranges GE, Sriram S. (1991) Successful treatment of experimental allergic encephalomyelitis with transforming growth factor-beta 1. *J Immunol* 147:1792–1796.

Johnson HM, Bazer FW, Szente BE, Jarpe MA. (1994) How interferons fight disease. *Sci Am* 40–47.

Johnson KP, Brooks BR, Cohen JA et al. (1995) Copolymer 1 reduces relapse rate and improves disability in relapsing-remitting multiple sclerosis: Results of a phase III multicenter, double-blind, placebo-controlled trial. *Neurology* 45:1268–1276.

Johnson RT, Griffin DE, Gendelman HE. (1985) Post-infectious encephalomyelitis. *Sem Neurol* 5:180–190.

Johnson RT, Richardson EP. (1968) The neurological manifestations of systemic lupus erythematosus. *Medicine (Baltimore)* 47:337–369.

Jones SM, Streletz LJ, Raab VE, Knobler RL, Lublin FD. (1991) Lower extremity motor evoked potentials in multiple sclerosis. *Arch Neurol* 48:944–948.

de Jong RN. (1970) Multiple sclerosis. History, definition and general considerations. In: Vinken PJ, Bruyn GW, eds. *Multiple Sclerosis and Other Demyelinating Diseases. Handbook of Clinical Neurology, Vol. 9*. Amsterdam, Holland: North Holland Publishing Company; 45–62.

Jung S, Toyka KV, Hartung HP. (1994) Impact of 15-deoxyspergualin on effector cells in experimental autoimmune diseases of the nervous system in the Lewis rat. *Clin Exp Immunol* 98:494–502.

Kaell AT, Shetty AM, Lee BCP, Lockshin MD. (1986) The diversity of neurological events in systemic lupus erythematosus. *Arch Neurol* 43:273–276.

Kanchandani R, Howe JG. (1982) Lhermitte's sign in multiple sclerosis: a clinical survey and review of the literature. *J Neurol Neurosurg Psychiat* 45:308–312.

Kappos L. (1990) *Immunsuppressive Therapie der multiplen Sklerose mit Azathioprin und Cyclosporin A. Langzeiteffekte, Risiken, kernspintomographische und immunologische Befunde*. Springer: New York: Schriftenreihe Neurol 32.

Kappos L. (1995) Interferon beta in the treatment of multiple sclerosis – closing remarks. *Multiple Sclerosis* 1:S64–S66.

Kappos L, Dommasch D. (1983) Quantitative assessment of the clinical status in multiple sclerosis – Development of new grading and documentation systems. In: *Annual Report 1983; 1*. Edited by Max-Planck-Society Clinical Research Unit for Multiple Sclerosis. 24.

Kappos L, Gold R, Kuenstler E et al. (1990a) Mitoxantrone in the treatment of rapidly progressive MS. A pilot study with serial gadolinium enhanced MRI. 42. Annual Meeting, American Academy of Neurology, Miami, April 30th–May 6th, 1990. *Neurology* 40(Suppl. 1):261.

Kappos L, Heun R, Mertens HG. (1990b) A 10-year matched-pairs study comparing azathioprine and no immunosuppression in multiple sclerosis. *Eur Arch Psychiat Clin Neurosci* 240:34–38.

Kappos L, Patzold U, Dommasch D, et al. (1988a) Cyclosporin versus azathioprine in the long-term treatment of multiple sclerosis – results of the German multi center study. *Ann Neurol* 23:56–63.

Kappos L, Radü EW, Haas J et al. (The DSG Study Group) (1995) Deoxyspergualin (DSG) in MS: second interim analysis of the European multicenter study. *Neurology* 242:(Suppl. 2), S23 (Abstract).

Kappos L, Staedt D, Keil W et al. (1987) An attempt to quantify magnetic resonance imaging in multiple sclerosis – correlation with clinical parameters. *Neurosurg Rev* 10:133–135.

Kappos L, Staedt D, Posers S et al. (1989) Clinical, MRI and immunological findings of the German Multicenter Study Cyclosporin A versus azathioprine in multiple sclerosis. In: Battaglia MA, ed. *Multiple Sclerosis Research*. Amsterdam: Elsevier. 275–284.

Kappos L, Staedt D, Ratzka M et al. (1988b) Magnetic resonance imaging in the evaluation of treatment in multiple sclerosis. *Neuroradiology* 30:299–302.

Kappos L, Staedt D, Rohrbach E et al. (1988c) Time course of gadolinium enhancement in MRI of patients with multiple sclerosis: effects of corticosteroid treatment. *J Neurol* 235:10.

Kappos L, Stolle U, Wilhelm U. (1985) Occurrence of cancer after long-term treatment with azathioprine in multiple sclerosis and myasthenia gravis. In: *Annual Report 1985;3*. Edited by Max Planck Society Clinical Research Unit for Multiple Sclerosis. 13–17.

Kappos L, Theobald K, Hartung H-P. (1992) 15-Deoxyspergualin, eine Hoffnung für MS-Betroffene? *Nervenarzt* 63:768–771.

Karussis DJ, Meiner Z, Lehmann D et al. (1995) Treatment of secondary progressive multiple sclerosis with the immunomodulator linomide: results of a double-blind placebo-controlled study with monthly MRI evaluation. *Neurology* 45(Suppl. 4): A417(Abstract).

Karussis DM, Lehmann D, Slavin S et al. (1993a) Inhibition of acute, experimental autoimmune encephalomyelitis by the synthetic immunomodulator linomide. *Ann Neurol* 34:654–660.

Karussis DM, Lehmann D, Slavin S et al. (1993b) Treatment of chronic-relapsing experimental autoimmune encephalomyelitis with the synthetic immunomodulator linomide (quinoline-3-carboxamide). *Proc Natl Acad Sci USA* 90:6400–6404.

Kaufmann SHE. (1990) Heat shock proteins and the immune response. *Immunol Today* 11:129–136.

Kempster PA, Iansek R, Balla JI, Dennis PM, Biegler B. (1987) Value of visual evoked response and oligoclonal bands in cerebrospinal fluid in diagnosis of spinal multiple sclerosis. *Lancet i:769–771.*

Kerlero de Rosbo N, Milo R, Lees MB, Burger D, Bernard CCA, Ben-Nun A. (1993) Reactivity to myelin antigens in multiple sclerosis. *J Clin Invest* 92:2602–2608.

Kermode AG, Tofts PS, Thompson AJ, et al. (1990) Heterogeneity of blood-brain-barrier changes in multiple sclerosis: An MRI study with gadolinium-DTPA enhancement. *Neurology* 40:229–235.

Kernell D, Wu Ch-P. (1967) Responses of the pyramidal tract to stimulate of the baboon's motor cortex. *J Physiol* 191:653–672.

Kesselring J, Miller DH, MacManus DG, et al. (1989a) Quantitative magnetic resonance imaging in multiple sclerosis: the effect of high dose intravenous methylprednisolone. *J Neurol Neurosurg Psychiat* 52:14–17.

Kesselring J, Miller DH, Robb SA, et al. (1990) Acute disseminated encephalomyelitis. MRI findings and the distinction from multiple sclerosis. *Brain* 113:291–302.

Kesselring J, Ormerod IEC, Miller DH, du Boulay EPGH, McDonald WI. (1989b) *Magnetic Resonance Imaging in Multiple Sclerosis – an Atlas of Diagnosis and Differential Diagnosis*. Stuttgart, Germany: Thieme.

Khoshbin S, Hallett M. (1981) Multiple evoked potentials and blinkreflex in multiple sclerosis. *Neurology* 31:138–144.

Kidd D, Thorpe JW, Thompson AJ et al. (1993) Spinal cord MRI using multi-array coils and fast spin echo. II. Findings in multiple sclerosis. *Neurology* 43:2632–2637.

Kies MW, Murphy JB, Alvord EC. (1960) Fractionation of guinea pig brain proteins with encephalitogenic activity. *Fed Proc* 19:207.

Kinn A-C, Larsson PO. (1990) Desmopressin: a new principle for symptomatic treatment of urgency and incontinence in patients with multiple sclerosis. *Scand J Nephrol* 24:109–112.

Kinlen LJ. (1985) Incidence of cancer in rheumatoid arthritis and other disorders after immunosuppressive treatment. *Am J Med* 78:44–49.

Kinnunen E, Wikström J. (1986) Prevalence and prognosis of epilepsy in patients with multiple sclerosis. *Epilepsia* 27:729–733.

Kirk J. (1991) Demyelination – background and mechanisms. *J Neuroimmun* 32:87–94.

Kissel JT, Levy RJ, Mendell JR, Griggs RC. (1986) Azathioprine toxicity in neuromuscular disease. *Neurology* 36:35–39.

Kjaer M. (1982) The value of a multimodal evoked potential approach in the diagnosis of multiple sclerosis. In: Courjon J, Mauguière F & Revol, eds. *Clinical Applications of Evoked Potentials in Neurology*. New York, NY: Raven Press; 507–512.

Knobler RL, Rodriguez M, Lampert PW, Oldstone MBA. (1983) Virologic models of chronic relapsing demyelinating disease. *Acta Neuropathol.* (suppl.) 9:31–37.

Knott M, Voss DE. (1981) *Komplexbewegungen. Bewegungsbahnung nach Dr. Kabat.* New York, NY: Gustav Fischer Verlag.

Kojima K, Berger T, Lassmann H, et al. (1994) Experimental autoimmune panencephalitis and uveoretinitis transferred to the Lewis rat by T lymphocytes specific for the S100β molecule, a calcium binding protein of astroglia. *J Exp Med* 180:817–829.

Koprowski H, Defreitas EC, Harper ME, et al. (1985) Multiple sclerosis and human T-cell lymphotropic viruses. *Nature 318*:154–160.

Korn-Lubetzki I, Kahana E, Cooper G, Abramsky O. (1984) Activity of multiple sclerosis during pregnancy and puerperium. *Ann Neurol* 16:229–231.

Kousmine C. (1986) *Die Multiple Sklerose ist heibar.* Paris, France: Delachaux & Niestlé.

Kovarsky J. (1983) Clinical pharmacology and toxicology of cyclophosphamide: emphasis on use in rheumatic diseases. *Semin Arthritis Rheum* 12:359–372.

Kraft GH, Freal JE, Coryell JK, Hanan CL, Chintnis N. (1981) Multiple sclerosis: early prognostic guidelines. *Arch Phys Med Rehabil* 62:54–58.

Krapf H, Mauch E, Fetzer U et al. (1995) Serial gadolinium-enhanced magnetic resonance imaging in patients with multiple sclerosis treated with mitoxantrone. *Neuroradiology* 37:113–119.

Kremer JM, Alarcon GS, Lightfoot RWJ. (1994) Methotrexate for rheumatoid arthritis: suggested guidelines for monitoring liver toxicity. *Arthritis Rheum* 37:316–328.

Krupp LB, Alvarez LA, LaRocca NG, Schienberg LC. (1988) Fatigue in multiple sclerosis. *Arch Neurol* 45:435–437.

Krupp LB, Sliwinski M, Masur DM et al. (1994) Cognitive functioning and depression in patients with chronic fatigue syndrome and multiple sclerosis. *Arch Neurol* 51:705–710.

Kupersmith MJ, Kaufmann D, Paty DW et al. (1994) Megadose corticosteroids in multiple sclerosis. *Neurology* 44:1–4.

Kurtzke JF. (1965) Further notes on disability evaluation in multiple sclerosis, with scale modifications. *Neurology* 15:654–661.

Kurtzke JF. (1980) Epidemiologic contribution to multiple sclerosis: an overview. *Neurology* 30(2):61–79.

Kurtzke JF. (1983a) Rating neurological impairment in multiple sclerosis: an expanded disability rating scale (EDSS). *Neurology* 13:1444–1452.

Kurtzke JF. (1983b) Epidemiology of multiple sclerosis. In: Hallpike JF, Adams CWM, Tourtellotte WW, eds. *Multiple Sclerosis.* London, England: Chapman and Hall; 47–95.

Kurtzke JF. (1985) Optic neuritis or multiple sclerosis. *Arch Neurol* 42:704–710.

Kurtzke JF, Beebe GW, Nagler B, et al. (1968) Studies on the natural history of multiple sclerosis. 4. Clinical features on the onset bout. *Acta Neurol Scand* 44:379–395.

Kurtzke JF, Beebe GW, Nagler B, Kurland LT, Auth TL. (1977) Studies on the natural history of multiple sclerosis. 8. Early prognostic features of the later course of the illness. *J Chron Dis* 30:819–830.

Kurtzke JF, Beebe GW, Nagler B, Nefzger MD, Auth TL, Kurland LT. (1970) Studies on the natural history of multiple sclerosis. 5. Long-term survival in young men. *Arch Neurol* 22:215–225.

Kurtzke JF, Bui-Quoc-Huong. (1974) Multiple sclerosis in a migrant population. *Eur Neurol* 12:1–12.

Kurtzke JF, Gudmundsson KR, Bergmann S. (1982) Multiple sclerosis in Iceland: 1. Evidence of a postwar epidemic. *Neurology* 32:143–150.

Kurtzke JF, Hyllested K. (1979) Multiple sclerosis in the Faroe Islands: 1. Clinical and epidemiological features. *Ann Neurol* 5:6–21.

Kurtzke JF, Hyllested K. (1988) Validity of the epidemics of multiple sclerosis in the Faroe Islands. *Neuroepidemiology* 7:190–227.

Lafontaine S, Rasminsky M, Saida T, Sumner AJ. (1982) Conduction block in rat myelinated fibres following acute exposure to anti-galactocerebroside serum. *J Physiol* 323:287–306.

Lai SM, Zhag ZX, Alter M, Sobel E. (1989) Worldwide trends in multiple sclerosis mortality. *Neuroepidemiology* 8:56–67.

Lampert PW. (1965) Demyelination and remyelination in experimental allergic encephalomyelitis. *J Neuropath Exp Neurol* 24:371–385.

Lampert PW. (1967) Electromicroscopic studies on ordinary and hyperacute experimental allergic encephalomyelitis. *Acta Neuropathol* 9:99–126.

Lando Z, Teitelbaum D, Arnon R. (1979) Effect of cyclophosphamide on suppressor cell activity in mice unresponsive to EAE. *J Immunol* 123:2156–2160.

Larner AJ. (1986) Aetiological role of viruses in multiple sclerosis: a review. *J R Soc Med* 79:412–417.

Lassmann H. (1983a) *Comparative Neuropathology of Chronic Experimental Allergic Encephalomyelitis and Multiple Sclerosis.* New York, NY: Springer-Verlag.

Lassmann H. (1983b) Chronic relapsing experimental allergic encephalomyelitis: Its value as an experimental model for multiple sclerosis. *J Neurol* 229:207–220.

Lassmann H, Bodka H, Schnaberth G. (1981a) Inflammatory demyelinating polyradiculitis in a patient with multiple sclerosis. *Arch Neurol* 38:99–102.

Lassmann H, Kitz K, Wisniewski HM. (1980) Structural variability of demyelinating lesions in different models of subacute and chronic experimental allergic encephalomyelitis. *Acta Neuropathol* 51:191–201.

Lassmann H, Kitz K, Wisniewski HM. (1981b) Ultrastructural variability of demyelinating lesions in experimental allergic encephalomyelitis and multiple sclerosis. *Acta Neuropathol* (Suppl. VII):173–175.

Lassmann H, Rössler K, Zimprich F, Vass K. (1991a) Expression of adhesion molecules and histocompatibility antigens at the blood brain barrier. *Brain Pathol* 1:115–123.

Lassmann H, Vass K, Brunner C, Wisniewski HM. (1986) Peripheral nervous system lesions in experimental allergic encephalomyelitis. Ultrastructural distribution of T-cells and Ia-antigen. *Acta Neuropathol* 69:193–204.

Lassmann H, Zimprich F, Rössler K, Vass K. (1991b) Inflammation in the nervous system. Basic mechanisms and immunological concepts. *Rev Neurol* 147:763–781.

Latov N, Braun PE, Gross RB, Sherman WH, Penn AS, Chess L. (1981) Plasma cell dyscrasia and peripheral neuropathy: identification of the myelin antigens that react with human paraproteins. *Proc Natl Acad Sci (USA)* 78:7139–7142.

Lauer K. (1986) Some comments on the occurrence of multiple sclerosis in the Faroe Islands. *J Neurol* 293:1–8.

Lazarte JA. (1950) Multiple sclerosis: prognosis for ambulatory and nonambulatory patients. *Ass Res Nerv Dis Proc* 28:512–523.

Lechner-Scott J, Brunnschweiler H, Kappos L. (The Study Steering Committee) (1995) Is it possible to achieve cross-cultural European agreement in the assessment of neurological deficits? First experiences in the European interferon-beta 1b trial for secondary progressive MS. *ECTRIMS (11th European Congress on Multiple Sclerosis), Jerusalem, 3–7:9*, 95 (Abstract).

Lee RG, Tatton WG. (1975) Motor responses to sudden limb displacements in primates with specific CNS lesions and in human patients with motor system disorders. *Can J Neurol Sci* 2:285–293.

Leibowitz U, Kahana E, Alter M. (1969) Survival and death in multiple sclerosis. *Brain* 92:115–130.

Leppert D, Hauser SL, Kishiyama JL et al. (1995a) Stimulation of matrix metalloproteinase-dependent migration of T cells by eicosanoids. *FASEB Journal (Bethesda)* 9:1473–1481.

Leppert D, Waubant E, Galardy R et al. (1995b) T cell gelatinases mediate basement membrane transmigration in vitro. *J Immunol* 154:4379–4389.

Leventhal LJ, Boyce EG, Zurier RB. (1993) Treatment of rheumatoid arthritis with gammalinoleic acid. *Ann Intern Med* 119:867–873.

Levin VA, Chelmicka-Szorc E, Arnason BGW. (1974) Peripheral segmental demyelination induced by intraneural diphtheria toxin injection. II. Sodium Na-24 and carbon-14 labelled insulin kinetics in diphtheria toxin injected nerve and effect of hydrocortisone *Arch Neurol* 30:163–168.

Levine S, Hirano A, Zimmerman H. (1965) Hyperacute allergic encephalomyelitis. Electron microscopic observations. *Am J Pathol* 47:209–221.

Levine S, Wenk EJ. (1965) A hyperacute form of allergic encephalomyelitis. *Am J Pathol* 47:61–88.

Leyden E. (1863) Über graue Degeneration des Rückenmarks. *Dtsch Klin* 35:121–128.

Lhermitte J, Bollack J, Nicolas M. (1924) Les douleurs à type de décharge électrique consecutives à la flexion céphalique dans la sclérose en plaques: un cas de forme sensitive de la sclérose multiple. *Rev Neurol* 2:56–62.

Lhermitte F, Marteau R, Gazengel J, Dordain G, Deloche G. (1973) The frequency of relapse in multiple sclerosis. *J Neurol* 205:47–59.

Lider O, Reshef T, Beraud E et al. (1988) Anti-idiotypic network induced by T-cell vaccination against experimental autoimmune encephalomyelitis. *Science* 239: 181–183.

Lidsky AA, Wisniewski HM, Madrid RE, Lassmann H. (1980) Visual evoked potentials and pathology on relapsing experimental allergic encephalomyelitis. *Docum Ophthal Proc Series* 23:113–120.

Likosky WH, Fireman B, Elnore R, et al. (1991) Intense immunosuppression in chronic progressive multiple sclerosis: the Kaiser study. *J Neurol Neurosurg Psychiat* 54:1055–1060.

Lilemark J, Albertioni F, Hassan M, Juliusson G. (1992) On the bioavailability of oral and subcutaneous 2-chlor-2'-deoxyadenosine in humans: alternative routes of administration. *J Clin Oncol* 10:1514–1518.

Lilius HG, Valtonen EJ, Wikström J. (1976) Sexual problems in patients suffering from multiple sclerosis. *J Chron Dis* 29:643–647.

Lim L, Ron MA, Ormerod IEC, et al. (1988) Psychiatric and neurological manifestations in systemic lupus erythematosus. *Quart J Med* 28:27–38.

Lindsey JW, Hodgkinson S, Mehta R et al. (1994) Phase I clinical trial of chimeric monoclonal anti-CD4 antibody in multiple sclerosis. *Neurology* 44:413–419.

Linington C, Berger T, Perry L, et al. (1993) T cells specific for the myelin oligodendrocyte glycoprotein mediate an unusual autoimmune inflammatory response in the central nervous system. *Eur J Immunol* 23:1364–1372.

Linington C, Bradl M, Lassmann H, Brunner Ch, Vass K. (1988) Augmentation of demyelination in rat acute allergic encephalomyelitis by circulating mouse monoclonal antibodies directed against myelin/oligodendroglia glycoprotein. *Amer J Pathol* 130:443–454.

Linington C, Engelhardt B, Kapocs G, Lassmann H. (1992a) Induction of persistently demyelinated lesions in the rat following the repeated adoptive transfer of encephalitogenic T cells and demyelinating antibody. *J Neuroimmunol* 40:219–224.

Linington C, Gunn CA, Lassmann H. (1990) Identification of an encephalitogenic determinant of myelin proteolipid protein for the rabbit. *J Neuroimmunol* 30:135–144.

Linington C, Izumo S, Suzuki M, Uyemura K, Meyermann R, Wekerle H. (1984a) A permanent rat T-cell line that mediates experimental allergic neuritis in the Lewis rat in vivo. *J Immunol* 133:1946–1950.

Linington C, Lassmann H, Ozawa K, Kosin S, Mongan L. (1992b) Cell adhesion molecules of the immunoglobulin supergene family as tissue specific autoantigens: Induction of experimental allergic neuritis (EAN) by PO protein specific T cell lines. *Eur J Immunol* 22:1813–1817.

Linington C, Webb M, Woodhams PL. (1984b) A novel myelin associated glycoprotein defined by a mouse monoclonal antibody. *J Neuroimmunol* 6:387–396.

Lipton HL. (1975) Theiler's virus infection in mice: an unusual biphasic disease process leading to demyelination. *Infect Immunol* 11:1147–1155.

Lipton HL, Friedman A. (1980) Purification of Theiler's murine encephalomyelitis virus and analysis of the structural virion polypeptides: Correlation of polypeptide profile with virulence. *J Virol* 33:1165–1172.

Lowenthal A, Raus J. (1987) Cellular and humoral immunological components of cerebrospinal fluid in multiple sclerosis. *NATO ASI Series A: Life Sciences* 129.

Lublin FP, Maurer PH, Berry RG, Tippet D. (1981) Delayed relapsing experimental allergic encephalomyelitis in mice. *J Immunol* 126:819–822.

Ludwin SK. (1978) Central nervous system demyelination and remyelination in the mouse. An ultrastructural study of cuprizone toxicity. *Lab Invest* 39:597–612.

Ludwin SK. (1980) Chronic demyelination inhibits remyelination in the central nervous system. An analysis of contributing factors. *Lab Invest* 43:382–387.

Ludwin SK. (1984) Proliferation of mature oligodendrocytes after trauma to the central nervous system. *Nature* 308:274–275.

Lumsden CE. (1970) The neuropathology of multiple sclerosis. In: Vinken PI, Bryun GW, eds. *Handbook of Clinical Neurology*. New York, NY: Elsevier; 9:217–309.

Lundberg PO. (1981) Sexual dysfunction in female patients with multiple sclerosis. *Int Rehab Med* 3:32–34.

Lygner PE, Andersen O, Bergström T, Vahlne A. (1988) Prospective epidemiological and virological study of the relationship between upper respiratory infections and multiple sclerosis. In: Confavreux C, Aimard G, Devic M, eds. *Trends in European Multiple Sclerosis Research*. New York, NY: Elsevier Science Publishers; 41–47.

Lyon-Caën O, Izquierdo G, Marteau R, Lhermitte F, Castaigne P, Hauw JJ. (1985) Late onset multiple sclerosis. A clinical study of pathologically proven cases. *Acta Neurol Scand* 72:56–60.

Lyon-Caën O, Jouvent R, Hauser S, et al. (1986) Cognitive function in recent-onset demyelinating diseases. *Arch Neurol* 43:1138–1141.

Lyons PR, Newman PK, Saunders M. (1988) Methylprednisolone therapy in multiple sclerosis: a profile of adverse effects. *J Neurol Neurosurg Psychiatry* 51:285–287.

Mackay RP, Myrianthopoulos NC. (1966) Multiple sclerosis in twins and their relatives. *Arch Neurol* 15:449–462.

Mackay RP, Hirano A. (1967) Forms of benign multiple sclerosis: report of two 'clinically silent' cases discovered at autopsy. *Arch Neurol* 17:588–600.

MacLeod AM, Thompson AW. (1991) FK 506: an immunosuppressant for the 1990s? *Lancet* 337:25–27.

Madrid RE, Wisniewski HM, Hashim GA, Moscarello MA, Wood DD. (1982) Lipophilin-induced experimental allergic encephalomyelitis in guinea pigs. *J Neurosci Res* 7:203–213.

Maertens de Noordhout A, Remacle JM, Pepin JL, Born JD, Delwaide PJ. (1991) Magnetic stimulation of the motor cortex in cervical spondylosis. *Neurology* 41:75–80.

Maida E, Summer K. (1979) Serum cortisol levels of multiple sclerosis patients during ACTH treatment. *J Neurol* 220:143–148.

Male D, Pryce G, Hughes C, Lantos P. (1990a) Lymphocyte migration into brain modelled in vitro: control by lymphocyte activation, cytokines and antigens. *Cell Immunol* 127: 1–11.

Male D, Pryce G, Rahman J. (1990b) Comparison of the immunological properties of rat cerebral and aortic endothelium. *J Neuroimmunol* 30:161–168.

Malmgren RM, Dudley JP, Visscher BR, Valdiviezo NL, Clark VA, Detels R. (1981) Mortality in persons with multiple sclerosis in the Seattle and Los Angeles areas. *JAMA* 246:2042–2046.

Malmgren RM, Valdiviezo NL, Visscher BR, et al. (1983) Underlying cause of death as recorded for multiple sclerosis patients: associated factors. *J Chron Dis* 36:699–705.

Marburg O. (1906) Die sogenannte akute Multiple Sklerose. *Jahrb Psychiatrie* 27:211–312.

Marie P. (1884) Sclérose en plaques et maladies infectieuses. *Progr Med (Paris)* 12:287–289.

Markham A, Faulds D. (1994) Methotrexate: a review of its pharmacodynamic and pharmacokinetic properties, and therapeutic efficacy in rheumatoid arthritis and other immunoregulatory disorders. *Clin Immunother* 1:217–224.

Martin R, McFarland HF, McFarlin DE. (1992a) Immunological aspects of demyelinating diseases. *Annu Rev Immunol* 10:153–187.

Martin R, Utz U, Coligan JE et al. (1992b) Diversity in fine specificity and T cell receptor usage of the human CD4+ cytotoxic T cell response specific for the immunodominant myelin basic protein peptide 87–106. *J Immunol* 148:1359–1366.

Martin R, Vergelli M, Conlon P et al. (1995) Altered peptide ligands modify functions of T cells specific for the immunodominant MBP peptide 87–99. *Neurology* 45(Suppl 4):A383(Abstract).

Martin R, Voskuhl R, Flerlage M et al. (1993) Myelin basic protein-specific T-cell responses in identical twins discordant or concordant for multiple sclerosis. *Ann Neurol* 34:524–535.

Martyn C. (1991) Epidemiology. In: Matthews WB, ed. *McAlpine's Multiple Sclerosis*, 2nd edition. London, England: Churchill Livingstone.

Marx J. (1995) How glucocorticoids suppress immunity. *Science* 270:232–233.

Mason D. (1991) Genetic variation in the stress response: susceptibility to experimental allergic encephalomyelitis and implications for human inflammatory demyelinating disease. *Immunol Today* 12:57–60.

Massa PT, ter Meulen V. (1987) Analysis of Ia induction on lewis rat astrocytes in vitro by virus particles and bacterial adjuvants. *J Neuroimmunol* 13:259–271.

Massa PT, Wege H, ter Meulen V. (1986) Analysis of murine hepatitis virus (JHM strain) tropism toward lewis rat glial cells in vitro. *Lab Invest* 55:318–327.

Masson C. (1987) Aspects neurologique de la maladie de Lyme. *Presse Med* 16:72–75.

Mastaglia FL, Black JL, Thickbroom G, Collins DWK. (1982) Saccadic eye movements in multiple sclerosis. *Neuro-ophthalmology* 2:225–236.

Mathiowetz V, Weber K, Kashman N, Volland G. (1985) Adult norms for the nine hole peg test of finger dexterity. *Occup Ther J Res* 5:24–38.

Matthews WB. (1966) Facial myokymia. *J Neurol Neurosurg Psychiat* 29:35–39.

Matthews WB. (1975) Paroxysmal symptoms in multiple sclerosis. *J Neurol Neurosurg Psychiat* 38: 617–623.

Matthews WB, ed. (1991) *McAlpine's Multiple Sclerosis*. 2nd ed. Edinburgh, Scotland: Churchill Livingstone.

Matthews WB, Acheson ED, Batchelor JQ, Weller RO, eds. (1991) *McAlpine's Multiple Sclerosis*. London, England: Churchill Livingstone.

Matthews WB, Wattam-Bell JRB, Poutney F. (1982) Evoked potentials in the diagnosis of multiple sclerosis: a follow-up study. *J Neurol Neurosurg Psychiat* 45:303–307.

Mattson DH, Roos RP, Arnason BGW. (1980) Isoelectric focusing of IgG eluted from multiple sclerosis and subacute sclerosing panencephalitis brains. *Nature* 287:335–337.

Mauch E, Kornhuber HH, Krapf H et al. (1992) Treatment of multiple sclerosis with mitoxantrone. *Eur Arch Psychiat Clin Neurosci* 242:96–102.

Mauch E, Kornhuber HH, Pfrommer U et al. (1989) Effective treatment of chronically progressive MS with low-dose cyclophosphamide with minor side-effects. *Eur Arch Psychiat Neurol Sci* 238:115–117.

McAlpine D. (1961) The benign form of multiple sclerosis: a study based on 241 cases seen within three years of onset and followed up until the tenth year or more of the disease. *Brain* 84:186–203.

McCarron RM, Kempski O, Spatz M, McFarlin DE. (1985) Presentation of myelin basic protein by murine cerebral vascular endothelial cells. *J Immunol* 134:3100–3103.

McCarron RM, Spatz M, Kempski O, Hogn RN, Muehl L, McFarlin DE. (1986) Interaction between myelin basic protein-sensitized T lymphocytes and murine cerebral vascular endothelial cells. *J Immunol* 137:3428–3435.

McCouch GP, Austin GM, Liu CN, Liu CY. (1958) Sprouting as a cause of spasticity. *J Neurophysiol* 21:205–216.

McDonald WI. (1974a) Pathophysiology in multiple sclerosis. *Brain* 97:179–196.

McDonald WI. (1974b) Remyelination in relation to clinical lesions of the central nervous system. *Br Med Bull* 30:186–189.

McDonald WI. (1983a) Multiple sclerosis: The present position. *Acta Neurol Scand* 68:65–76.

McDonald WI. (1983b) Doyne lecture: The significance of optic neuritis. *Trans ophthal Soc UK* 103:230–246.

McDonald WI. (1986) The pathophysiology of multiple sclerosis. In: McDonald WI, Silberberg DH, eds. *Multiple Sclerosis*. London: Butterworths; 112–133.

McDonald WI. (1992) Multiple sclerosis: diagnostic optimism. *Brit Med J* 304:1259–1260.

McDonald WI. (1993) The dynamics of multiple sclerosis. The Charcot Lecture. *J Neurol* 240:28–36.

McDonald WI, Barnes D. (1989) Lessons from magnetic resonance imaging in multiple sclerosis. *TINS* 12:376–379.

McDonald WI, Barnes D. (1992) The ocular manifestations of multiple sclerosis. 1. Abnormalities of the afferent visual system. *J Neurol Neurosurg Psychiat* 55:747–752.

McDonald WI, Miller DH, Barnes D. (1992) The pathological evolution of multiple sclerosis. *Neuropathol Appl Neurobiol* 18:319–334.

McDonald WI, Sears TA. (1970a) The effects of experimental demyelination on conduction in the central nervous system. *Brain* 93:583–598.

McDonald WI, Halliday AM. (1977) Diagnosis and classification of multiple sclerosis. *Br Med Bull* 33:4–8.

McDonald WI, Miller DH, Thompson AJ. (1994) Are magnetic resonance findings predictive of clinical outcome in therapeutic trials in multiple sclerosis? The dilemma of Interferon-beta. *Ann Neurol* 36:14–18.

McDonald WI, Sears TA. (1970b) Focal experimental demyelination in the central nervous system. *Brain* 575–582.

McDonald WI, Silberberg DH. (1986) The diagnosis of multiple sclerosis. In: McDonald WI, Silberberg DH, eds. *Multiple Sclerosis*. London: Butterworths; 1–10.

McEwen BS, Dekloet ER, Rostene W. (1986) Adrenal steroid receptors and actions in the nervous system. *Physiol Rev* 66:1121–1188.

McFarland HF, Frank JA, Albert PE, et al. (1992) Using gadolinium-enhanced magnetic resonance imaging lesions to monitor disease activity in multiple sclerosis. *Ann Neurol* 32:758–766.

McFarland HF, Greenstein J, McFarlin DE, Eldrige R, Xu X-H, Krebs H. (1984) Family and twin studies in multiple sclerosis. *Ann NY Acad Sci* 436: 118–124.

McFarlin DE, McFarland HF. (1982) Multiple sclerosis. *N Engl J Med* 307:1183–1188 and 1246–1251.

McFarling DA, Susac JO. (1979) 'Hoquet diabolique': intractable hiccup as a manifestation of multiple sclerosis. *Neurology* 29:797–801.

McHenry LC. (1969) Garrinson's *History of Neurology*. Springfield, Ill: Charles C Thomas Publisher.

Medaer R. (1979) Does the history of multiple sclerosis go back as far as the 14th century? *Acta Neurol Scand* 60:189–192.

Medaer R, Stinissen P, Truyen L et al. (1995) Depletion of myelin-basic-protein autoreactive T cells by T-cell vaccination: pilot trial in multiple sclerosis. *Lancet* 346:807–808.

Mehta PD, Miller JA, Tourtellotte WW. (1982) Oligoclonal IgG bands in plaques from multiple sclerosis brains. *Neurology* 32:372–376.

Meienberg O, Flammer J, Ludin HP. (1982) Subclinical visual field defects in multiple sclerosis. *J Neurol* 227:125–133.

Meienberg O, Müri R, Rabineau PA. (1986) Clinical and oculographic examinations of saccadic eye movements in the diagnosis of multiple sclerosis. *Arch Neurol* 43:438–443.

Meinck HM, Schönle PW, Conard B. (1989) Effect of canabinoids on spasticity and ataxia in multiple sclerosis. *J Neurol* 236:120–122.

Meinl E, Weber F, Drexler K et al. (1993) Myelin basic protein-specific T lymphocyte repertoire in multiple sclerosis. *J Clin Invest* 92:2633–2643.

Mellman I, Plutner H. (1984) Internalization and degradation of macrophage Fc-receptors bound to polyvalent immune complexes. *J Cell Biol* 98: 1170–1177.

Melvold RW, Jokinen DM, Knobler RL, Lipton HL. (1987) Variations in genetic control of susceptibility to Theiler's murine encephalomyelitis virus (TMEV)-induced demyelinating disease. *J Immunol* 138:1429–1433.

Mertin J. (1980) Dietary polyunsaturated fatty acids and immunosuppression. In: Davison AN, Cuzner ML, eds. *The Suppression of Experimental Allergic Encephalomyelitis and Multiple Sclerosis.* New York, NY: Academic Press; 171–187.

Mertin J. (1985) Drug treatment of patients with multiple sclerosis. In: Vinken P, Bruyn GW, Klawans HL, Koestsier JC, eds. *Handbook of Clinical Neurology,* revised series 3, vol. 47, *Demyelinating Diseases.* Amsterdam, Holland: Elsevier Science Publishers; 187–212.

Mertin J. (1994) Rehabilitation in multiple sclerosis. *Ann Neurol* 36(Suppl):S130–S133.

Mertin J, Meade CJ. (1977) Relevance of fatty acids in multiple sclerosis. *Brit Med Bull* 33:67–71.

Mertin J, Mertin LA. ((1988) Modulation of *in vivo* immune responses following changes in the intake of essential fatty acids. *Prog Allergy* 44:172–206.

Mertin J, Paeth B. (1994) Physiotherapy and multiple sclerosis – application of the Bobath concept. *MS Management* 1:10–13.

Mertin J, Stackpoole A. (1981) Anti-PGE antibodies inhibit in vivo development of cell-mediated immunity. *Nature* 294:456–457.

Mertin J, Stackpoole A, Shumway S. (1985) Nutrition and immunity: The immunoregulatory effect of n-6 essential fatty acids is mediated through prostaglandin E. *Int Arch Allergy Appl Immunol* 77:390–395.

Merton PA, Morton HB. (1980) Stimulation of the cerebral cortex in the intact human subject. *Nature* 285:227.

Meyermann RM, Lampert PW, Korr H, Wekerle H. (1987) The blood brain barrier – the strict border to lymphoid cells. In: Cervos-Navarro J, Ferszt R, eds. *Stoke and Microcirculation.* New York, NY: Raven Press; 289–296.

Mickel HS. (1975) Multiple sclerosis: a new hypothesis. *Perspect Biol Med* 18:363–374.

Milanese C, La Mantia L, Salmaggi A, Eolie M. (1993) A double blind study of azathioprine efficacy in multiple sclerosis: final report. *J Neurol* 240:295–298.

Millar JHD, Vas CJ, Noronka MJ et al. (1967) Long-term treatment of multiple sclerosis with corticotrophin. *Lancet* ii:429–431.

Millar JHD, Zilkha KJ, Langman MJS, et al. (1973) Double-blind trial of linoleate supplementation of the diet in multiple sclerosis. *Brit Med J* 1:765–768.

Miller A, Al Sabbagh A, Santos LMB et al. (1993) Epitopes of myelin basic protein that trigger TGF-beta release after oral tolerization are distinct from encephalitogenic epitopes and mediate epitope-driven bystander suppression. *J Immunol* 151:7307–7315.

Miller A, Lider O, Weiner HL. (1991) Antigen driven bystander suppression following oral administration of antigens. *J Exp Med* 174:791–798.

Miller DH, Barkhof F, Berry I, Kappos L, Scotti G, Thompson AJ. (1991) Magnetic resonance imaging in monitoring the treatment of multiple sclerosis: concerted action guidelines. *J Neurol Neurosurg Psychiat* 54:683–688.

Miller DH, Hammond SR, McLeond JG, Purdie G, Skegg DC. (1990) Multiple sclerosis in Australia and New Zealand: Are the determinants genetic or environmental? *J Neurol Neurosurg Psychiat* 53:903–905.

Miller DH, Hornabrook RW, Dagger J, Fong R. (1986) Ethnic and HLA patterns related to multiple sclerosis in Wellington, New Zealand. *J Neurol Neurosurg Psychiat* 49:43–46.

Miller DH, Kesselring J, Thompson AJ, McDonald WI, Paty DW. (In press) *Magnetic Resonance Imaging in Multiple Sclerosis.* New York, NY: Cambridge University Press.

Miller DH, Lai HM, Lewellyn-Smith N et al. (1995) Phase II trial of anti-CD4-antibodies in the treatment of multiple sclerosis. *Neurology* 242(Suppl. 2):S23(Abstract).

Miller DH, Newton MR, van der Poel JC, et al. (1988a) Magnetic resonance imaging of the optic nerve in optic neuritis. *Neurology* 38:175–179.

Miller DH, Ormerod IEC, Gibson A, du Boulay EPGH, Rudge P, McDonald WI. (1987) MRI brain scanning in patients with vasculitis: differentiation from multiple sclerosis. *Neuroradiology* 29:226–231.

Miller DH, Rudge P, Johnson G, et al. (1988) Serial gadolinium enhanced magnetic resonance imaging in multiple sclerosis. *Brain* 111:927–939.

Miller HJ, Newell DJ, Ridley A. (1961) MS: Treatment of acute exacerbations with ACTH. *Lancet* ii:1120–1122.

Milligan NM, Newcombe R, Compston DAS. (1987) A double-blind controlled trial of high dose methylprednisolone in patients with multiple sclerosis: 1. clinical effects. *J Neurol Neurosurg Psychiatry* 50:511–516.

Mills KR, Murray NMF. (1985) Cortical spinal tract conduction times in multiple sclerosis. *Ann Neurol* 18:601–605.

Milner P, Lovelidge CA, Taylor WA, Hughes RC. (1987) P0 myelin protein produces experimental allergic neuritis in Lewis rats. *J Neurol Sci* 79: 275–285.

Minderhoud JM, Leemhuis JG, Kremer J, Laban E. Smits PML. (1984) Sexual disturbances arising from multiple sclerosis. *Acta Neurol Scand* 70:299–306.

Miro J, Amado JA, Pesquera C, Lopez-Cordovilla JJ, Berciano J. (1990a) Assessment of the hypothalamic–pituitary–adrenal axis function after corticosteroid therapy for MS relapses. *Acta Neurol Scand* 81:524–528.

Miro J, Pena Sagredo JL, Berciano J, Insua S, Leno C, Velarde R. (1990b) Prevalence of primary Sjögren's syndrome in patients with multiple sclerosis. *Ann Neurol* 27:582–584.

Miyawaki T, Taga K, Nagaoki T et al. (1984) Circadian changes of T-lymphocyte subsets in human peripheral blood. *Clin Exp Immunol* 55:618–622.

Montesano R, Mossaz A, Vassalli P, Orci L. (1983) Specialization of the macrophage plasma membrane at sites of interaction with opsonized erythrocytes *J Cell Biol* 96:1227–1233.

Moore GRW, Neumann PE, Suzuki K, Litjmaer HN, Traugott U, Raine CS. (1985) Balo's concentric sclerosis – new observations on lesion development. *Ann Neurol* 17:604–611.

Moore KW, O'Garra A, De Waal Malefyt R et al. (1993) Interleukin-10. *Ann Rev Immunol* 11:165–190.

Moreau T, Thorpe JW, Miller DH et al. (1994) Preliminary evidence from magnetic resonance imaging for reduction in disease activity after lymphocyte depletion in multiple sclerosis. *Lancet* 344:298–301.

Morgan BP, Campell AK, Compston DAS. (1984) Terminal component of complement (C9) in cerebrospinal fluid of patients with multiple sclerosis. *Lancet* ii:251–254.

Morgan SL, Baggott JE, Vaughn WH. (1994) Supplementation with folic acid during methotrexate therapy for rheumatoid arthritis: a double-blind placebo-controlled trial. *Ann Intern Med* 121:833–841.

Morris RE. (1991) ±15-deoxyspergualin: a mystery wrapped in an enigma. *Clin Transplantation* 5:530–533.

Morrissey SP, Miller DH, Kendall BE, et al. (1993) The signifance of brain magnetic resonance imaging abnormalities at presentation with clinically isolated syndromes suggestive of multiple sclerosis. A 5-year follow-up study. *Brain* 116:135–146.

Moser HW, Moser AE, Singh I, O'Neill P. (1984) Adrenoleukodystrophy: survey of 303 cases: biochemistry, diagnosis, and therapy. *Ann Neurol* 16:628–641.

Motomura S, Tabira T, Kuroiwa Y. A clinical comparative study of multiple sclerosis and neuro-Behcet syndrome. *J Neurol Neurosurg Psychiat* 43:210–213.

Moulin D, Paty DW, Ebers GC. (1983) The predictive value of cerebrospinal fluid electrophoresis in 'possible' multiple sclerosis. *Brain* 106:809–816.

Moulin DE, Foley KM, Ebers GC. (1988) Pain syndromes in multiple sclerosis. *Neurology* 38:1830–1834.

Mumford CJ, Campston A. (1993) Problems with rating scales for multiple sclerosis: a novel approach – the CAMBS score. *J Neurol* 240:209–215.

Müller E. (1904) *Die Multiple Sklerose des Gehirns und Ruckenmarks*. Jena, Germany: Gustav-Fischer-Verlag.

Müller R. (1951) Course and prognosis of disseminated sclerosis in relation to age at onset. *Arch Neurol Psychiat* 66:561–570.

Multiple Sclerosis Study Group. (1988) The efficacy and toxicity of cyclosporine immunosuppression in MS: a preliminary report of a randomized blinded, placebo controlled clinical trial. *Ann Neurol* 24:169.

Müri R, Meienberg O. (1985) The clinical spectrum of internuclear ophthalmoplegia in multiple sclerosis. *Arch Neurol* 42:851–855.

Murray M, Goldberger ME. (1974) Restitution of function and collateral sprouting in the cat spinal cord: the partially hemisected animal. *J Comp Neurol* 158:19–36.

Murray TJ, Murray SJ. (1984) Characteristics of patients found not to have multiple sclerosis. *Can Med Assoc J* 131:336–337.

Mussini JM, Hauw JJ, Escourolle R. (1977) Immunofluorescence studies of intracytoplasmic immunoglobulin binding lymphoid cells (CILC) in the central nervous system. Report of 32 cases including 19 multiple sclerosis. *Acta Neuropathol* 40:227–232.

Myers LW. (1992) Treatment of multiple sclerosis with ACTH and corticosteroids. In: Rudick RA, Goodkin DE, eds. *Treatment of Multiple Sclerosis*. New York: Springer Verlag; 135–156.

Myers LW, Ellison GW, Merrill JE et al. (1995) Pentoxifylline – not a promising treatment for multiple sclerosis. *Neurology* 45(Suppl. 4): A419(Abstract).

Nadler SG, Tepper MA, Schacter B, Mazzucco CE. (1992) Interaction of the immunosuppressant deoxyspergualin with a member of the Hsp70 family of heat shock proteins. *Science* 258:484–486.

Nagai Y, Momoi T, Saito M, Mitsuzawa E, Ohtani S. (1976) Ganglioside syndrome: a new autoimmune neurological disorder, experimentally induced with brain gangliosides. *Neurosci Lett* 2:107–111.

Naparstek Y, Cohen IR, Fuks Z, Vladavsky I. (1984) Activated T-lymphocytes produce a matrix-degrading heparan sulfate endoglycosidase. *Nature*. 310:241–244.

Nataf S, Louboutin JP, Chabannes D et al. (1993) Pentoxifylline inhibits experimental allergic encephalomyelitis. *Acta Neurol Scand* 88:97–99.

Nelson D, Vates TS, Thomas R. (1973) Complications from intrathecal steroid therapy in patients with multiple sclerosis. *Acta Neurologica Scandinavica* 49:176–588.

Nelson LM, Hamman RF, Thompson DS, et al. (1986) Higher than expected prevalence of multiple sclerosis in northern Colorado: dependence on methodologic issues. *Neuroepidemiology* 5:17–28.

Neu I. (1982) Intrathekale Gabe eines Depot-Kortikosteroids. Anwendung bei infektiösen und entzündlichen Erkrankungen des zentralen Nervensystems. *Muench Med Wochenschr* 124:67–68.

Newman NJ, Lessell S. (1990) Isolated pupil-sparing third-nerve palsy as the presenting symptom of multiple sclerosis. *Arch Neurol* 47:817–818.

Niewodniczy A, Posniak-Patewicz E. (1973) Negative results following use of indomethacin in treatment of multiple sclerosis. *Neurol Neurochir Pol* 7:291.

Nishimura K, Tokunaga T. (1989) Mechanism of action of 15-deoxyspergualin. I. Suppressive effect on the induction of alloreactive secondary cytotoxic T-lymphocytes in vivo and in vitro. *Immunology* 68:66–71.

Nordin M, Nyström B, Wallin U, Hagbarth KE. (1984) Ectopic sensory discharges and paresthesiae in patients with disorders of peripheral nerves, dorsal roots and dorsal columns. *Pain* 20:231–245.

Noronha ABC, Richman DP, Arnason BGW. (1980) Detection of in vivo stimulated cerebrospinal-fluid lymphocytes by flow cytometry in patients with multiple sclerosis. *N Engl J Med* 303:713–717.

Noseworthy J, Paty DW, Wonnacott T, Feasby T, Ebers GC. (1983) Multiple sclerosis after age 50. *Neurology* 33:1537–1544.

Noseworthy JH, Ebers GC, Vandervoort MK et al. (1994a) The impact of blinding on the results of a randomized, placebo-controlled multiple sclerosis clinical trial. *Neurology* 44:16–20.

Noseworthy JH, Hopkins MB, Vandervoort MK et al. (1993) An open-trial evaluation of mitoxantrone in the treatment of progressive MS. *Neurology* 43:1401–1406.

Noseworthy JH, O'Brien PC, Van Engelen BGM, Rodriguez M. (1994b) Intravenous immunoglobulin therapy in multiple sclerosis: progress from remyelination in the Theiler's virus model to a randomized, double-blind, placebo-controlled clinical trial. *J Neurol Neurosurg Psychiatry* 57(Suppl.):11–14.

Noseworthy JH, Rodriguez M, An KN et al. (1994c) I.v. Ig treatment in multiple sclerosis: pilot study results and design of a placebo-controlled, double-blind clinical trial. *Ann Neurol* 36:325.

Noseworthy JH, Vandervoort MK, Hopkins MB, Ebers GC. (1989) A referendum on clinical trial research in multiple sclerosis: the opinion of the participants in the Jekyll Island Workshop. *Neurology* 39:977–981.

Noseworthy JH, Vandervoort MK, Wong CJ, Ebers GC. (The Canadian Cooperative MS Study Group). (1990) Interrater variability with the extended disability status scale (EDSS) and functional systems (FS) in a multiple sclerosis clinical trial *Neurology* 40:971–975.

Nuwer MR. (1990) Evoked potentials. In: Cook SD, ed. *Handbook of Multiple Sclerosis.* New York, Basel: Marcel Dekker, Inc. 271–290.

Nyland H, Matre R, Mork S, Bjerke JR, Naess A. (1982) T-lymphocyte subpopulations in multiple sclerosis lesions. *New Engl J Med* 307:1643–1644.

Oesch P, Kesselring J. (In press) Bewegungs messang in der Neurorehabilitation. *Neurol & Rehabil.*

Offenbacher H, Fazekas F, Schmidt R, et al. (1993) Assessment of MRI criteria for a diagnosis of MS. *Neurology* 43:905–909.

Offner H, Jones R, Vandenbark AA. (1988) Attenuated T-lymphocyte lines as vaccinating agents against experimental autoimmune encephalomyelitis. *Ann N Y Acad Sci* 540:540–542.

Oger JJF, Antel JP, Arnason BGW. (1982) Effects of imuran therapy on in vitro immune function of MS patients. *Ann Neurol* 11:177–182.

Ohta M, Ohta K, Mori F, Nishitani H, Saida T. Sera from patients with multiple sclerosis react with human T-cell lymphotropic virus Gag proteins but not ENV proteins – Western blotting analysis. *J Immunol* 137:3440–3443.

Oksenverg JR, Begovich AB, Erlich HA, Steinman L. (1993) Genetic factors in multiple sclerosis. *JAMA* 270:2362–2369.

Oksenberg JR, Stuart S, Begovich AB, et al. Limited heterogeneity of rearranged T-cell receptor V alpha transcripts in brains in multiple sclerosis patients. *Nature* 345:344–346.

Olgiati R, Jacquet J, di Prampero PE. (1986) Energy cost of walking and exertional dyspnoea in multiple sclerosis. *Am Rev Respir Diseases* 134:1005–1010.

Olsson T. (1992) Immunology of multiple sclerosis. *Curr Opinion Neurol Neurosurg* 5:195–202.

Olsson T. (1994) Role of cytokines in multiple sclerosis and experimental autoimmune encephalomyelitis. *Eur J Neurol* 1:7–19.

Olsson T, Zhi WW, Höjeberg B, et al. (1990) Autoreactive T lymphocytes in multiple sclerosis determined by antigen induced secretion of interferon-gamma. *J Clin Invest* 86:981–985.

Oppenheimer DR. (1978) The cervical cord in multiple sclerosis. *Neuropath Appl Neurobiol* 4:151–162.

Optic Neuritis Study Group. (1991) The clinical profile of optic neuritis. Experience of the Optic Neuritis Treatment Trial. *Arch Ophthalmol* 109:1673–1678.

Ormerod IEC, Harding AE, Miller DH, et al. (1994) Magnetic resonance imaging in degenerative ataxic disorders. *J Neurol Neurosurg Psychiat* 57:51–57.

Ormerod IEC, Miller DH, McDonald WI, et al. (1987) The role of NMR imaging in the assessment of multiple sclerosis and isolated neurological lesions: a quantitative study. *Brain* 110:1579–1616.

Österberg A, Boivie J, Henrikson A et al. (1993) Central pain in multiple sclerosis. *Pain* (Suppl.).

Osterman PO. (1976) Paroxysmal itching in multiple sclerosis. *Br J Dermatol* 95:555–558.

Osterman PO, Westerberg CE. (1975) Paroxysmal attacks in multiple sclerosis. *Brain* 98:189–202.

Ozawa K, Suchanek G, Breitschopf H, et al. (1994) Patterns of oligodendroglia pathology in multiple sclerosis. *Brain* 117:1311–1322.

Panitch H, Ciccone C. (1981) Induction of recurrent experimental allergic encephalomyelitis with myelin basic protein. *Ann Neurol* 9:433–438.

Panitch HS. (1992) Interferons in multiple sclerosis: a review of the evidence. *Drugs* 44:946–962.

Panitch HS, Hirsch RL, Haley AS, Johnson KP. (1987a) Exacerbations of multiple sclerosis in patients treated with interferon gamma. *Lancet* i:893–894.

Panitch HS, Hirsch RL, Schindler J, Johnson KP. (1987b) Treatment of multiple sclerosis with gamma interferon: exacerbations associated with activation of the immune system. *Neurology* 37:1097–1102.

Parkin PJ, Hierons R, McDonald WI. (1984) Bilateral optic neuritis. A long-term follow-up. *Brain* 107:951–964.

Parsons CL. (1983) The bladder in multiple sclerosis. In: Hallpike JF, Adams CWM, Tourtellotte WW, eds. *Multiple Sclerosis. Pathology, Diagnosis and Management.* London, England: Chapman and Hall; 579–602.

Paterson P. (1960) Transfer of allergic encephalomyelitis in rats by means of lymph node cells. *J Exp Med* 111:119–135.

Patterson VH, Heron JR. (1980) Visual field abnormalities in multiple sclerosis. *J Neurol Neurosurg Psychiat* 43:205–208.

Paty DW, Li DKB (UBC MS/MRI Study Group, IFNβ Multiple Sclerosis Study Group). (1993) Interferon beta-1b is effective in relapsing-remitting multiple sclerosis. II. MRI analysis results of a multicenter, randomized double-blind, placebo-controlled trial. *Neurology* 43:662–667.

Paty DW, Poser CM. (1984) Clinical symptoms and signs. In: Poser CM et al., eds. *The Diagnosis of Multiple Sclerosis.* New York, NY: Thieme Stratton Inc; 27–43.

Paty DW, Willoughby E, Whitaker J. (1992) Assessing the outcome of experimental therapies in multiple sclerosis patients. In: Rudick RA, Goodkin DE, eds. *Treatment of Multiple Sclerosis.* London Berlin Heidelberg New York: Springer-Verlag. 47–90.

Paulley JW. (1976) Psychological management of multiple sclerosis. *Psychother Psychosom* 27:26–40.

Pedersen L, Trojaborg W. (1981) Visual, auditory and somatosensory pathway involvement in hereditary cerebellar ataxia, Friedreich's ataxia and familial spastic paraplegia. *Electroenceph Clin Neurophysiol* 52:283–297.

Pederson-Bjergaard J, Ersboll J, Sorensen HM et al. (1985) Risk of acute nonlymphocytic leukemia and preleukemia in patients treated with cyclophosphamide for non-Hodgkin's lymphoma. *Ann Intern Med* 103:195–200.

Pender MP, McCombe A, Yoong G, Nguyen KB. (1992) Apoptosis of alpha/beta T lymphocytes in the nervous system in experimental autoimmune encephalomyelitis: its possible implications for recovery and aquired tolerance. *J Autoimmun* 5:401–410.

Penn I. (1986) The occurrence of malignant tumors in immunosuppressed states. *Prog Allergy* 37:259–300.

Perkin GD, Rose FC. (1979) *Optic Neuritis and its Differential Diagnosis.* Oxford, England: Oxford University Press.

Pette M, Fujita K, Kitze B et al. (1990a) Myelin basic protein-specific T lymphocyte lines from MS patients and healthy individuals. *Neurology* 40:1770–1776.

Pette M, Fujita K, Wilkinson D et al. (1990b) Myelin autoreactivity in multiple sclerosis: Recognition of myelin basic protein in the context of HLA-DR2 products by T lymphocytes of multiple sclerosis and healthy donors. *Proc Natl Acad Sci USA* 87:7968–7972.

Peyser JM, Rao SM, LaRocca NG, Kaplan E. (1990) Guidelines for neuropsychological research in multiple sclerosis. *Arch Neurol* 47:94–97.

Phadke JG. (1987) Survival pattern and cause of death in patients with multiple sclerosis: results from an epidemiological survey in North East Scotland. *J Neuro Neurosurg Psychiat* 50:523–531.

Phadke JG, Best PV. (1983) Atypical and clinically silent multiple sclerosis: a report of 12 cases discovered unexpectedly at necropsy. *J Neurol Neurosurg Psychiat* 46:414–420.

Plunkett W, Saunder PP. (1991) Metabolism and action of purine nucleosid analogs. *Pharmacol Ther* 49:239–268.

Pollack M, Calder C, Allpress S. (1977) Peripheral nerve abnormality in multiple sclerosis. *Ann Neurol* 2:41–48.

Pollard JD, King RHM, Thomas PK. (1975) Recurrent experimental allergic neuritis. An electron microscopic study. *J Neurol Sci.* 24:365–383.

Polman CH, Bertelsmann FW, Van Loenen AC, Koetsier JC. (1994) 4-Aminopyridine in the treatment of patients with multiple sclerosis. *Arch Neurol* 51:292–296.

Polman CH, Dahlke F, Thompson AJ et al. (1995) Interferon beta-1b in secondary progressive multiple sclerosis – outline of the clinical trial. *Multiple Sclerosis* 1(Suppl. 1):S51–S54.

Polman CH, Koetsier JC, Wolters EC. (1985) Multiple sclerosis: incorporation of results of laboratory techniques in the diagnosis. *Clin Neurol Neurosurg* 87:187–192.

Poser CM. (1980) Exacerbations, activity, and progression in multiple sclerosis. *Arch Neurol* 37:471–474.

Poser CM. (1986) Pathogenesis of multiple sclerosis. A critical reappraisal. *Acta Neuropathol* 71:1–10.

Poser CM. (1993) The pathogenesis of multiple sclerosis. Additional considerations. *J Neurol Sci* 115(suppl):S3–S15.

Poser CM, Benedikz J, Hibberd PL. (1992) The epidemiology of multiple sclerosis: the Iceland model. Onset-adjusted prevalence rate and other methodological considerations. *J Neurol Sci* 111:143–152.

Poser CM, Paty DW, Scheinberg LC, et al. (1983) New diagnostic criteria for multiple sclerosis: Guidelines for research protocols. *Ann Neurol* 13:227–231.

Poser CM, Paty DW, Scheinberg LC, McDonald WI, Ebers GC, eds. *The Diagnosis of Multiple Sclerosis.* New York, NY: Thieme-Stratton Inc.

Poser S. (1986) *Multiple Sklerose.* Darmstadt, Germany: Wissenschaftliche Buchgesellschaft.

Poser S, Poser W, Schlaf G, et al. (1986) Prognostic indicators in multiple sclerosis. *Acta Neurol Scand* 74:387–392.

Poser S, Raun NE, Poser W. (1982) Age at onset, initial symptomatology and the course of multiple sclerosis. *Acta Neurol Scand* 66:355–362.

Poser S, Wikström J, Bauer HJ. (1981) Multiple Sklerose und verwandte Krankheiten. In: Hopf HCH, Poeck K, Schliack H, eds. *Neurologie in Praxis und Klinik,* Band II. New York, NY: Georg Thieme Verlag; 5.0–5.31.

Poskanzer DC, Walker AM, Prenney LB, Sheridan JL. (1981) The etiology of multiple sclerosis: temporal-spatial clustering indicating two environmental exposures before onset. *Neurology* 31:708–713.

Potvin AR, Tourtellotte WW. (1976) The neurological examination: advancements in its quantification. *Arch Phys Med Rehabil* 56:425–437.

Potvin AR, Tourtellotte WW. (1985). *Quantitative Examination of Neurologic Functions,* Vols. I and II. Boca Raton, Florida: CRC Press.

Powell MB, Mitchell D, Lederman J, et al. (1990) Lymphotoxin and tumor necrosis factor-alpha production by myelin basic protein-specific T cell clones correlates with encephalitogenicity. *Int Immunol* 2:539–544.

Powell T, Sussman JG, Davies Jones GA. (1992) MR imaging in acute multiple sclerosis: ringlike appearance in plaques suggesting the presence of paramagnetic free radicals. *Am J Neuroradiol* 13:1544–1546.

Pozzilli C, Bernardi S, Mansi L, et al. (1988) Quantitative assessment of blood-brain barrier permeability in multiple sclerosis using 68-Ga-EDTA and positron emission tomography. *J Neurol Neurosurg Psychiat* 51:1058–1062.

Pratt RTC. (1951) An investigation on the psychiatric aspects of disseminated sclerosis. *J Neurol Neurosurg Psychiat* 14:326–336.

Prineas JW. (1975) Pathology of early lesions in multiple sclerosis. *Hum Path* 6:531–554.

Prineas JW. (1979) Multiple sclerosis: presence of lymphatic capillaries and lymphoid tissue in the brain and spinal cord. *Science* 203:1123–1125.

Prineas JW. (1986) The neuropathology of multiple sclerosis. In: Koetsier JC, ed. *Handbook of Clinical Neurology*, Vol. 3 47. New York, NY: Elsevier; 213–257.

Prineas JW, Barnard RO, Kwon EE, Sharer LR, Cho ES. (1993a) Multiple sclerosis: remyelination of nascent lesions. *Ann Neurol* 33:137–151.

Prineas JW, Barnard RO, Revesz T, Kwon EE, Sharer L, Cho ES. (1993b) Multiple sclerosis. Pathology of recurrent lesions. *Brain* 116:681–693.

Prineas JW, Connell F. (1978) The fine structure of chronically active multiple sclerosis plaques. *Neurology* 28:68–75.

Prineas JW, Connell F. (1979) Remyelination in multiple sclerosis. *Ann Neurol* 5:22–31.

Prineas JW, Kwon EE, Sternberger NH, Lennon VA. (1984) The distribution of myelin associated glycoprotein and myelin basic protein in actively demyelinating multiple sclerosis lesions. *J Neuroimmunol* 6:251–264.

Prineas JW, Kwon EE, Goldenberg PZ, et al. (1989) Multiple sclerosis: Oligodendrocyte proliferation and differentiation in fresh lesions. *Lab Invest* 61:489–503.

Prineas JW, Raine CS. (1976) Electron microscopy and immunoperoxidase studies in early multiple sclerosis lesions. *Neurology* 26:29–32.

Prineas JW, Wright RG. (1978) Macrophages, lymphocytes and plasma cells in the perivascular compartment in chronic multiple sclerosis. *Lab Invest* 38:409–421.

Prosiegel M, Michael C. (1993) Neuropsychology and multiple sclerosis: diagnostic and rehabilitative approaches. *J Neurol Sci* 115(Suppl):1–4.

Putnam TJ. (1933) The pathogenesis of multiple sclerosis: a possible vascular factor. *N Engl J Med* 209:786–790.

Racke MK, Dhib-Jalbut S, Canella B, Albert PS, Raine CS, McFarlin DE. (1991) Prevention and treatment of chronic relapsing experimental allergic encephalomyelitis by transforming growth factor-beta 1. *J Immunol* 146:3012–3017.

Raine CS. (1976) On the development of CNS lesions in natural distemper encephalomyelitis. *J Neurol Sci* 30:13–28.

Raine CS. (1986) Experimental allergic encephalomyelitis and experimental allergic neuritis. In: Koetsier JC, ed. *Handbook of Clinical Neurology*, Vol. 3 47. New York, NY: Elsevier; 429–466.

Raine CS, Bornstein MB. (1970a) Experimental allergic encephalomyelitis: a light and electron microscopic study of remyelination and sclerosis in vitro. *J Neuropath Exp Neurol* 29:552–574.

Raine CS, Bornstein MB. (1970b) Experimental allergic encephalomyelitis: an ultrastructural study of experimental demyelination in vitro. *J Neuropath Exp Neurol* 29:177–191.

Raine CS, Lee SC, Scheinberg LC, Duijvestin AM, Cross AH. (1990) Adhesion molecules on endothelial cells of the central nervous system: an emerging area in the neuroimmunology of multiple sclerosis. *Clin Immunol Immunopathol* 57:173–187.

Raine CS, Scheinberg L, Waltz JM. (1981) Multiple sclerosis: oligodendroglia survival and proliferation in an active established lesion. *Lab Invest* 45:534–546.

Raine CS, Traugott U, Stone SH. (1978) Glial bridges and Schwann cell migration during chronic demyelination in the CNS. *J Neurocytol* 7:541–553.

Rao SM. (1986) Neuropsychology of multiple sclerosis. *J Clin Exp Neuropsychol* 8:503–542.

Rao SM. (1995) Neuropsychology of multiple sclerosis. *Current Opinion in Neurology* 8:216–220.

Rao SM, Hammeke TA, McQuillen MP, Khatri BO, Lloyd D. (1984) Memory disturbance in chronic progressive multiple sclerosis. *Arch Neurol* 41:625–631.

Rasminsky M. (1973) The effects of temperature on conduction in demyelinated single nerve fibres. *Arch Neurol* 28:287–292.

Rasminsky M. (1978) Ectopic generation of impulses and cross talk in spinal nerve roots in 'dystrophic' mice. *Ann Neurol* 13:351–357.

Rawlinson DG, Braun CW. (1981) Granulomatous angiitis of the nervous system, first seen as relapsing myelopathy. *Arch Neurol* 38:129–131.

Reder AT, Thapar M, Jensen MA. (1994) A reduction in serum glucocorticoids provokes experimental allergic encephalomyelitis: implications for treatment of inflammatory brain disease. *Neurology* 44:2289–2294.

Reik L, Smith L, Khan A, Nelson W. (1985) Demyelinating encephalopathy in Lyme disease. *Neurology* 35:267–269.

Reulen JPH, Danders EACM, Hogenhuis LAH. (1983) Eye movement disorders in multiple sclerosis and optic neuritis. *Brain* 106:121–140.

Reynolds EH. (1992) Multiple sclerosis and vitamin B_{12} metabolism. *J Neurol Neurosurg Psychiat* 55:339–340.

Reynolds E, Linnell JC, Faludy JE. (1991) Multiple sclerosis associated with Vitamin B_{12} deficiency. *Arch Neurol* 48:808–811.

Rieckmann P, Albrecht M, Kitze B et al. (1995a) Tumor necrosis factor-alpha messenger RNA expression in patients with relapsing-remitting multiple sclerosis is associated with disease activity. *Ann Neurol* 37:82–88.

Rieckmann P, Albrecht M, Kitze B et al. (1994) Cytokine mRNA levels in mononuclear blood cells from patients with multiple sclerosis. *Neurology* 44:1523–1526.

Rieckmann P, Weber F, Günther A et al. (1995b) Soluble forms of intercellular adhesion molecule-1 (ICAM-1) block cellular adhesion and cytokine production in multiple sclerosis. *Neurology* 45(Suppl 4):A164(Abstract).

Rindfleisch E. (1863) Histologisches Detail zu der grauen Degeneration von Gehirn und Rückenmark. *Virchows Arch Path Anat* 26:474–483.

Riser M, Géraud J, Rascol A, Benazet AM, Segria MG. (1971) L'évolution de la sclérose en plaques (étude de 203 observations suivies au-delà de 10 ans). *Rev Neurol* 124:479–484.

Rivers TM, Sprunt DH, Berry GP. (1933) Observations on attempts to produce acute disseminated encephalomyelitis in monkeys. *J Exp Med* 58:39–53.

Rohrbach E, Kappos L, Staedt D et al. (1988a) Intrathecal versus oral corticosteroid therapy of spinal symptoms of multiple sclerosis. A double-blind controlled trial. American Academy of Neurology, 40th Annual Meeting, Cincinnati, April 25–29, 1988. *Neurology* 38(Suppl. 1):256.

Rohrbach E, Kappos L, Staedt D et al. (1988b) Intrathecal versus oral corticosteroid therapy of spinal symptoms in multiple sclerosis. A double-blind controlled trial. In: Confavreux C, Aimard G, Devic M, eds. *Trends in European Multiple Sclerosis Research*. Amsterdam: Excerpta Medica. 414.

Ron MA, Callanan MM, Warrington EK. (1991) Cognitive abnormalities in multiple sclerosis: a psychometric and MRI study. *Psychol Med* 21:59–68.

Rose AS, Kuzma JW, Kurtzke JF et al. (1970) Cooperative study in the evaluation of therapy in multiple sclerosis: ACTH versus placebo. Final report. *Neurology* 20:1–59.

Roser W, Hagberg G, Mader I et al. (1995) Proton MRS of gadolinium-enhancing plaques and metabolic changes in normal-appearing white matter. *Magn Reson Imaging* 33:811–817.

Rössler K, Neuchrist C, Kitz K, Scheiner O, Kraft D, Lassmann H. (1992) Expression of leukocyte adhesion molecules at the human blood brain barrier. *J Neurosci Res* 31:365–374.

Rostami AM. (1991) Plasmapheresis in acute attacks of multiple sclerosis: The cons. *J Clin Apheresis* 6:205–206.

Roth GA, Röyttä M, Yu RK, Raine CS, Bornstein MB. (1985) Antisera to different glycolipids induce myelin alterations in mouse spinal cord tissue cultures. *Brain Res* 339:9–18.

Rothfelder U, Neu I, Pelkar. (1982) Therapie der Multiplen Sklerose mit Immunglobulin G. *Muench Med Wochenschr* 124:74–78.

Rowe PM. (1994) Clinical potential for TGF-beta. *Lancet* 344:72–73.

Rudge P. (1985) Diskussionbemerkung. In: Hommes OR, Mertin J, Tourtellotte WW, eds. *Immunotherapies in Multiple Sclerosis*. Sutton, England: Stuart Phillips Publishers; 128.

Rudge P, Koetsier JC, Martin J, et al. (1988) Randomised double blind control trial of cyclosporin (Sandimmun) in multiple sclerosis. *J Neurol Neurosurg Psychiat* 52:559–565.

Rudick RA, Schitter RB, Schwetz KM, Herndon RM. (1986) Multiple sclerosis: the problem of incorrect diagnosis. *Arch Neurol* 43:578–583.

Runmarker B, Andersen O. (1993) Prognostic factors in a multiple sclerosis incidence cohort with twenty-five years of follow-up. *Brain* 116:117–134.

Sadovnick AD, Armstrong H, Rice GP, et al. (1993) A population-based study of multiple sclerosis in twins: update. *Ann Neurol* 33:281–285.

Sadovnik AD, Baird PA, Ward RH. (1988) Multiple sclerosis: Updated risks for relatives. *Am J Med Gen* 29:533–541.

Saida T, Saida K, Dorfman SH, et al. (1979) Experimental allergic neuritis induced by sensitization with galactocerebroside. *Science* 204:1103–1106.

Salier JP, Sesbo IR, Martin-Mondihre C, et al. (1986) Combined influences of Gm and HLA phenotypes upon multiple sclerosis susceptibility and severity. *J Clin Invest* 78:533–538.

Samra Y, Hertz M, Lindner A. (1985) Urinary bladder tumors following cyclophosphamide therapy: a report of two cases with a review of the literature. *Med Pediatr Oncol* 13:86–91.

Sandberg-Wollheim M, Bynke H, Cronqvist S, Holtas S, Platz P. (1990) A long-term prospective study of optic neuritis: evaluation of risk factors. *Ann Neurol* 27:386–393.

Sandberg-Wollheim M, Hommes OR, Hughes RAC et al. (1995) Recombinant human interferon beta in the treatment of relapsing-remitting and secondary progressive multiple sclerosis. *Multiple Sclerosis* 1(Suppl. 1):S48–S50.

Sanders EA, Arts RJ. (1986) Paraesthesias in multiple sclerosis. *J Neurol Sci* 74:297–305.

Sanders EACM, Reulen JPH, Van der Velde EA, Hogenhuis LAH. (1986) The diagnosis of multiple sclerosis. Contribution of nonclinical tests. *J Neurol Sci* 72:273–285.

Sanders ME, Koski CL, Robbins D, Shin ML, Frank MM, Joiner KA. (1986) Activated terminal complement in cerebrospinal fluid in Guillain-Barré syndrome and multiple sclerosis. *J Immunol* 136:4456–4459.

Sarkari NBS. (1968) Involuntary movements in multiple sclerosis. *Br Med J* ii:738–740.

Schauf CL, Davis FA. (1974) Impulse conduction in multiple sclerosis: a theoretical basis for modification by temperature and pharmacological agents. *J Neurol Neurosurg Psychiat* 37:152–161.

Schauf CL, Davis FA, Sack DA, Reed BJ, Kesler RL. (1976) Neuroelectric blocking factors in human and animal sera evaluated using the isolated frog spinal cord. *J Neurol Neurosurg Psychiat* 39:680–685.

Scheinmann RI, Cogswell PC, Lofquist AK, Baldwin ASJ. (1995) Role of transcriptional activation of I-kappa-B-alpha in mediation of immunosuppression by glucocorticoids. *Science* 270:283–286.

Schiepers C, Vanderberghe R, Van Hecke P et al. (1995) FDG-PET, MRI and NMR spectroscopy of normal-appearing white matter (NAWM) in multiple sclerosis. *Neurology* 45(Suppl 4):A282(Abstract).

Schiffer RB. (1987) The spectrum of depression in multiple sclerosis: an approach to clinical management. *Arch Neurol* 44:596–599.

Schiffer RB, Herndon RM, Stabrowski A. (1988) Effects of dietary trace metals on experimental allergic encephalomyelitis in SJL mice. *Ann Neurol* 24:141.

Schiffer RB, Slater RJ. (1985) Neuropsychiatric features of multiple sclerosis. Recognition and management. *Sem Neurol* 5:127–133.

Schimrigk K, Schmitt D. (1988) *Multiple Sklerose.* Weinheim Basel: VHC Verlagsgesellschaft mbH.

Schlesinger H. (1909) Sur Frage der akuten multiplen Sklerose. *Arbeiten aus dem Wiener Neurologischen Institut* 410–434.

Schmid UD, Walker G, Schmid-Sigron J, Hess CW. (1991) Transcutaneous magnetic and electrical stimulation over the cervical spine: excitation of plexus roots rather than spinal roots. *Electroencephalogr Clin Neurophysiol* (suppl), 43:369–384.

Schrader H, Gotlibsen OB, Skomedal GN. (1980) Multiple sclerosis and narcolepsy/cataplexy in a monozygotic twin. *Neurology* 30:105–108.

Schriefer TN, Hess CW, Mills KR, Murray NM. (1989) Central motor conduction studies in motor neurone disease using magnetic brain stimulation. *Electroencephalogr Clin Neurophysiol* 74:431–437.

Schroth WS, Tenner SM, Rappaport BA, Mani R. (1992) Multiple sclerosis as a cause of atrial fibrillation and electrocardiographic changes. *Arch Neurol* 49:422–424.

Schubert DS, Foliart RH. (1993) Increased depression in multiple sclerosis patients. A meta-analysis. *Psychosomatics* 34:124–130.

Schuller E, Govaerts A. (1987) First results of immunotherapy with immunoglobulin G in multiple sclerosis patients. *Exp Neurol* 22:205–212.

Schumacher GA, Beebe GW, Kebler RF et al. (1965) Problems of experimental trials of therapy in multiple sclerosis, report by the panel on the evaluation of experimental trials in therapy in multiple sclerosis. *Ann N Y Acad Sci* 122:552–568.

Schwerer B, Lassmann H, Kitz K, Bernheimer H. (1986) Ganglioside GM1, a molecular target for immunological and toxic attacks: similarity of neuropathological lesions induced by ganglioside antiserum and cholera toxin. *Acta Neuropathol* 72:55–61.

Scolding NJ, Morgan PB, Houston A, Campell AK, Linington C, Compston DA. (1989) Normal rat serum cytotoxicity against syngeneic oligodendrocytes. Complement activation and attack in the absence of anti-myelin antibodies. *J Neurol Sci* 289:399–400.

Seitelberger F. (1969) Histochemistry of demyelinating diseases proper including allergic encephalomyelitis and Pelizäus Merzbacher's disease. In: Cummings JN, ed. *Modern Scientific Aspects of Neurology.* London, England: Edward Arnold; 146–185.

Seitelberger F. (1973) Pathology of multiple sclerosis. *Ann Clin Res* 5:337–344.

Seitbelberger F, Jellinger K, Tschabitscher H. (1958) Zur Genese der akuten Entmarkungsenzephalitis. *Wien Klin Wochenschr* 70:453–459.

Selmaj K, Brosnan CF, Raine CS. (1991a) Colocalization of lymphocytes bearing gamma delta T-cell receptor and heat shock protein HSP65+ oligodendrocytes in multiple sclerosis. *Proc Natl Acad Sci (USA)* 88:6452–6456.

Selmaj KW, Raine CS. (1988) Tumor necrosis factor mediates myelin and oligodendrocyte damage in vitro. *Ann Neurol* 23:339–346.

Selmaj K, Raine CS, Cannella B, Brosnan CF. (1991b) Identification of lymphotoxin and tumor necrosis factor in multiple sclerosis lesions. *J Clin Invest* 87:949–954.

Selmaj K, Raine CS, Cross AH (1991c) Anti-tumor necrosis factor therapy abrogates autoimmune demyelination. *Ann Neurol* 30:694–700.

Sharief MK, Hentges R. (1991) Association between tumor necrosis factor-alpha and disease progression in patients with multiple sclerosis. *N Engl J Med* 325:467–472.

Shaw SY, Laursen RA, Lees MB. (1986) Analogous amino acid sequences in myelin proteolipid and viral proteins. *FEBS Letters* 207:266–270.

Sheldon JJ, Siddhartan R, Tobias J, Siermata WA, Soila K, Viamonte M. (1985) MR imaging of multiple sclerosis: Comparison with clinical and CT examinations in 74 patients. *AJR* 145:957–964.

Shenkenberg TD, Von Hoff DD. (1986) Possible mitoxantrone-induced amenorrhea. *Cancer Treat Rep* 70:659–661.

Shibasaki H, McDonald WI, Kuroiwa Y. (1981) Racial modification of clinical picture of multiple sclerosis: comparison between British and Japanese patients. *J Neurol Sci* 49:253–271.

Shimizu Y, Newman W, Tanaka Y, Shaw S. (1992) Lymphocyte interactions with endothelial cells. *Immunol Today* 13:106–112.

Shiroky JB, Neville C, Esdaile JM. (1993) Low-dose methotrexate with leucovorin (folinic acid) in the management of rheumatoid arthritis: results of a multicenter randomized, double-blind, placebo-controlled trial. *Arthritis Rheum* 36:795–803.

Sibley WA. (1992) *Therapeutic Claims in Multiple Sclerosis.* New York: Demos.

Sibley WA, Bamford CR, Clark K. (1984) Triggering factors in multiple sclerosis. In: Poser CM, ed. *The Diagnosis of Multiple Sclerosis.* New York, NY: Thieme Stratton Inc; 14–24.

Sibley WA, Bamford CR, Clark K. (1985) Clinical viral infections and multiple sclerosis. *Lancet* i:1313–1315.

Siemerling E, Raecke E. (1914) Beitrag zur Klinik und Pathologie der multiplen Sklerose mit besonderer Berücksichtigung ihrer Pathogenese. *Arch Psychiat Nervenkr* 53:385–564.

Sigal NH, Dumond FJ. (1992) Cyclosporin A, FK-506 and rapamycin: Pharmacologic probes of lymphocyte signal transduction. *Ann Rev Immunol* 10:519–560.

Sipe JC, Knobler RL, Braheny SL et al. (1984) A neurologic rating scale (NRS) for use in multiple sclerosis. *Neurology* 34:1368–1372.

Sipe JC, Romine J, Koziol J et al. (1995) Cladribine treatment of chronic progressive (C/P) MS: a double-blind, crossover study with 2+ years' observation. *Neurology* 45(Suppl 4):A418(Abstract).

Sipe JC, Romine JS, Koziol JA et al. (1994) Cladribine in treatment of chronic progressive multiple sclerosis. *Lancet* 344:9–13.

Skias DD, Reder AT. (1995) IL-10 inhibits EAE. *Neurology* 45(Suppl 4):A349(Abstract).

Smith KJ, Blakemore WF, McDonald WI. (1979) Central remyelination restores secure conduction. *Nature* 280:395–396.

Smith KJ, Bostock H, Hall SM. (1982) Saltatory conduction precedes remyelination in axons demyelinated with lysophosphatidycholine. *J Neurol Sci* 54:13–31.

Smith KJ, McDonald WI. (1982) Spontaneous and evoked electrical discharges from a central demyelinating lesion. *J Neurol Sci* 55:39–47.

Smith ME, Stone LA, Albert PS, et al. (1993) Clinical worsening in multiple sclerosis is associated with increased frequency and area of gadopenetate dimeglumine-enhancing magnetic resonance imaging lesions. *Ann Neurol* 33:480–489.

Snyder BD, Lakatua DJ, Doe RP. (1981) ACTH-induced cortisol production in multiple sclerosis. *Ann Neurol* 10:388–389.

Sobel RA, Mitchell ME, Fondren G. (1990) Intercellular adhesion molecule I (ICAM-1) in cellular immune reactions in the human central nervous system. *Amer J Pathol* 136:1309–1316.

Solari A, Amato MP, Bergamaschi R, et al. (1993) Accuracy of self-assessment of the minimal record of disability in patients with multiple sclerosis. *Acta Neurol Scand* 87:43–46.

Sommer N, Löschmann P-A, Northoff GH et al. (1995) The antidepressant rolipram suppresses cytokine production and prevents autoimmune encephalomyelitis. *Nature Medicine* 1:244–248.

Spielman RS, Nathanson N. (1982) The genetics of susceptibility to multiple sclerosis. *Epidemiol Rev* 4:45–65.

Spielmeyer W. (1922) *Histopathologie des Nervensystems*. New York, NY: Springer-Verlag.

Spina CA. (1984) Azathioprine as an immune modulating drug: clinical applications. *Clin Immunol All* 4:415–446.

Spiro HM. (1993) Is the steroid ulcer a myth? (Editorial). *N Engl J Med* 309:45–48.

Spurkland A, Ronningen KS, Vandvik B, Thorsby E, Vartdal F. (1991) HLA-DQA1 and HLA-DQB1 genes may jointly determine susceptibility to develop multiple sclerosis. *Hum Immunol* 30:69–75.

Sriram S. (1994) Longitudinal study of frequency of HPRT mutant T cells in patients with multiple sclerosis. *Neurology* 44:311–315.

Stefoski D, Davis FA, Fitzsimmons WE, Luskin SS, Rush J, Parkhurst GW. (1991) 4-aminopyridine in multiple sclerosis: prolonged administration. *Neurology* 41:1344–1348.

Stefoski D, Davis FA, Schauf CL. (1985) Acute improvement in exacerbating MS produced by intravenous administration of mannitol. *Ann Neurol* 18:443–450.

Stein EC, Schiffer RB, Hall WJ, Young N. (1987) Multiple sclerosis and the workplace—report of an industry-based cluster. *Neurology* 37:1672–1677.

Steiner G. (1931) Regionale Verteilung der Entmarkungsherde in ihrer Bedeutung für die Pathogenese der multiplen Sklerose. In: *Krankheitserreger und Gewebsbefund bei Multipler Sklerose*. New York, NY: Springer-Verlag; 108–120.

Stenager E, Knudsen L, Jensen K. (1991) Acute and chronic pain syndromes in multiple sclerosis. *Acta Neurol Scand* 84:197–200.

Stenager EN, Stenager E, Koch Henriksen N, et al. (1992) Suicide and multiple sclerosis: an epidemiological investigation. *J Neurol Neurosurg Psychiat* 55:542–545.

Stern BJ, Krumholz A, Johns C, Scott P, Nissim J. (1985) Sarcoidosis and its neurological manifestations. *Arch Neurol* 42:909–917.

Stewart GJ, McLeod JG, Basten A, Bashir HW. (1981) HLA family studies and susceptibility to multiple sclerosis: a common gene, dominantly expressed. *Human Immunol* 3:13–29.

Stöhrer M, Palmtag H, Madersbacher H. (1984) *Blasenlähmung. Sexualität und Blasenfunktion bei Rückenmarkverletzten und Erkrankungen des Nervensystems*. New York, NY: Georg Thieme Verlag.

Stone LA, Frank JA, Albert PS et al. (1995) The effect of interferon-beta on blood–brain barrier disruptions demonstrated by contrast-enhanced magnetic resonance imaging in relapsing-remitting multiple sclerosis. *Ann Neurol* 37:611–619.

Sun J, Link H, Olsson T, et al. (1991a) T and B cell responses to myelin-oligodendroglia glycoprotein in multiple sclerosis. *J Immunol* 146:1490–1495.

Sun JB, Olsson T, Wang WZ, et al. (1991b) Autoreactive T- and B-cells responding to myelin proteolipid protein in multiple sclerosis and controls. *Eur J Immunol* 21:1461–1468.

Sun D, Quin Y, Chluba J, Epplen JT, Wekerle H. (1988) Suppression of experimental induced autoimmune encephalomyelitis by cytolytic T-T cell interactions. *Nature* 332:843–845.

Sun D, Wekerle H. (1986) Ia-restricted encephalitogenic T lymphocytes mediating EAE lyse autoantigen-presenting astrocytes. *Nature* 320:70–72.

Surridge D. (1969) An investigation into some psychiatric aspects of multiple sclerosis. *Br J Psychiat* 115:749–764.

Suzuki K, Andrews JM, Waltz JM, Terry RD. (1969) Ultrastructural studies of multiple sclerosis. *Lab Invest* 20:444–454.

Swank RL, Brewer Dugan, B. (1990) Effect of low saturated fat diet in early and late cases of multiple sclerosis. *Lancet* i:37–39.

Swingler RJ, Compston DAS. (1986) The distribution of multiple sclerosis in the United Kingdom. *J Neurol Neurosurg Psychiat* 49:1115–1124.

Takeoka T, Shinohara Y, Furumi K, Mori K. (1983) Impairment of blood cerebrospinal fluid barrier in multiple sclerosis. *J Neurochem* 41:1102–1108.

Teitelbaum D, Milo R, Arnon R, Sela M. (1992) Synthetic copolymer 1 inhibits human T-cell lines specific for myelin basic protein. *Proc Natl Acad Sci USA* 89:137–141.

Tenser RB. (1976) Myokymia and facial contraction in multiple sclerosis. *Arch Intern Med* 136:81–83.

Tenser RB, Hay KA, Aberg JA. (1993) Immunoglobulin G immunosuppression of multiple sclerosis. *Arch Neurol* 50:417–420.

The Canadian Cooperative Multiple Sclerosis Study Group. (1991) The Canadian cooperative trial of cyclophosphamide and plasma exchange in progressive multiple sclerosis. *Lancet* 337:441–446.

The IFNβ Multiple Sclerosis Study Group. (1993) Interferon beta-1b is effective in relapsing-remitting multiple sclerosis. I. Clinical results of a multicenter, randomized, double-blind, placebo-controlled trial. *Neurology* 43:655–661.

The IFNβ Multiple Sclerosis Study Group, The University of British Columbia MS/MRI Analysis Group. (1995) Interferon beta-1b in the treatment of multiple sclerosis. *Neurology* 45:1277–1285.

The Multiple Sclerosis Study Group. (1990) Efficacy and toxicity of cyclosporine in chronic progressive multiple sclerosis: a randomized, double-blinded, placebo-controlled clinical trial. *Ann Neurol* 27:591–605.

The Quality Standards Subcommittee of the American Academy of Neurology. (1994) Practice advisory on selection of patients with multiple sclerosis for treatment with Betaseron. *Neurology* 44:1537–1540.

Thomke F, Hopf HC. (1992) Abduction nystagmus in internuclear ophthalmoplegia. *Acta Neurol Scand* 86:365–370.

Thompson AJ, Brazil J, Feighery C, et al. (1985) CSF myelin basic protein in multiple sclerosis. *Acta Neurol Scand* 72:577–583.

Thompson AJ, Hutchinson M, Brazil J, Feighery C, Martin EA. (1986) A clinical and laboratory study of benign multiple sclerosis. *Quart J Med* 58:69–80.

Thompson AJ, Kennard C, Swash M, et al. (1989a) Relative efficacy of intravenous methylprednisolone and ACTH in the treatment of acute relapse in MS. *Neurology* 39:969–971.

Thompson AJ, Kermode AG, Wicks D, et al. (1991) Major differences in the dynamics of primary and secondary progressive multiple sclerosis. *Ann Neurol* 29:53–62.

Thompson AJ, Kermode AG, MacManus DG, et al. (1989b) Pathogenesis of progressive multiple sclerosis. *Lancet* i:1322–1323.

Thompson AJ, Kermode AG, Wicks D, et al. (1991) Major differences in the dynamics of primary and secondary progressive multiple sclerosis. *Ann Neurol* 29:53–62.

Thompson DS, Nelson LM, Burns A, Burks JS, Franklin GM. (1986) The effects of pregnancy in multiple sclerosis: A retrospective study. *Neurology* 36:1097–1099.

Thompson EJ, Riches PG, Kohn J. (1983) Antibody synthesis within the central nervous system: comparison of CSF indices and electrophoresis. *J Clin Pathol* 36:312–315.

Thompson RHS. (1975) Unsaturated fatty acids in multiple sclerosis. In: Davison AN, Humphrey JH, Liversedge AL, McDonald WI, Porterfield JS, eds. *Multiple Sclerosis Research.* London, England: Her Majesty's Stationary Office; 184–191.

Thorpe JW, Kidd D, Kendall BE, et al. (1993) Spinal cord MRI using multi-array coils and fast spin echo. I. Technical aspects and findings in healthy controls. *Neurology* 43:2652–2661.

Tola MR, Granieri E, Casetta I, et al. (1993) Retinal periphlebitis in multiple sclerosis: a marker of disease activity? *Eur Neurol* 33:93–96.

Tourtellotte WW, Baumhefner RW, Potvin AR, et al. (1980) Multiple sclerosis de novo CNS IgG synthesis: effect of ACTH and corticosteroids. *Neurology* 30:1155–1162.

Tourtellotte WW, Baumhefner RW, Potvin JH, Potvin AR, Poser S. (1983) Comprehensive management of multiple sclerosis. In: Hallpike JF, Adams CWM, Tourtellotte WW, eds. *Multiple Sclerosis: Pathology, Diagnosis and Management.* London, England: Chapman and Hall; 513–578.

Tourtellotte WW, Haeven AF. (1965) Use of oral corticosteroids in the treatment of multiple sclerosis: A double-blind study. *Arch Neurol* 12:536–545.

Tourtellottee WW, Walsh MJ. (1984) Cerebrospinal fluid profile in multiple sclerosis. In: Poser CM et al, eds. *The Diagnosis of Multiple Sclerosis.* New York, NY: Thieme Stratton Inc; 165–178.

Traugott U. (1984) Characterization and distribution of lymphocyte subpopulations in multiple sclerosis plaques versus autoimmune demyelinating lesions. *Springer Semin Immunopathol* 8:71–95.

Traugott U. (1987) Multiple sclerosis: relevance of class I and class II MHC-expressing cells to lesion development. *J Neuroimmunol* 16:283–302.

Traugott U, Lebon P. (1988) Multiple sclerosis: involvement of interferons in lesion pathogenesis. *Ann Neurol* 24:243–251.

Traugott U, Reinherz EL, Raine CS. (1982) Monoclonal anti T-cell antibodies are applicable to the study of inflammatory infiltrates in the central nervous system. *J Neuroimmunol* 3:365–373.

Traugott U, Reinherz EL, Raine CS. (1983a) Multiple sclerosis: Distribution of T-cell subsets within active chronic lesions. *Science* 219:308–310.

Traugott U, Reinherz EL, Raine CS. (1983b) Multiple sclerosis: distribution of T-cells, T-cell subsets and Ia-positive macrophages in lesions of different ages. *J Neuroimmunol* 4:201–221.

Traugott U, Scheinberg LC, Raine CS. (1985) On the presence of Ia-positive endothelial cells and astrocytes in multiple sclerosis lesions and its relevance to antigen presentation. *J Neuroimmunol* 8:1–14.

Troiano R, Cook SD, Dowling PC. (1987) Steroid therapy in multiple sclerosis. *Arch Neurol* 44:803–807.

Trojaborg W, Petersen E. (1979) Visual and somatosensory evoked cortical potentials in multiple sclerosis. *J Neurol Neurosurg Psychiat* 42:323–330.

Trotter JL, Clark BH, Collins KG, Wegenscheide CL, Scarpellini JAD. (1987) Myelin proteolipid protein induces demyelinating disease in mice. *J Neurol Sci* 79:173–188.

Trotter JL, Hickey WF, van der Veen RC, Sulze L. (1991) Peripheral blood mononuclear cells from multiple sclerosis patients recognize myelin proteolipid protein and selected peptides. *J Neuroimmunol* 33:55–62.

Trouillas P, Courjon J. (1972) Epilepsy with multiple sclerosis. *Epilepsia* 13:325–333.

Tsukada N, Koh CS, Yanagisawa N, Okano O, Behan WHM, Behan PO. (1987) A new model for multiple sclerosis: Chronic experimental allergic encephalomyelitis induced by immunization with cerebral endothelial cell membrane. *Acta Neuropathol* 73:259–266.

Uchimura I, Shiraki H. (1957) A contribution to the classification and the pathogenesis of demyelinating encephalomyelitis. *J Neuropath Exp Neurol* 16:139–208.

Uhthoff W. (1890) Untersuchungen über die bei der multiplen Herdsklerose vorkommenden Augenstörungen. *Arch Psychiat Nervenkr* 21:55–116, 303–410.

Ulrich J, Groebke-Lorenz W. (1983) The optic nerve in multiple sclerosis: a morphological study with retrospective clinicopathological correlations. *Neuroophthalmology* 3:149–159.

Valentiner W. Über die Sklerose des Gehirns und des Rückenmarks. *Dtsch Klin* 8:147–151, 158–162, 167–169.

Valli A, Sette A, Kappos L et al. (1993) Binding of myelin basic protein peptides to HLA class II molecules and their recognition by T cells from multiple sclerosis. *J Clin Invest* 91:616–628.

Vandenbark AA, Nilaver G, Konat G, Teal P, Offner H. (1986) Chronic neurologic dysfunction and demyelination induced in Lewis rats by repeated injections of encephalitogenic T-lymphocyte line. *J Neurosci Res* 16:643–656.

Vandevelde M, Bichsel P, Cerruti Sola S, Steck A, Kristensen F, Higgins RJ. (1983) Glial proteins in canine distemper virus-induced demyelination. A sequential immunocytochemical study. *Act Neuropathol* 59:269–276.

Vandevelde M, Higgins RJ, Kristensen B, Kristensen F, Steck AJ, Kihm U. (1982) Demyelination in experimental canine distemper infection: Immunological, pathologic and immunohistological studies. *Acta Neuropathol* 56:285–293.

Vandevelde M, Kristensen B. (1977) Observations on the distribution of canine distemper virus in the central nervous system of dogs with demyelinating encephalitis. *Acta Neuropathol* 40:233–236.

Van Diemen HAM, Polman CH, Van Dongen TMMM et al. (1992) The effect of 4-aminopyridine on clinical signs in multiple sclerosis: A randomized, placebo-controlled, double blind, cross-over study. *Ann Neurol* 32:123–130.

Vanguri P, Koski CL, Silverman B, Shin ML. (1982) Complement activation by isolated myelin: Activation of the classical pathway in the absence of myelin-specific antibodies. *Immunol* 79:3290–3294.

Van Oosten BW, Truyen L, Barkhof F, Polman CH. (1995) Multiple sclerosis therapy. A practical guide. *Drugs* 49:200–212.

Vartdal F, Sollid LM, Vandvik B, Markussen G, Thorsby E. (1989) Patients with multiple sclerosis carry DQB1 genes which encode shared polymorphic amino acid sequences. *Hum Immunol* 25:103–110.

Vas CJ. (1969) Sexual impotence and some autonomic disturbances in men with multiple sclerosis. *Acta Neurol Scand* 45:166–182.

Vass K, Lassmann H. (1990) Intrathecal application of interferon gamma progressive appearance of MHC antigens within the rat nervous system. *Amer J Pathol* 137:789–800.

Vass K, Lassmann H, Wekerle H, Wisniewski HM. (1986) Distribution of Ia-antigen in the lesions of rat acute experimental allergic encephalomyelitis. *Acta Neuropathol (Berl)* 70:149–160.

Vassalli P. (1992) The pathophysiology of tumor necrosis factors. *Ann Rev Immunol* 10:411–452.

Venetz U, Casanova G, Hess Ch W, Ludin H-P. (1989) Kombinierte urodynamisch-elektromyographische Untersuchung bei Patienten mit multipler Sklerose und Blasenstörungen. *Nervenarzt* 60:163–167.

Ventre JJ, Guillot M, Confavreux C et al. (1985) Les effets indesirables de l'azathioprine (imurel). A propos de 313 maldes traites pour une sclerose en plaques. Revue de la litterature. *Therapie* 40:195–202.

Verdier-Taillefer MH, Zuber M et al. (1991) Observer disagreement in rating neurologic impairment in multiple sclerosis: facts and consequences. *Eur Neurology* 31:117–119.

Vergith TS. (1986) Mechanism of active expiration in tetraplegic subjects. *N Engl J Med* 315:1233 (letter).

Vermote R, Ketelaer P, Carton H. (1986) Pain in multiple sclerosis patients. A prospective study using the McGill pain questionnaire. *Clin Neurol Neurosurg* 88:87–91.

Villani F, Galimberti M, Crippa F. (1989) Evaluation of ventricular function by echocardiography and radionuclide angiography in patients treated with mitoxantrone. *Drugs Exp Clin Res* 15:501–506.

Visscher BR, Liu KS, Clark VA, Detels R, Malmgren RM, Dudley JP. (1984) Onset symptoms as predictors of mortality and disability in multiple sclerosis. *Acta Neurol Scand* 70:321–328.

von Pulfrich C. (1922) Die Stereoskopie im Dienste der isochromen und heterochromen Photometrie. *Naturwissenschaften* 10:553–751.

Waksman BH. (1989) Multiple sclerosis. *Curr Opinion Immunol* 1:733–739.

Waksman BH, Adams RD. (1955) Allergic neuritis: An experimental disease of rabbits induced by injection of peripheral nervous tissue and adjuvants. *J Exp Med* 102:213–234.

Waksman BH, Reynolds WE. (1984) Multiple sclerosis as a disease of immune regulation. *Proc Soc Exp Biol Med* 175:228–294.

Waldmann TA. (1992) Immune receptors: targets for therapy of leukemia/lymphoma, autoimmune diseases and for the prevention of allograft rejection. *Ann Rev Immunol* 10:675–704.

Wallace GL, Holmes S. (1993) Cognitive-linguistic assessment of individuals with multiple sclerosis. *Arch Phys Med Rehabil* 74:637–643.

Wallen WC, Houff SA, Iivanainen M, Calabrese VP, De Vries GH. (1981) Suppressor cell activity in patients with multiple sclerosis. *Neurology* 31:668–674.

Walsh MJ, Tourtellotte WW. (1983) The cerebrospinal fluid in multiple sclerosis. In: Hallpike JF, Adams CWM, Tourtellotte WW, eds. *Multiple Sclerosis.* London, England: Chapman and Hall; 275–358.

Ware JE, Sherbourne CD. (1992) The MOS 36-item short-form health survey (SF-36). *Medical Care* 30:473–483.

Warren KG, Catz I. (1986) Diagnostic value of cerebrospinal fluid anti-myelin basic protein in patients with multiple sclerosis. *Ann Neurol* 20:20–25.

Warren KG, Gordon PA, McPherson TA. (1982) Plasma exchange of malignant multiple sclerosis. *Can J Neurol Sci* 9:27–30.

Warren S, Greenhill S, Warren KG. (1982) Emotional stress and the development of multiple sclerosis. Case-control evidence of a relationship. *J Chron Dis* 35:861–865.

Watanabe R, Wege H, ter Meulen V. (1983) Adoptive transfer of EAE-like lesions from rats with coronavirus induced demyelinating encephalomyelitis. *Nature* 305:150–153.

Watson CP, Chiu M. (1979) Painful tonic seizures in multiple sclerosis: localization of the lesion. *J Canad Sci Neurol* 6:359–361.

Waxman SG (1982) Membranes, myelin and the pathophysiology of multiple sclerosis. *N Engl J Med* 306:1529–1533.

Waybright EA, Gutman L, Chou SM. (1979) Facial myokymia. Pathological features. *Arch Neurol* 36:244–245.

Weber F, Rieckmann P. (1995) Pathogenese und Therapie der multiplen Sklerose. *Nervenarzt* 66:150–155.

Wechsler IS. (1922) Statistics of multiple sclerosis including a study of the infantile, congenital and hereditary forms and the mental and psychic symptoms. *Arch Neurol Psychiat* 8:59–75.

Weiner HL, Bhan AK, Burks J, et al. (1984) Immunohistochemical analysis of the cellular infiltrates in multiple sclerosis lesions. *Neurology* (suppl) 34:112.

Weiner HL, Dau PC, Khatri BO et al. (1989) Double-blind study of true vs. sham plasma exchange in patients treated with immunosuppression for acute attacks of multiple sclerosis. *Neurology* 39:1143–1149.

Weiner HL, Fallis RJ, Aoun M, Hafler DA. (1986) Immunologic effects in progressive MS patients treated with anti-T11 and anti-T4 monoclonal antibodies. *Neurology* 36(Suppl 1):284–285.

Weiner HL, Friedman A, Miller A et al. (1994) Oral tolerance: immunologic mechanisms and treatment of animal and human organ-specific autoimmune diseases by oral administration of autoantigens. *Annu Rev Immunol* 12:809–837.

Weiner HL, Mackin GA, Matsui M et al. (1993a) Double-blind pilot trial of oral tolerization with myelin antigens in multiple sclerosis. *Science* 259:1321–1324.

Weiner HL, Mackin GA, Orav EJ et al. (1993b) Intermittent cyclophosphamide pulse therapy in progressive multiple sclerosis: final report of the Northeast Cooperative Multiple Sclerosis Treatment Group. *Neurology* 43:910–918.

Weinshenker BG, Bass B, Rice GPA, et al. (1989) The natural history of multiple sclerosis: a geographically based study. I. Clinical course and disability. *Brain* 112:133–146.

Weinshenker BG, Rice GPA, Noseworthy JH et al. (1991) The natural history of multiple sclerosis: a geographically based study. 4. Applications to planning and interpretation of clinical therapeutic trials. *Brain* 114:1057–1067.

Weinstock-Guttman B, Ransohoff RM, Kinkel RP, Rudick RA (1995) The interferons: biological effects, mechanisms of action, and use in multiple sclerosis. *Ann Neurol* 37:7–15.

Weiss W, Standlan EM. (1992) Design and statistical issues related to testing experimental therapy in multiple sclerosis. In: Rudick RA, Goodkin DE, eds. *Treatment of Multiple Sclerosis.* New York, NY: Springer Verlag; 91–122.

Wekerle H, Engelhardt B, Risau W, Meyermann R. (1991) Interaction of T-lymphocytes with cerebral endothelial cells in vitro. *Brain Pathology* 1:107–114.

Wekerle H, Fierz W. (1985) T-lymphocyte autoimmunity in experimental autoimmune encephalomyelitis. *Concepts Immunopathol* 2:102–127.

Wekerle H, Schwab M, Linington C, Meyerman R. (1986) Antigen presentation in the peripheral nervous system: Schwann cells present endogenous myelin autoantigens to lymphocytes. *Eur J Immunol* 16:1551–1557.

Weller RO, Kida S, Zhang ET. (1992) Pathways of fluid drainage from the brain—morphological aspects and immunological significance in rat and man. *Brain Pathology* 2:262–277.

Wenning GK, Wiethölter H, Schnauder G. (1994) Recovery of the hypothalamic–pituitary–adrenal axis from suppression by short-term, high-dose intravenous prednisolone therapy in patients with MS. *Acta Neurol Scand* 89:270–273.

Wheeler JS, Siroky MB, Pavlakis AJ, Goldstein I, Krane RJ. (1983) The changing neurologic pattern in multiple sclerosis. *J Urol* 130:1123–1126.

Whitaker JN, Kachelhofer RD, Bradley EL et al. (1995a) Urinary myelin basic protein-like material as a correlate of the progression of multiple sclerosis. *Ann Neurol* 38:625–632.

Whitaker JN, McFarland HF, Rudge P, Reingold SC. (1995b) Outcomes assessment in multiple sclerosis clinical trials: a critical analysis. *Multiple Sclerosis* 1:37–47.

Whitlock FA, Siskind MM. (1980) Depression as a major symptom of multiple sclerosis. *J Neurol Neurosurg Psychiat* 43:861–865.

WHO. (1981) Azathioprine. In: *Evaluation of the carcinogenic risks to humans. Some antineoplastic and immunosuppressive agents.* (IARC Vol. 26). Edited by WHO. Lyon: IARC monographs. 47–78.

Wickramasinghe SM, Dodsworth H, Rault RMJ, Hulme B. (1974) Observations on the incidence and cause of macrocytosis in patients on azathioprine therapy following renal transplantation. *Transplant Proc 18*:443–446.

Wicks DAG, Tofts PS, Miller DH et al. (1992) Volume measurement of multiple sclerosis lesions with magnetic resonance images. *Neuroradiology 34*:475–479.

Wiederkehr F, Imfeld H, Vonderschmitt DJ. (1986) Two-dimensional gel electrophoresis, isoelectric focusing and agarose gel electrophoresis in the diagnosis of multiple sclerosis. *J Clin Chem Clin Biochem 211*:1017–1021.

Wikström J, Kinnunen E, Porras J. (1984) The age-specific prevalence ratio of familial multiple sclerosis. *Neuroepidemiology 3*:74–81.

Wikström J, Poser S, Ritter G. (1980) Optic neuritis as an initial symptom in multiple sclerosis. *Acta Neurol Scand 61*:178–185.

Wilcox CE, Ward AVM, Evans A, Baker D, Rothlein R, Turk JL. (1990) Endothelial cell expression of the intercellular adhesion molecule-1 (ICAM-1) in the central nervous system in guinea pigs during acute and chronic relapsing experimental allergic encephalomyelitis. *J Neuroimmunol 30*:43–51.

Wiles CM, Omar L, Swan AV et al. (1994) Total lymphoid irradiation in multiple sclerosis. *J Neurol Neurosurg Psychiatry 57*:154–163.

Williams ES, Jones DR, McKeran RO. (1991) Mortality rates from multiple sclerosis: geographical and temporal variations revisited. *J Neurol Neurosurg Psychiat 54*:104–109.

Willoughby EW, Grochowski E, Li DK, Oger J, Kastrukoff LF, Paty DW. (1989) Serial magnetic resonance scanning in multiple sclerosis: a second prospective study in relapsing patients. *Ann Neurol 25*:43–49.

Willoughby EW, Paty DW. (1988) Scale for rating impairment in multiple sclerosis. *Neurology 38*:1793–1798.

Wisniewski HM. (1977) Immunopathology of demyelination in autoimmune diseases and virus infection. *Brit Med Bull 33*:54–59.

Wisniewski HM, Bloom BR. (1975) Primary demyelination as a non-specific consequence of a cell-mediated immune reaction. *J Exp Med 141*:346–359.

Wisniewski HM, Brostoff SW, Carter H, Eylar EH. (1974) Recurrent experimental allergic polyganglioradiculoneuritis. *Arch Neurol 30*:347–358.

Wisniewski HM, Keith AB (1977) Chronic relapsing experimental allergic encephalomyelitis—an experimental model of multiple sclerosis. *Ann Neurol 1*:144–148.

Wisniewski HM, Lassmann H, Rosnan CF, Mehta PD, Lidsky AA, Madrid RE. (1982) Multiple sclerosis: Immunological and experimental aspects. In: Matthews WB, Glaser GH, eds. *Recent Advances in Clinical Neurology (3)*. London, England: Churchill Livingstone; 95–124.

Wisniewski HM, Oppenheimer D, McDonald WI. (1976) Relation between myelination and function in multiple sclerosis and EAE. *J Neuropathol Exp Neurol 35*:327.

Wist ER, Hennerici M, Dichgans J. (1978) The Pulfrich spatial frequency phenomenon: a psychophysical method competitive to visual evoked potentials in the diagnosis of multiple sclerosis. *J Neurol Neurosurg Psychiat 41*:1069–1077.

Witte AS, Cornblath OR, Schatz NJ, Lisak RP. (1986) Monitoring azathioprine therapy in myasthenia gravis. *Neurology 36*:1533–1534.

Wolfgram F. (1979) What if multiple sclerosis isn't an immunological or viral disease? The case of a circulating toxin. *Neurochem Res 4*:1–14.

Wolinsky JS. (1992) Treatment of multiple sclerosis with cyclosporine A. In: Rudick RA, Goodkin DE, eds. *Treatment of Multiple Sclerosis*. New York, NY: Springer Verlag; 217–232.

Wolinsky JS. (1995) Copolymer 1: A most reasonable alternative therapy for early relapsing-remitting multiple sclerosis with mild disability. *Neurology 45*:1245–1247.

Wolinsky JS, Narayana PA. (1991) Proton magnetic resonance spectroscopy and multiple sclerosis. *Lancet 337*:362.

Wong GHW, Bartlett PF, Clark Lewis I, Battye F, Schrader JW. (1984) Inducible expression of H-2 and Ia-antigens on brain cells. *Nature 310*:688.

Woodroofe MN, Bellamy AS, Feldman M, Davison AN, Cuzner ML. (1986) Immunocytochemical characterization of the immune reaction in the central nervous system in multiple sclerosis. Possible role for microglia in lesion growth. *J Neurol Sci 74*:135–152.

Wucherpfennig KW, Newcombe J, Li H, Keddy C, Cuzner ML, Hafler DA. (1992a) T cell receptor V alpha-V beta repertoire and cytokine gene expression in active multiple sclerosis lesions. *J Exp Med 175*:993–1003.

Wucherpfennig KW, Newcombe J, Li H, Keddy C, Cuzner ML, Hafler DA. (1992b) Gamma-delta T-cell receptor repertoire in acute multiple sclerosis lesions. *Proc Natl Acad Sci 89*:4588–4592.

Wynn DR, Rodriguez M, O'Fallon WM, Kurland LT. (1990) A reappraisal of the epidemiology of multiple sclerosis in Olmsted County, Minnesota. *Neurology 40*:780–786.

Yao DL, Webster H de F, Hudson LD, et al (1994) Concentric sclerosis (Balo): Morphometric and in situ hybridization study of lesions in six patients. *Ann Neurol 35*:18–30.

Yates SK, Brown WF. (1981) The human jaw jerk. Electrophysiologic methods to measure the latency: normal values and changes in multiple sclerosis. *Neurology 31*:632–634.

Yednock TA, Cannon C, Fritz LC, Sanchez-Madrid F, Steinmann L, Karin N. (1992) Prevention of experimental autoimmune encephalomyelitis by antibodies against alpha-4-beta-1 integrin. *Nature 356*:63–66.

Yetkin FZ, Haughton VM, Papke RA, Fischer ME, Rao SM. (1991) Multiple sclerosis: specificity of MR for diagnosis. *Radiology 178*:447–451.

Youl BD, Turano G, Miller DH, et al. (1991) The pathophysiology of optic neuritis: an association of gadolinium leakage with clinical and electrophysiological deficits. *Brain 114*:2437–2450.

Young IR, Hall AS, Pallis CA, Bydder GM, Legg NJ, Steiner RE. (1981) Nuclear magnetic resonance imaging of the brain in multiple sclerosis. *Lancet ii*:1063–1066.

Yudkin PL, Ellison GW, Ghezzi A, et al. (1991) Overview of azathioprine treatment in multiple sclerosis *Lancet ii*:1051–1055.

Zabriskie JB, Mayer L, Fu M, Cam V, Plank C. (1985) T-cell subsets in multiple sclerosis: Lack of correlation between helper and suppressor T-cells and the clinical state. *J Clin Immunol 5*:7-12.

Zamvil S, Nelson P, Trotter J, et al. (1985) T-cell clones specific for myelin basic protein induce chronic relapsing paralysis and demyelination. *Nature 317*:355–358.

Zander H. (1986) Clinical and immunogenetic data of 33 double case families with multiple sclerosis. In: Hommes OR, ed. *Multiple Sclerosis Research in Europe.* Lancaster, England: MTP Press; 333–336.

Zanetta JP, Warter JM, Kuchler S, et al. (1990) Antibodies to cerebellar soluble lectin CSL in multiple sclerosis. *Lancet 335*:1482–1484.

Zettl UK, Gold R, Toyka KV, Hartung H-P. (1995) Intravenous glucocorticosteroid treatment augments apoptosis of inflammatory T cells in experimental autoimmune neuritis (EAN) of the Lewis rat. *J Neuropathol Exp Neurol 54*:540–547.

Zhang J, Medaer R, Stinissen P et al. (1993) MHC-restricted depletion of human myelin basic protein-reactive T cells by T cell vaccination. *Science 261*:1451–1454.

Zimprich F, Winter J, Wege H, Lassmann H. (1991) Corona virus induced primary demyelination: indications for the involvement of a humoral immune response. *Neuropath Appl Neurobiol 17*:469–484.

Zurbriggen A, Vandevelde M, Dumas M. (1986) Secondary degeneration of oligodendrocytes in canine distemper. *Lab Inv 54*:424–431.

Index